Prentice Hall Health

outline review

of Medical Technology/ Clinical Laboratory Science

Donna L. Leach, Ed.D., MT (ASCP) DLM
Winston-Salem State University
Winston-Salem, North Carolina

Denny G. Ryman, Ed.D., MT (ASCP)
Winston-Salem State University
Winston-Salem, North Carolina

Consulting Editor
Linda Graves, Ed.D., MT (ASCP)
Program Director
Medical Laboratory Technology
University of Maine at Presque Isle
Presque Isle, Maine

Associate Consulting Editor
Frank J. Scarano, Ph.D., CLS (M)
Department of Medical Laboratory Science
University of Massachusetts, Dartmouth

Associate Consulting Editor
Deanna D. Klosinski, Ph.D., MT (ASCP), DLM
Consultant/Educator Medical Sciences
Adjunct Associate Professor, Michigan State University,
East Lansing, Michigan
Instructor, Baker College
Owosso, Michigan

PEARSON
Prentice
Hall

Upper Saddle River, New Jersey 07458

Library of Congress Cataloging-in-Publication Data

Leach, Donna L.
 Prentice Hall health's outline review of medical techology/clinical
laboratory science / Donna L. Leach, Denny G. Ryman.
  p. ; cm.
 title: Outline review of medical technology/clinical laboratory
science.
 Includes index.
 ISBN 0-13-018404-7
 1. Medical laboratory technology—Outlines, syllabi, etc.
 [DNLM: 1. Technology, Medical—Outlines. 2. Clinical Laboratory
Techniques--Outlines. QY 18.2 L434p 2004] I. Title: Outline review of
medical technology/clinical laboratory science. II. Ryman, Denny G. III.
Title.
 RB37.5 .L43 2004
 616.07'56'076--dc21

                                        2003009826

Publisher: Julie Levin Alexander
Assistant to Publisher: Regina Bruno
Acquisitions Editor: Mark Cohen
Assistant Editor: Melissa Kerian
Editorial Assistant: Mary Ellen Ruitenberg
Marketing Manager: Nicole Benson
Product Information Manager: Rachele Strober
Director of Production and Manufacturing:
 Bruce Johnson
Managing Production Editor: Patrick Walsh
Production Liaison: Alexander Ivchenko

Production Editor: Jessica Balch, Pine Tree Composition
Manufacturing Manager: Ilene Sanford
Manufacturing Buyer: Pat Brown
Design Director: Cheryl Asherman
Design Coordinator: Maria Guglielmo-Walsh
Cover and Interior Designer: Janice Bielawa
Composition: Pine Tree Composition, Inc.
Manager of Media Production: Amy Peltier
New Media Project Manager: Stephen Hartner
Printing and Binding: Banta Book Group
Cover Printer: Phoenix Color Corp.

Pearson Education, Ltd., *London*
Pearson Education Australia Pty. Limited, *Sydney*
Pearson Education Singapore Pte. Ltd.
Pearson Education North Asia Ltd., *Hong Kong*
Pearson Education Canada, Ltd., *Toronto*
Pearson Educación de Mexico, S.A. de C.V.
Pearson Education—Japan, *Tokyo*
Pearson Education Malaysia, Pte. Ltd.
Pearson Education, Upper Saddle River, New Jersey

10 9 8 7 6
ISBN 0-13-018404-7

Contents

Introduction

 SUCCESS ACROSS THE BOARDS:
THE PRENTICE HALL HEALTH REVIEW SERIES

Prentice Hall Health is pleased to present *Success Across the Boards,* our new review series. These authoritative texts give you expert help in preparing for certifying examinations. Each title in the series comes with its own technology package, including a CD-ROM and a Companion Website. You will find that this powerful combination of text and media provides you with expert help and guidance for achieving success across the boards.

This book is designed as an outline for students looking for an all-in-one review and summary of the major topics within a medical technology curriculum. It is also an ideal resource for preparing for a Medical Technology Certification or Licensure Examination.

Prentice Hall Health's Outline Review of Medical Technology/Clinical Laboratory Science is a comprehensive text containing concise and authoritative content. A set of review questions at the end of each chapter will help simulate the testing experience. This format not only tests your knowledge of the subject matter, but also facilitates additional study. Included free with this book is a 100-question self-assessment test on CD-ROM. Visit the companion website at **www.prenhall.com/review** for an additional 50-question comprehensive practice examination.

The book is organized into 11 chapters corresponding to the areas tested on medical technology certification examinations. The chapters include:

1. Urinalysis and Body Fluids

2. Hematology

3. Coagulation

4. Clinical Chemistry

5. Immunology and Serology

6. Immunohematology

7. Bacteriology

8. Clinical Parasitology

9. Clinical Mycology

10. Clinical Virology

11. Management, Laboratory Principles, Education, and Research

As you can see, each chapter represents a specific discipline in the medical technology field. Each chapter presents an outline review of important concepts, followed by review questions. The CD-ROM is organized around the same chapter sequence, so once you complete each book chapter, you should turn your attention to the corresponding CD-ROM module before moving on to the next chapter.

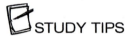
STUDY TIPS

Review Materials

Choose review materials that contain the information you need to study. Save time by making sure that you aren't studying anything you don't need to. Before the exam, the best study preparation would be to use this Outline Review to identify your strengths and weaknesses. The references at the end of each rationale will direct you to additional resources for more in-depth study.

Set a Study Schedule

Use your time-management skills to set a schedule that will help you feel as prepared as you can be. Consider all the relevant factors—the materials you need to study, how many months, weeks, or days until the test date, and how much time you can study each day. If you establish your schedule ahead of time and write it in your date book, you will be much more likely to follow it.

Take Practice Tests

Practice as much as possible, using the questions in this book, on the accompanying CD, and the Web site. These questions were designed to follow the format of questions that appear on the exam you will take, so the more you practice with these questions, the better prepared you will be on test day.

The printed practice test in the back of the book and the practice tests on the CD will give you a chance to the experience the exam before you actually have to take it and will also let you know how you're doing and where you need to do better. For best results, we recommend you take a practice test 2 to 3 weeks before you are scheduled to take the actual exam. Spend the next weeks targeting those areas in which you performed poorly by reviewing questions in those areas.

Practice under test-like conditions—in a quiet room, with no books or notes to help you, and with a clock telling you when to stop. Try to come as close as you can to duplicating the actual test situation.

TAKING THE EXAMINATION

Prepare Physically

When taking the exam, you need to work efficiently under time pressure. If your body is tired or under stress, you might not think as clearly or perform as well as you usually do. If you can, avoid staying up all night. Get some sleep so that you can wake up rested and alert.

Eating right is also important. The best advice is to eat a light, well-balanced meal before a test. When time is short, grab a quick-energy snack such as a banana, orange juice, or a granola bar.

The Examination Site

The examination site should be located prior to the required examination time. It is wise to find the site and parking facilities the day before the test. Parking fee information should be obtained so that sufficient money can be taken along on the examination day.

Allow plenty of time for travel to the site in case of unexpected mishaps such as traffic snarls. During travel, think positive thoughts (e.g. "My preparation for the exam was thorough, so I'll be able to answer the questions easily"). Maintain a confident attitude to prevent unnecessary stress.

Materials

Be sure to take all required identification materials, registration forms, and any other items required by the testing organization or center. Read information and instructions supplied by the testing organizations thoroughly to be sure you have all necessary materials before the day of the exam.

Read Test Directions

Read the examination directions thoroughly! Because some board examinations have different test sections with different question formats, it is important to be aware of changes in directions. Read each set of directions completely before starting a new section of questions.

The examination is computerized. The computer is capable of keeping track of questions you have skipped, answered, and number remaining. Be sure to read and re-read each question before closing the program.

Selecting the Right Answer

Keep in mind that only one answer is correct. First read the stem of the question with each possible choice provided and eliminate choices that are obviously incorrect. Be cautious about choosing the first answer that might be correct; all possibilities should be considered before the final choice is made; the best answer should be selected.

If a question is complicated, try to break it down into small sections that are easy to understand. Pay special attention to qualifiers such as only, except, etc. For example, negative words in a question can confuse your understanding of what the question asks ("Which of the following is not. . .").

Intelligent Guessing

If you don't know the answer, eliminate those answers that you know or suspect are wrong. Your goal is to narrow down your choices. Here are some questions to ask yourself:

- Is the choice accurate in its own terms? If there's an error in the choice, for example, a term that is incorrectly defined—the answer is wrong.
- Is the choice relevant? An answer may be accurate, but it may not relate to the essence of the question.
- Are there any distractors, such as *always, never, all, none,* or *every*? Qualifiers make it easy to find an exception that makes a choice incorrect.

Mark answers you aren't sure of, and go back to them at the end of the test.

Ask yourself whether you would make the same guesses again. Chances are that you will leave your answers alone, but you may notice something that will make you change your mind—a qualifier that affects meaning or a remembered fact that will enable you to answer the question without guessing.

Watch the Clock

Keep track of how much time is left and how you are progressing. Wear a watch or bring a small clock with you to the test room. A wall clock may be broken, or there may be no clock at all.

Some students are so concerned about time that they rush through the exam and have time left over. In such situations, it's easy to leave early. The best approach, however, is to take your time. Stay until the end so that you can check your answers.

KEYS TO SUCCESS ACROSS THE BOARDS

- Study, Review, and Practice
- Keep a positive, confident attitude
- Follow all directions on the examination
- Do your best

Good luck!

You are encouraged to visit **http://www.prenhall.com/success** *for additional tips on studying, test-taking, and other keys to success. At this stage of your education and career you will find these tips helpful.*

Reviewers

Karen S. Chandler, MA, MT (ASCP)
Program Coordinator and Associate Professor
Medical Technologist Program
University of Texas—Pan American
Edinburg, Texas

Margaret L. Charette, MEd, MT (ASCP) SC
Program Director
Medical Laboratory Technician Program
University of Maine at Augusta
Augusta, Maine

Beverly A. Kirby, MT (ASCP)
Medical Technology Rural Education Coordinator
Adjunct Assistant Professor
West Virginia University
Medical Technology Program
Morgantown, West Virginia

Virginia Kotlarz, PhD, CLS (NCA), MT (ASCP)
Department Chair
Clinical Laboratory Sciences
Daemen College
Amherst, New York

Jay W. Wilborn, MEd, BSMT
Program Director
Clinical Laboratory Science
Garland County Community College
Hot Springs, Arkansas

Urinalysis and Body Fluids

contents

➤ COMPREHENSIVE KEY CONCEPTS

1. Discuss factors that can affect the formation and composition of urine, and recognize how these factors can be detected by physical examination, chemical analysis, and microscopic analysis. In addition, correlate disease states with abnormal urine findings.

2. Describe the various factors that can cause false negatives and positives when performing urine chemical strip testing, and list various confirmation tests for positive urine chemical strip testing. Also correlate chemical with microscopic results.

I. INTRODUCTION TO URINALYSIS

A. Introduction

1. Urinalysis is the practice of examining urine for diagnostic purposes; it aids in following the course or treatment of disease.

B. Importance of Urine

1. Urine transports most of the body's waste products.
2. Urine chemical changes are directly related to pathological conditions.
3. A complete urinalysis is composed of multiple tests, including physical, microscopic, and chemical analysis.
4. Urinalysis is used for diabetic monitoring, drug screening, and initial diagnosis of inborn errors of metabolism.

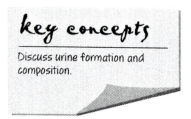

key concepts

Discuss urine formation and composition.

C. Urine Composition

1. Urine contains **mostly water** and various amounts of urea and organic/inorganic compounds.
2. Composition varies according to diet, physical activity, and disease processes. Composition is directly related to the amount and type of waste material that is to be excreted.
3. Urine **organic** substances
   a. **Urea** accounts for roughly 50 percent of all dissolved solids in the urine.
   b. Other organic substances in relatively large amounts include **creatinine** and **uric acid.**
   c. Organic substances in small amounts include **NH_4, glucose,** and **albumin (protein).**
   d. Urine **inorganic** substances (listed in order of highest to lowest average concentration):
      1) **Chloride, sodium,** and **potassium.**
      2) Other inorganic substances in minute amounts include hormones, vitamins, and medications.
   e. Substances not normally part of the original plasma filtrate may include bacteria, crystals, and other cellular formed elements.

II. THE KIDNEY AND URINE FORMATION

A. Renal Anatomy (See Chapter 4 Clinical Chemistry Sections XXI, Electrolytes and Water Balance and XXII, Renal Function)

1. **Renal biochemistry**
   a. **Renin** is secreted by the kidneys and stimulates the production of **angiotensin I** (a hormone in the inert form).
   b. **Angiotensin I** stimulates the production of **angiotensin II** in the active form.
   c. **Angiotensin II** regulates renal blood flow in three ways:
      1) **Vasoconstriction** of renal arterioles
      2) **Reabsorption** of sodium in the proximal tubules
      3) **Release** of aldosterone that retains sodium

III. RENAL PATHOLOGY AND RENAL FUNCTION TESTS
A. Renal Pathology
1. **Acute glomerulonephritis:** inflammation of the glomerulus seen in children and young adults that can follow a Group A Streptococcus respiratory infection
2. **Rapidly progressive glomerulonephritis:** a more serious form of acute glomerulonephritis resulting in renal failure
3. **Acute interstitial nephritis:** an infection of the nephrons
4. **Chronic glomerulonephritis (Berger's disease):** results in a long-term progressive lost of renal function
5. **Membranous glomerulonephritis:** thickening of the glomerular capillary basement membrane
6. **Nephrotic syndrome:** may be caused by renal blood pressure irregularities, resulting in proteinuria and lipiduria
7. **Focal segmental glomerulosclerosis:** affects a specific number of glomeruli, not the entire glomerulus; often seen in HIV patients
8. **Acute pyelonephritis:** an infection of the renal tubules caused by a urinary tract infection
9. **Chronic pyelonephritis:** chronic inflammation of the tubules and interstitial tissue
10. **Renal failure:** tubular necrosis caused by nephrotoxic agents and other disease processes, resulting in a failure of the kidneys to filter blood

B. Renal Function Tests
1. **Renal tubular reabsorption tests** are used to detect early renal disease. Also known as **concentration tests.** Examples of these tests include:
   a. **Osmolarity** measures the number of particles present in a solution.
   b. **Specific gravity** depends on the number of particles present in a solution and the density of these particles. Osmolarity and specific gravity evaluate renal concentrating ability, monitor the course of renal disease, and monitor fluid and electrolyte therapy.
   c. **Tubular secretion or renal blood flow test** which uses **p-aminohippuric acid (PAH):** a substance that is infused into the patient. This substance is completely removed from the blood by functional renal tissue. If renal problems exist, the PAH will not be removed completely.

    d. **Osmolar/Free Water Clearance**
      1) Used in the diagnosis of various types of diabetes
      2) Measures renal clearance of solutes and substance-free water

2. **Glomerular tests** are used to assess renal waste removal and solute reabsorbing abilities. *Note:* Urea is not normally used in clearance testing because of tubular reabsorption, diet, and urine rate of flow problems.

    a. **Creatinine clearance** is widely used in renal clearance testing.
      1) Creatinine levels are not changed by diet (normal) or urine rate of flow, and are not reabsorbed by renal tubules. **P:** plasma creatinine, **C:** urine creatinine, **V:** urine flow in mL/min, and **SA:** body surface area. 1.73 m^2/SA is average body surface area.
      2) Creatinine clearance formula:

$$C \ (mL/min) = \frac{U \times V}{P} \times \frac{1.73 \ m^2}{SA}$$

      3) 24-hour timed urine is the specimen of choice.
      4) Reference values differ according to age and sex.
        Males: 105 ± 20mL/min
        Females: 95 ± 20mL/min

IV. URINE VOLUME AND SAMPLE HANDLING

A. Volume of Urine — determined by the body's state of hydration. The normal output of urine is between 600–2,000mL/24hrs.

1. **Factors that affect urine volume**
    a. Fluid intake and loss
    b. Diuretic and antidiuretic hormone levels
    c. Excretion of dissolved solids including **glucose** and **salts**

2. **Examples of pathological conditions that affect urine volume**
    a. **Oliguria:** a decrease in urine output due to dehydration, i.e., vomiting, diarrhea, perspiration, and burns
    b. **Anuria:** no urine output as a result of kidney damage or renal failure
    c. **Nocturia:** increased urine output at night
      1) Caused by a reduction in bladder capacity resulting from pregnancy, stones, or prostate enlargement
      2) Increased fluid intake at night
    d. **Polyuria:** increased daily output, may exceed 3L/day
      1) Polyuria is usually caused by **diabetes mellitus, diabetes insipidus, diuretics** (block water reabsorption), **caffeine,** and **alcohol** (suppresses secretion of antidiuretic hormones).
      2) Polyuria resulting from solute diuresis can also be caused by increased sodium intake.

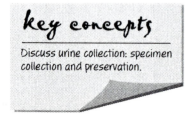

key concepts

Discuss urine collection: specimen collection and preservation.

B. Specimen Collection and Handling
1. Urine is a biohazard and must be treated with universal precautions.
2. Use dry cups with lids.
3. Label container with name, date, and time of collection.
4. Test within **one hour** or preserve.

5. **Preservation of urine**
    a. Refrigeration will prevent bacterial decomposition but will **increase** specific gravity and amorphous phosphates/urates.
    b. Before testing, urine must be brought to room temperature.
    c. Chemical preservatives can be bactericidal, but will preserve formed elements and will not interfere with chemical testing.
    d. Changes in unpreserved urine:
        1) **Increased** pH, nitrites, bacteria, and turbidity
        2) **Decreased** urobilinogen, glucose, ketones, and bilirubin
        3) Formed element destruction
        4) Change in color
6. **Specimen types and collection times**
    a. **Random:** used for routine screening; time of collection is not a consideration.
    b. **Fasting:** used for diabetic monitoring.
    c. **Glucose tolerance test:** used for the diagnosis of diabetes and diabetic monitoring, usually collected at 1-hour intervals.
    d. **24-hour:** collection over a period of 24 hours for **creatinine clearance** or other analytes, including Na, K.
    e. **Catheterized (cath) urine:** urine collected from a tube placed through the urethra into the bladder.
    f. **Void:** collected by the patient during routine urination, same as a random sample.
    g. **Midstream clean catch:** the pubic area is cleansed with a soap and urine is collected in the middle of urination.
    h. **Suprapubic aspiration:** a needle is inserted into the bladder through the abdominal wall.
    i. **Three glass-collection:** used for **prostate** infection diagnosis. The third sample is used for white blood cell (WBC) analysis and bacterial count and should contain increased WBCs and bacteria in prostatitis.
    j. **Pediatric collection:** uses small, clear plastic bags with adhesive to adhere to the genital area.
    k. **2-hour postprandial:** void two hours after eating; used to monitor sugar content.

V. PHYSICAL EXAMINATION OF THE URINE

A. **Color, Appearance, and Odor** — varies from colorless to any color shade (black, red, green, etc.). Changes in color can be due to normal metabolism, disease, diet, and physical activity. The normal color of urine (yellow) is derived from **urochrome,** which is a pigmented substance excreted at a constant rate. Urobilin and uroerythrin also add to the normal yellow color. Increased urochrome production can result from thyroid disease or a fasting urine sample. In general, pale yellow samples are dilute, whereas dark yellow samples are concentrated.

1. **Abnormal urine color**
    a. Dark yellow/amber
        1) Increased bilirubin from liver problems such as hepatitis
        2) Infections causing fever and dehydration
        3) High specific gravity due to concentrated urine

      b. Intense yellow/orange

         1) **Pyridium** (phenazoyridine)—medication prescribed for urinary tract infections (UTIs), the resulting thick orange urine masks chemical and microscopic analysis.

         2) Bilirubin and urobilin—yellow foam may indicate excess bilirubin while urobilin does not produce foam.

      c. Red

         1) Blood—glomerular bleeding can also produce brown/black urine

         2) Hemoglobin, erythrocytes

         3) Myoglobin (muscle trauma)

         4) Porphyrins

      d. Green/purple

         1) Medications and dyes such as indican and phenols

         2) Infections caused by *Pseudomonas*

Note: Many abnormal colors are nonpathogenic in nature and are the result of food, drugs, or vitamins.

2. **Appearance of urine (clarity):** Visual inspection of urine uses the following terminology: clear, hazy, slightly cloudy, cloudy, turbid, milky, bloody.

    a. **White cloudy:** amorphous phosphates and carbonates

    b. **Cloudy:** amorphous urates, calcium oxalate crystals, uric acid crystals

    c. **Hazy:** epithelial cells, mucus

    d. **Turbid:** WBCs, RBCs, bacteria, and epithelial cells

3. **Urine odor:** urine odor is not generally a part of the routine urinalysis but may provide useful information to the physician.

    a. Urea breakdown: ammonia

    b. Strong odor: bacterial infection

    c. Sweet or fruity odor: ketone bodies (diabetic ketosis)

    d. Maple syrup odor: maple syrup urine disease

    e. Various odors: different foods

B. Specific Gravity

1. Specific gravity determines the kidney's ability to reabsorb essential chemicals and water from the glomerular filtrate. Reabsorption is the first renal function to become impaired. Specific gravity also determines dehydration and antidiuretic hormone abnormalities.

2. Specific gravity is the density of a substance compared with the density of a similar volume of distilled water at a similar temperature and can be influenced by the number of particles present and by particle size.

3. **Specific gravity instruments**

    a. **Urinometer** is a float attached to a scale. The level to which the urinometer sinks represents the specimen's mass or specific gravity. Requires 10–15mL of urine and must be corrected for temperature. Rarely used.

    b. **Refractometer** measures a refractive index, which is a comparison of the velocity of light in air with the velocity of light in a solution. Uses a small volume of urine and does not require temperature corrections.

  c. **Specific gravity (S.G.) values**

    1) **Normal** random urine ranges from 1.001 to 1.035 with the average falling between 1.015 to 1.025.

    2) **Isosthenuric** urine: 1.010 (fixed S.G. indicates a loss of concentrating and diluting ability)

    3) **Hyposthenuric** urine: less than 1.010

    4) **Hypersthenuric** urine: greater than 1.010

 4. **Conditions associated with specific gravity value**

  a. **Low specific gravity:** indicates a loss of the kidney's ability to concentrate urine or seen in such diseases as diabetes insipidus, glomerulonephritis, and pyelonephritis.

  b. **High specific gravity:** adrenal insufficiency, hepatic disease, congestive heart failure, and dehydration due to vomiting, diarrhea, or strenuous exercise

  c. **Interference:** x-ray contrast media

C. Terms Associated with Urology

 1. **Diuretics** are medications that increase urine output and block water reabsorption.

 2. **Diabetes mellitus** is an insulin defect that affects glucose metabolism, resulting in hyperglycemia.

 3. **Diabetes insipidus** is decreased production and inhibited function of antidiuretic hormone (ADH) causing water not to be reabsorbed from urine.

VI. CHEMICAL EXAMINATION OF URINE

A. Reagent Strips — used for the following tests: pH, protein, glucose, ketones, blood, bilirubin, urobilinogen, nitrite, leukocytes, and specific gravity. Reagent strips are the method of choice for the chemical analysis of urine.

 1. **Basic use:** reagent strips are chemical-containing absorbent pads that react with urine, producing a chemical reaction that results in a color change. The color is characteristic of positive reactions for various substances. Color intensity is semiquantitative for these substances. Confirmatory tests are then performed for some analytes.

 2. **Sources of error** include excess time in the urine, runover between chemicals, not following specific reaction times to read results, and not testing samples at room temperature.

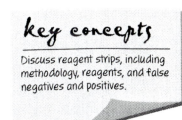

key concepts

Discuss reagent strips, including methodology, reagents, and false negatives and positives.

B. Chemical Tests and Clinical Significance

 1. **pH**

  a. Kidneys regulate the acid/base balance of the body (hydrogen ion concentration) by secreting NH_3 ions, hydrogen phosphate, weak acids, and by reabsorbing bicarbonate.

  b. The pH of urine ranges from **4.5–8.0** and between **5.0–6.0** with the first morning void. The following urine pHs may indicate various diseases and conditions:

    1) **Acidic pH (<6.0):** high protein diets, after normal sleep, respiratory/metabolic acidosis, uncontrolled diabetes mellitus.

2) **Alkaline pH (>7.0):** excreted after meals in response to HCl gastric acid, increased consumption of vegetables, renal tubular acidosis, respiratory/metabolic alkalosis, and UTIs.

c. The **pH reagent strip** uses methyl red and bromthymol blue to detect changes in pH. At pH 5.0 the strip is orange; as the pH increases, the strip will go from orange to yellow to green, and finally to blue at pH 9.0.

2. **Protein**

a. Uses **tetrabromphenol blue** to detect protein.

b. Principle: "protein error of indicators": indicator is yellow in the absence of protein and blue when abnormal amounts of protein are present.

c. Urine protein is very diagnostic for renal disease.

d. Normal urine will contain less than 10mg/dl of protein or 100mg/24hr. Protein types include albumin, microglobulins, and Tamm-Horsfall.

e. Protein can come from nonrenal sources such as the prostate, seminal, and vaginal secretions.

f. **Proteinuria** does not always indicate renal disease but may indicate tubular reabsorption problems, increased low molecular weight proteins, and glomerular membrane damage caused by toxic agents, lupus, or *streptococcal glomerulonephritis*. A positive protein can also indicate an increase in low molecular weight serum proteins.

g. **Bence Jones protein** is produced due to a proliferative disorder of plasma cells as seen in multiple myeloma. Bence Jones proteins are light chain monoclonal immunoglobulins. Sulfosalicyclic acid is also used to detect Bence Jones proteins.

h. **Benign proteinuria** can occur in cold temperatures, exercise, fever, dehydration, late pregnancy, and orthostatic/postural proteinuria in young adults (going from supine to upright).

i. **Protein precipitation tests:** sulfosalicylic acid causes the protein to precipitate out in urine. The amount of precipitant is quantitated from 1+ to 4+.

j. **Reaction interference**

1) False positives: urine pH > 9 resulting from alkaline medicine and keeping the dipstick in urine too long

2) False negatives: dilute urine

3. **Glucose**

a. Glucose testing is used to detect and monitor diabetes mellitus.

b. **Glycosuria** is the presence of urine glucose and is seen in the following conditions: diabetes mellitus, impaired tubular reabsorption seen in Fanconi's syndrome, advanced tubular renal disease, central nervous system (CNS) damage, thyroid disorders, and pregnancy.

c. **Methodology of glucose testing**

1) **Reagent strip:** glucose + oxygen reacts with glucose oxidase to form gluconic acid and H_2O_2. The H_2O_2 +

chromogen reacts with peroxidase to form an oxidized colored chromagen + water.

    a) False positives: strong oxidizing agents, i.e., bleach

    b) False negatives: ascorbic acid

  2) **Copper reduction test** (Benedict's, Clinitest tablet): a reduction reaction where glucose or other substances reduce copper sulfate to cuprous oxide. Cuprous oxide reacts with a reducing substance when heated to form cuprous ions plus an oxidized substance, which forms a color reaction.

    a) False positives: antibiotics, ascorbic acid and other reducing agents

    b) False negatives: none

4. **Ketones**

  a. Include three intermediate products of fat metabolism: **acetone, acetoacetic acid,** and **beta-hydroxybutyric acid.**

  b. Normal urine contains no ketones when metabolized fat is broken down completely, but when fat reserves are needed for energy, ketones will show up in the urine.

  c. **Ketonuria** the presence of ketones in the urine.

  d. **Clinical significance:** diabetes mellitus, insulin dosage monitoring, electrolyte imbalance, and dehydration due to excessive carbohydrate loss such as vomiting, starvation, exercise, and rapid weight loss.

  e. **Methodology of ketone testing**

    1) Reagent strips use **sodium nitroprusside (nitroferricyanide)** to measure **acetoacetic acid.** The addition of glycine permits the measurement of acetone and acetoacetic acid.

      a) **Reaction interference (false positives)** are minimal but may result from pigmented urine, dyes, phenylketones, and bacterial breakdown of acetoacetic acid.

    2) **Acetest** is a nitroprusside and glycine tablet used to detect ketones; which gives an enhanced color reaction and permits serial dilutions to be done. Reaction interference parallels the reagent strip method.

5. **Blood**

  a. Reagent strip test detects hematuria and hemoglobinuria.

  b. **Types of blood/hgb in the urine**

    1) **Hematuria** (intact RBCs in the urine)

      a) Renal calculi, glomerulonephritis, pyelonephritis, tumors, trauma, toxins, exercise, menstruation, and pregnancy.

    2) **Hemoglobinuria** (hemoglobin in the urine)

      a) Transfusion reactions, hemolytic anemia, severe burns, infections, and exercise.

    3) **Myoglobin** (hemoglobin-like protein found in muscle tissue)

      a) Positive reaction with chemical test for blood; can be seen in muscle trauma, coma, convulsions, muscle-wasting diseases, and extensive exercise.

        b) **Screen for myoglobin** uses ammonium sulfate, which precipitates hemoglobin out of the urine; the urine is then filtered and tested with a reagent strip. Positive reaction: myoglobin; negative reaction: hemoglobin

   c. **Reagent strip methodology (strip)**

      1) Detects pseudo H_2O_2 found in hemoglobin; H_2O_2 plus chromogen reacts with hemoglobin peroxidase to form oxidized chromogen and water.

      2) Urine hemoglobin gives a speckled pattern on the reagent strip when intact RBCs lyse and free hemoglobin in the urine will form a uniform color on the strip.

   d. **Reaction interferences**

      1) False positive: vegetable peroxidase and *Escherichia coli* peroxidase.

      2) False negative: ascorbic acid and nitrites produced in enteric UTIs, and high protein levels.

6. **Bilirubin**

   a. Detects **bilirubinuria,** which is a degradation product of hemoglobin.

   b. Bilirubin is a pigmented yellow compound.

   c. Hemoglobin is broken down into iron, protein, and **protoporphyrin** which is converted to bilirubin by reticuloendothelial system cells and combines with albumin, which goes to the liver.

   d. In the liver, bilirubin is conjugated with **glucuronic acid** to form **bilirubin diglucuronide** which goes to the intestines and is reduced to **urobilinogen** via bacterial action and excreted in the feces as **urobilin.**

   e. **Bilirubinuria** may result from hepatitis, cirrhosis, biliary obstruction, and early liver disease.

   f. Bile duct obstruction is positive for bilirubin but normal for urobilinogen.

   g. Hemolytic disease will cause urobilinogen to be positive and negative for bilirubin.

   h. **Reagent strip** uses diazonium salt reaction (bilirubin → azobilirubin) methodology. The **Ictotest** tablet is a confirmatory test for bilirubin.

   i. **Reaction interferences**

      1) False positive: pigmented urine, i.e., medications Indican and Lodine

      2) False negative: specimen is too old, has too much exposure to light (bilirubin exposed to light is converted to biliverdin which does not react with diazonium salts), ascorbic acid, and nitrite

7. **Urobilinogen**

   a. Urobilinogen—bile pigment from hemoglobin breakdown (the reduction of bilirubin by bacteria in the small intestine)

   b. Urobilinogen in the urine can indicate early liver disease, bile duct obstruction, and hemolytic diseases.

    c. **Reagent strip** uses Ehrlich's reagent (paradimethylaminoben-zaldehyde) to detect urobilinogen.

    d. **Reaction interferences**

       1) False positive: pigmented urine

       2) False negative: improper storage

    e. Other tests

       1) **Ehrlich's tube** method

       2) **Watson-Schwartz** method that differentiates between uro-bilinogen and porphobilinogen

8. **Nitrite**

    a. Rapid test for UTIs

    b. A positive nitrite can indicate cystitis and pyelonenephritis.

    c. Used for evaluation of UTI antibiotic therapy

    d. **Reagent strip** detects the ability of certain bacteria to reduce nitrate (normal in urine) to nitrite (abnormal in urine).

    e. **Reaction interferences**

       1) False positive: old urine samples and pigmented urine

       2) False negative: ascorbic acid, antibiotics, bacteria that do not reduce nitrite, diet low in nitrates, inadequate time in bladder for reduction of nitrate to nitrite, and heavy bacteria reduce nitrate all the way to nitrogen which does not react.

9. **Leukocytes**

    a. Indicate possible urinary tract infections.

    b. Do not quantitate the number of WBCs.

    c. When positive, a urine microscopic is done.

    d. The strip method detects lysed leukocytes that would not be found under the microscope.

    e. **Reagent strip reactions:** indoxylcarbonic acid ester reacts with leukocyte esterase to form indoxyl and diazonium salt, forming a purple color.

    f. **Reaction interferences**

       1) False positive: pigmented urine

       2) False negative: increased glucose and protein; yellow-pigmented substances; high specific gravity (which prevents the release of leukocyte esterases); lymphocytes (do not contain leukocyte esterase)

10. **Specific gravity**

    a. Gives an approximate specific gravity value.

    b. **Clinical significance:** monitors hydration and dehydration, loss of renal tubular concentrating ability, and diabetes insipidus

    c. **Reagent strip reaction:** change in pH of methylvinyl ether maleic anhydride. Detects pH lowering caused by hydrogen ion concentration. Causes a change in color of bromthymol blue.

    d. **Reaction interferences**

       1) Increased protein or ketones increases the specific gravity.

       2) Urine pH of greater than 6.5, add .005 to the reading.

VII. MICROSCOPIC EXAMINATION OF URINE

A. **Microscopic Examination of Urine** — must be done to identify insoluble substances from the blood, kidney, lower urogenital tract, and external contaminants.

1. **Formed elements:** erythrocytes, leukocytes, epithelial cells, bacteria, yeast, fungal elements, parasites, mucus, sperm, crystals, and artifacts

2. **Standard rules for microscopics**
   a. Examine urine while fresh or when properly preserved.
   b. 12mL of urine is standard for centrifugation leaving 0.5mL of sediment for viewing.
   c. Report RBCs/WBCs using high power fields (HPF); report casts and crystals using low power field (LPF).
   d. All formed elements must be identified and quantitated.

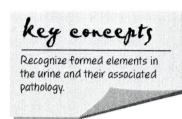

key concepts

Recognize formed elements in the urine and their associated pathology.

B. **Normal Urines** — 0–2 RBCs (HPF), 0–5 WBCs (HPF), 0–2 hyaline casts (LPF), several epithelial cells (HPF), and mucus

C. **Urine Formed Elements**

1. **Erythrocytes**
   a. Number of cells counted is related to extent of renal damage, glomerular membrane damage, or urogenital tract vascular damage.
   b. RBCs associated with infections, toxins, cancer, circulatory problems, renal calculi, menstrual contamination, trauma, and exercise.
   c. RBCs in normal urine appear as colorless disks; in concentrated urine they shrink and appear crenated; in dilute or alkaline urine, RBCs swell or lyse and appear as ghost cells.
   d. RBCs can be confused with yeast cells (budding) or oil droplets (highly refractile). Acetic acid can be used to lyse RBCs, and only yeast or oil will remain.

2. **Leukocytes**
   a. **Pyuria** is increased WBCs in the urine and may indicate infection in the urogenital tract. Leukocytes in the urine may indicate the following:
      1) Bacterial infections, pyelonephritis, cystitis, prostatitis, and urethritis
      2) Nonbacterial pyuria resulting from glomerulonephritis, lupus, and tumors
   b. WBCs appear in the urine with cytoplasmic granules and lobed nuclei.
      1) WBCs lyse in dilute alkaline urine and will produce **glitter cells,** which have a sparkling appearance and exhibit Brownian movement.
      2) **Eosinophils** in the urine may indicate a drug-induced nephritis or renal rejection.

3. **Epithelial cells**
   a. **Squamous:** very common in the urine and usually not clinically significant. Squamous epithelial cells line the vagina and lower

urethra. They have abundant, irregular cytoplasm and a central nucleus the size of an RBC.

b. **Transitional:** line the renal pelvis, bladder, and upper urethra. Smaller than squamous epithelial cells, are spherical/polyhedral, and have a central nucleus. No associated pathology except in large numbers, which may indicate renal carcinoma.

c. **Renal tubular:** most significant epithelial cell in the urine. Is round, larger than a WBC, and has an eccentric nucleus. Can indicate renal cancer, renal tubular damage, pyelonephritis, toxic reactions, and viral infection. Types of renal tubular cells include:

 1) **Bubble cells:** can be seen in renal necrosis and may contain large nonlipid filled vacuoles.

 2) **Oval fat bodies:** renal tubular epithelial cells that have absorbed lipids which are highly refractile.

d. **Miscellaneous cells: histocytes** in the urine may indicate lipid-storage disease.

4. **Casts**

a. Casts are the only formed elements in the urine that are **unique** to the kidney.

 1) Different casts represent different clinical conditions.

 2) **Cylindroiduria** is the term for casts in the urine.

 3) Casts are formed within the lumen of the distal tubule and collecting duct, and their shape is representative of the tubular lumen.

 4) Casts may have formed elements attached to their surface such as bacteria, crystals, etc.

 5) **Tamm-Horsfall** mucoprotein is the major constituent of casts, and is poorly detected by reagent strips methods.

5. **Types of casts**

a. **Hyaline cast:** the most commonly seen cast, 0–2 per high field is normal. Increased hyaline casts follow exercise, dehydration, heat, and emotional stress. Disease association: glomerulonephritis, renal disease, and heart failure.

 1) Appearance: colorless, and shows varied morphology

b. **RBC cast:** cellular casts containing erythrocytes may indicate renal disease or contact sports: bleeding within the nephron, damage to the glomerulus and renal capillaries.

 1) Appearance: yellow to brown color, contains hemoglobin or intact erythrocytes

c. **WBC cast:** a cellular cast that contains WBCs. Indicates infection or inflammation within the nephron (pyelonephritis). Bacterial cultures are indicated.

 1) Appearance: refractile. WBCs contain granules with multi-lobed nuclei.

d. **Epithelial cell cast:** contains epithelial cells, indicates renal tubular damage.

e. **Granular cast:** seen with hyaline casts following stress and exercise. May represent glomerular precipitants such as cellular casts or proteins, or nonpathogenic conditions such as stress and exercise.

1) Appearance: can be coarsely or finely granular (differentiation holds no clinical significance). Finely granular casts appear gray or pale yellow. Coarsely granular casts contain larger granules that may appear black.

f. **Waxy cast:** contains surface protein, granules adhere to the cast matrix. Found in renal failure.

1) Appearance: high refractive index, colorless to yellow with a smooth appearance

g. **Fatty cast:** seen with oval fat bodies in disorders with lipiduria.

1) Appearance: highly refractile, contains yellow-brown fat droplets. Positive identification of fatty casts is by Sudan III stain or polarized light, which shows a characteristic **Maltese cross formation.**

h. **Broad cast:** are formed in the collecting ducts due to anuria; all types of casts can occur in the broad form. Suggests renal failure.

6. **Bacteria:** are not present in normal sterile urine. Most labs only report bacteria in the urine in conjunction with WBCs.

7. **Yeast:** can be confused with erythrocytes, look for budding yeast forms. Seen in UTIs and diabetes mellitus.

8. **Parasites:** the most common parasite in the urine is ***Trichomonas vaginalis.*** Another parasite sometimes found in the urine is **pinworm ova,** which is usually due to fecal contamination.

9. **Sperm:** seen in urine following intercourse or nocturnal emissions. No clinical significance except in forensic cases.

10. **Mucus:** protein material produced by urogenital glands and epithelial cells. Not considered clinically significant. Appearance: thread-like structures with low refractive index, must view under reduced light. Can be confused with hyaline casts.

11. **Crystals**

a. Crystals are formed by the precipitation of urine salts, which can be altered by temperature, pH, and urine concentration. Will appear more frequently if urine stands at room temperature for prolonged time periods or is refrigerated. Urine pH is important in determining the type of crystal formation.

b. **Crystal formation:** the glomerular ultrafiltrate passes through the renal tubules, then the solutes in the ultrafilrate are concentrated. If an increased amount of a solute is present, the ultrafiltrate becomes saturated, leading to the solute precipitating into a characteristic crystal form. Crystal formation is enhanced when urine flow through the renal tubules is inhibited. The reduced flow allows time for concentration of the solutes in the ultrafiltrate.

c. **Crystal identification:** crystals differ in their solubility. **All clinically significant crystals are in acidic and neutral urine.**

12. **Types of acidic urine crystals**

a. **Amorphous urates**

1) Formed from the urate salts of Na, K, Mg, and Ca.

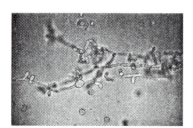

Yeast

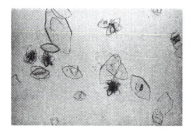

Uric acid

2) No clinical significance.

3) Small, yellow-to-brown granules usually in large amounts, which may make other urine elements difficult to see.

4) Refrigerated samples will produce more amorphous urates.

5) Amorphous urates will dissolve in alkaline pH or by heating above 60°C.

b. **Uric acid**

1) Seen in **gout** or cytotoxic drug use.

2) Appears yellow to orange/brown but can be colorless.

3) Pleomorphic (many) shapes include diamond, cube-shaped (four-sided), rhombic plates, prisms, and needles which may be clustered together to form rosettes.

c. **Sodium urate**

1) A form of uric acid crystal, appearing as light-yellow slender prisms, may be single or in clusters, and has no clinical importance.

d. **Calcium oxalate**

1) Most urine oxalate is from oxalic acid, which is a metabolite of ascorbic acid.

2) Often found in normal urine after eating tomatoes, asparagus, spinach, berries, and oranges.

3) Octahedral, envelope, or dumbbell shaped.

4) Can indicate chronic renal disease. Also seen in poison centers where children have ingested ethylene glycol (antifreeze).

e. **Bilirubin**

1) Formed when urine bilirubin exceeds its solubility.

2) Most often seen in liver disease.

3) Bilirubin crystals are abnormal and confirmed when the chemical screen is positive.

4) Fine needles, granules, or plates are yellow to brown in color.

f. **Cystine**

1) Abnormal crystal: congenital cystinosis or cystinuria. The crystals accumulate within renal tubules as calculi, which can result in renal damage.

2) Colorless, hexagonal plates.

3) Confirm with **cyanide-nitroprusside** for a purple color.

g. **Tyrosine**

1) Abnormal crystal: severe liver disease

2) Sheaths of fine delicate needles that are colorless or yellow

h. **Leucine**

1) Abnormal crystal: yellow to brown spheres with concentric circles and radial striations. Found with tyrosine crystals.

2) Resemble fat globules and are often described a buttonlike.

3) Seen in liver disease, including cirrhosis, hepatitis, and liver atrophy. Also seen in maple syrup urine disease.

i. **Cholesterol**

1) Abnormal crystal: large amounts of urinary cholesterol, in addition to protein, fatty casts, or oval fat bodies.

2) Clear, flat, rectangular plates with notched corners.

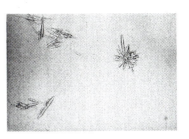

Uric acid

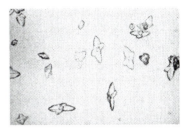

Uric acid

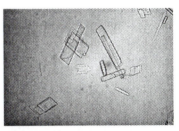

Uric acid

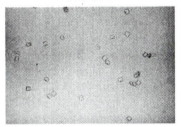

Calcium oxalate

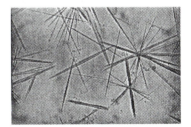

Tyrosine

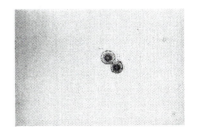

Leucine

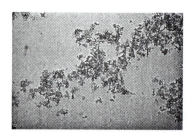

Amorphous phosphate

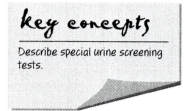

Ammonium biurate

j. **Crystals from medications**
   1) Medicine is excreted by the kidneys, any buildup can result in renal damage.
      a) **Ampicillin** crystals are long, colorless, thin prisms or needles.
      b) **Sulfonamide** crystals appear as bundles of needles that resemble sheaves of wheat or fan formations.

13. **Alkaline urine crystals**
    a. **Amorphous phosphate**
       1) Identical in appearance to amorphous urates and are generally colorless
       2) Amorphous phosphates are soluble in acetic acid (amorphous urates are insoluble in acetic acid) and will not dissolve when heated above 60°C.
       3) Not clinically significant
    b. **Triple phosphate**
       1) Normal crystal may be associated with renal calculi or UTIs.
       2) 3–6 sided prisms (coffin-lids)
    c. **Calcium phosphate**
       1) Normal crystal present in two forms:
          a) **Dicalcium phosphate** or "stellar phosphates"; colorless, thin prisms arranged in star-shaped patterns
          b) **Calcium phosphate:** irregular, granular sheets or plates that can be very large
    d. **Ammonium biurate**
       1) Normal crystal seen in old urine samples, will convert to uric acid crystals if acetic acid is added
       2) Yellow to brown spheres with striation on the surface, also can show irregular (thorny) projections (thorn apple)
    e. **Calcium carbonate**
       1) Appear as small, colorless crystals or dumbbells
       2) Have no clinical significance

VIII. **SPECIAL URINE SCREENING TESTS (usually performed in special chemistry)**
   A. **Phenylketonuria (PKU):** indicates defective metabolic conversion of phenylalanine to tyrosine which is caused by a gene failure to produce phenylalanine hydroxylase.
      1. Occurs in 1:10,000 births and if undetected will result in severe mental retardation.
      2. PKU screening tests are required in all fifty states for newborns (at least 24 hours old).
      3. The urine gives off a mousy odor associated with phenylpyruvate due to the increased ketones.
      4. When the PKU is positive, the diet is changed to eliminate all phenylalanine from the diet.
      5. As the child grows, an alternative phenylalanine pathway develops and dietary restrictions are eased.
      6. **Types of PKU testing** (all positive screening tests are confirmed by HPLC)

    a. **Guthrie** bacterial inhibition test: uses blood from a heel stick. Blood is placed on disks on culture media streaked with *Bacillus subtilis.* If phenylalanine is present in the sample, B-2-thienylalanine, which is an inhibitor of *B. subtilis,* will be counteracted, resulting in *B. subtilis* growth around the disks (positive PKU).

    b. Urine test uses **ferric chloride** (tube or reagent strip); a positive test is blue-gray to green-gray.

        1) **Microfluorometric assay** is a new method for direct measurement of phenylalanine in dried blood filter discs.

        2) It is a quantitative test (Guthrie is semiquantitative).

        3) It is not affected by antibiotics.

        4) A pretreated (trichloroacetic acid) patient sample extract is reacted in a microtiter plate containing ninhydrin, succinate, leucylalanine, and copper tartrate.

        5) The sample is measured at 360nm and 530nm.

B. Miscellaneous Special Urine Screening Tests

  1. **Tyrosinemia**

    a. Excess tyrosine or its by-products (p-hydroxyphenylpyruvic acid or p-hydroxyphenyllactic acid) in the urine.

    b. An inherited or metabolic defect.

    c. Disease states include **transitory tyrosinemia** seen in premature infants with an underdeveloped liver and **acquired severe liver disease,** which will produce tyrosine and leucine crystals.

    d. Screening tests include the nitroso-naphthol test and the Millon's test (contains mercury).

  2. **Alkaptonuria**

    a. Results from a genetic defect resulting in failure to produce homogentistic acid oxidase.

    b. This condition produces brown pigment deposits in body tissue that can lead to arthritis, liver, and cardiac problems.

    c. Screening test includes:

        1) Ferric chloride tube test (blue color)

        2) Benedict's test (yellow color)

        3) Alkalization of fresh urine (urine darkens)

  3. **Melanuria**

    a. Increased melanin in the urine.

    b. Indicates malignant melanoma.

    c. Screening test includes ferric chloride (gray/black precipitate) and sodium nitroprusside (red color).

  4. **Maple syrup urine disease**

    a. Characteristic of this disorder is maple syrup smell of the urine, breath, and skin.

    b. Caused by low levels of branched-chained keto acid decarboxylase, which inhibits the metabolism of leucine, isoleucine, and valine.

    c. If untreated, the disease causes severe mental retardation, convulsions, acidosis, and hypoglycemia. Death occurs during the first year.

    d. A modified Guthrie test is used to screen for this disorder.

IX. BODY FLUIDS (most CSF analysis is performed in chemistry, hematology, and microbiology)

key concepts

Discuss the significance of body fluids in the diagnosis of disease.

A. Cerebrospinal Fluid (CSF) — supplies nutrients to nervous tissue, removes wastes, and is a barrier and cushion to the brain and spinal cord against trauma. 20 mL of CSF is produced each hour. Total adult volume: 140–170mL, neonates: 10–60mL.

1. **Specimen collection** is by lumbar puncture between 3–4 or 4–5 lumbar vertebrae. The order of draw is:
   a. Tube #1: chemistry and serology
   b. Tube #2: microbiology
   c. Tube #3: hematology
   d. Extra tubes: freeze
2. **Cerebrospinal fluid appearance**
   a. **Clear and colorless:** normal
   b. **Cloudy:** indicates WBCs, RBCs, bacteria, seen in meningitis or hemorrhage
   c. **Bloody:** subarachnoid hemorrhage or traumatic tap
   d. **Xanthochromic** (yellow): increased Hgb, bilirubin, protein, immature liver in infants (normal newborn)
3. **Cerebrospinal fluid microscopic:** normal CSF contains 0–5 WBC/microliter
   a. **Lymphocytes:** seen in normal fluids; increased in viral, syphilitic, or fungal meningitis
   b. **PMNs:** bacterial meningitis (cerebral abscess)
   c. **Early cell forms:** acute leukemia
   d. **Plasma cells:** multiple sclerosis or lymphocytic reactions
4. **India ink:** used to detect *Cryptococcus neoformans*
5. **Gram stain:** used to detect bacteria

B. Seminal Fluid (Sperm) — used to evaluate infertility, postvasectomy, and forensic medicine cases

1. **Specimen collection**
   a. Collect in sterile containers after 3-day period of no sex for infertility studies, postvasectomy requires no waiting period.
   b. No plastic containers that will inhibit motility.
   c. No condom collection (may contain spermicidal agents).
   d. Keep at room temperature; transport within one hour.
2. **Types of sperm analysis**
   a. **Volume:** 2–5 mL
   b. **Viscosity:** normal is no clumps or strings; rate 0–4 with 0 being watery and 4 being gel-like. Must have specimen that is completely liquefied which takes about 30 minutes.
   c. **Appearance:** normal is a milky color, may be red, cloudy, etc.
   d. **pH:** 7.2–7.8 is normal (>7.8 could indicate infection).
   e. **Sperm count:** normal is 20–160 million/mL, borderline is 10–20 million/mL, sterile is less than 10 million/mL.
   f. **Motility:** based on the percentage of movement, 50–60 percent with a motility grade of 3 or 4 as normal (0–immotile; 4–motile with strong forward progression)

g. **Shape:** normal; abnormal forms—double head, giant head, amorphous head, pinhead, double tail, coiled tail, and spermatid

C. Synovial Fluid

1. Synovial fluid is a plasma ultrafiltrate and is often called joint fluid.
2. Synovial fluid functions as a lubricant and nutrient transport to articular cartilage.
3. Different joint disorders change the chemical and structural composition of synovial fluid, including inflammation, infection, bleeding, and crystal-associated disorders.
4. Normal color of synovial fluid is clear to straw colored.
5. Laboratory analysis (nonchemistry) includes color, differential count, gram stain with culture, and crystal identification with a polarizing microscope.
   a. Most crystals found in synovial fluid are associated with gout or calcium/phosphate deposits.

D. Gastric Analysis — collection is nasal or oral intubation. Analysis involves physical appearance, volume, titratable acidity, and pH. Most uses of gastric analysis are toxicology.

E. Miscellaneous Body Fluids

1. **Amniotic fluid**
   a. Protective fluid that surrounds the fetus
   b. Mostly used for genetic studies but may be used to check for fetal bleeding, infection, or estimation of **meconium** (dark green secretions of the fetal intestinal glands) content that in large amounts is associated with meconium aspiration syndrome.
2. **Peritoneal fluid**
   a. Fluid contained within the peritoneum (serous membrane that covers the walls of the abdomen and pelvis)
   b. Laboratory analysis includes cell counts, gram stains, and gross color examination.
3. **Pleural and pericardial fluid**
   a. Pleural fluid is contained within the pleural cavity and pericardial fluid surrounds the heart.
   b. Aspiration of pleural/pericardial/peritoneal fluid is termed thoracentesis.
   c. Laboratory analysis includes cell counts, gram stains, and gross color examination.

F. Fecal Analysis — used in the detection of gastrointestinal (GI) bleeding, liver and billary duct disorders, malabsorption syndromes, microbiology, and parasitology.

1. **Types of fecal analysis**
   a. **Color and consistency**
      1) **Black (tarry) stool:** GI bleeding
      2) **Steatorrhea:** fat malabsorption, bulky and frothy with a pale-to-dark yellow color
      3) **Diarrhea:** watery
      4) **Ribbonlike stools:** bowel obstruction

5) **Mucus:** inflammation of the intestinal wall (colitis)

b. **Fecal leukocytes:** determines cause of diarrhea

1) Neutrophils: bacterial intestinal wall infections or ulcerative colitis, abscesses

2) No neutrophils: toxin producing bacteria, viruses, and parasites

c. **Qualitative fecal fat:** detects fat malabsorption disorders by staining fecal fats with **Sudan III or oil red O.** Increased fecal fat (> 100/HPF).

d. **Muscle fibers:** look for undigested striated muscle fibers, which may indicate pancreatic insufficiency seen in cystic fibrosis (maldigestion).

e. **Occult blood:** Used for early detection of colorectal cancer; old name is guaiac test.

1) Most frequently performed fecal analysis

   a) Upper GI → black tarry stools

   b) Lower GI → bloody red stools

2) Several chemicals used that vary in sensitivity

   a) Benzidine — most senstivive but no longer used (carcinogenic)

   b) Orthotoluidine

   c) Gum guaiac — least sensitive, most common

reaction uses pseudoperoxidase activity of Hb reacting with H_2O_2 to oxidize a colorless compound to a colored compound

Hb → H_2O_2 → orthotoluidine → blue oxidized indicator

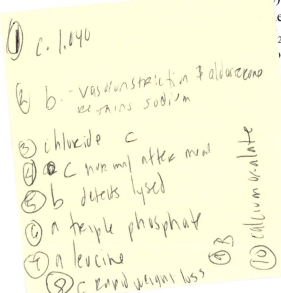

① c. 1.040

② b. - vasoconstriction & aldosterone retains sodium

③ chloride c

④ ⓒ normal after meal

⑤ b detects lysed

⑥ a triple phosphate

⑦ a leucine

⑧ c rapid weight loss

⑨ b

⑩ calcium oxalate

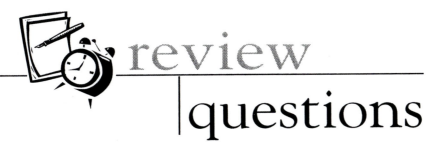

review questions

DIRECTIONS Each of the questions or incomplete statements below is followed by suggested answers or completions. Select the **one answer** that is best in each case.

1. After running 10 miles in a race, the patient seeks medical care at the local emergency room because of excessive vomiting and diarrhea. The most probable urine specific gravity would be:
   a. 1.002
   b. 1.010
   c. 1.040
   d. 1.000

2. Which statement is correct regarding Angiotensin II?
   a. It is a hormone secreted by the kidneys and is inert.
   b. It causes vasoconstriction of renal arterioles and releases aldosterone that retains sodium ions.
   c. It causes reabsorption of potassium ions in the proximal tubules.
   d. It acts to correct renal blood flow by releasing aldosterone that retains potassium.

3. The major inorganic substance in urine is:
   a. sodium
   b. potassium
   c. chloride
   d. mucus

4. A pH of more than 7.0 may indicate:
   a. gall bladder infection
   b. uncontrolled diabetes mellitus
   c. normal response following a meal
   d. viral infection

5. Which statement is correct for the leukocyte strip test?
   a. When negative a urine microscopic is performed.
   b. Detects lysed leukocytes.
   c. Indicates possible viral UTIs.
   d. May indicate high concentrations of bilirubin.

6. Which crystal is not found in acidic urine?
   a. triple phosphate
   b. sulfonamide
   c. cystine
   d. tyrosine

7. Which crystal is not found in alkaline urine?
   a. leucine
   b. calcium phosphate
   c. ammonium biurate
   d. none of the above

8. Ketonuria may indicate:
   a. menstruation.
   b. hemolytic anemia.
   c. rapid weight loss.
   d. none of the above.

9. Joe is a teacher who stands most of the day at the blackboard; he also has diabetes mellitus, which is usually controlled, but isn't today. In addition, Joe is getting over Hepatitis A from food he ate at a local pub. Choose the urinalysis result that best fits this case.

a. positive bilirubin, negative glucose, and acid urine pH
b. positive glucose, positive bilirubin, and acid pH
c. high urine specific gravity, negative bilirubin, and negative blood
d. normal urine pH with all negative urine chemistries

10. Which of the following can indicate chronic renal disease and is also seen in patients who have ingested ethylene glycol?
   a. cystine
   b. calcium oxalate
   c. calcium phosphate
   d. triple phosphate

2

Hematology

contents

➤ COMPREHENSIVE KEY CONCEPTS

1. Correlate erythrocyte, leukocyte, platelet indices, special stain analysis, and slide differential characteristics to disease states, including anemia, hemoglobinopathies, and myeloproliferative disorders.

2. Discuss hematopoiesis in regard to organs involved, erythrocyte, leukocyte, platelet maturation, hemoglobin synthesis, and disease processes that can inhibit hematopoiesis.

―――――――――

I. FUNDAMENTAL HEMATOLOGY PRINCIPLES

A. Blood Composition

1. **Whole blood** includes erythrocytes, leukocytes, platelets, and plasma. Leukocytes and platelets make up the **buffy coat.**
2. **Plasma** is the liquid portion of unclotted blood and **serum** is the fluid that remains after a clot has formed.
   a. Plasma is composed of 90% water and contains protein, enzymes, hormones, lipids, and salts.
   b. Plasma normally appears hazy and pale yellow (contains coagulation proteins), and serum normally appears clear and straw colored (contains no coagulation proteins).

B. Basic Hematology Terminology

a-	without
-blast	young/nucleated
-cyte	cell
-chromic	color
dys-	abnormal
-emia	blood
ferro-	iron
hyper-	increased
hypo-	decreased
iso-	equal
macro-	large
micro-	small
myelo-	marrow
mega-	large
normo-	normal
-oid	like
-osis	increased
-penia	decreased
-plasia	formation
-poiesis	cell production
poly-	many
pro-	before

C. Formed Elements and Sizes

1. Thrombocytes (platelets)	2–4μm	disk-shaped
2. Erythrocytes (RBCs)	7–8μm	biconcave
3. Normal Lymphocytes	6–9μm	round
a. Atypical lymphcyte	10–22μm	variable/irregular

4. Basophils	8–10μm	round
5. Neutrophils	10–15μm	round
a. Band neutrophil	10–15μm	round
6. Eosinophils	12–16μm	round
7. Monocytes	12–22μm	variable/irregular

D. RBC Indices and Platelet Index

1. **MCV: mean corpuscular volume**. Normal range is 80–95 femto-liters (fL), and is an indicator of the average volume of individual erythrocytes (RBCs). Calculate using the hemaotcrit (Hct) and RBC counts:

$$MCV(fL) = \frac{Hct\ (\%) \times 10}{RBC\ count\ (\times 10^{12}/L)}$$

   a. **Increased** in megaloblastic anemias, hemolytic and aplastic anemias, liver disease, and hypothyroidism
   b. **Decreased** in any condition that results in the production of microcytes, such as iron deficiency anemia
   c. May be **normal** in anemia of chronic disorders, sideroblastic anemia, and myelofibrosis

2. **MCH: mean corpuscular hemoglobin**. Normal range is 26–34 picograms (pg), and is an indicator of the average weight of hemoglobin (hemoglobin) in individual RBCs. Calculate using the hemoglobin and RBC counts:

$$MCH\ (pg) = \frac{Hemoglobin\ (g/dL) \times 10}{RBC\ count\ (\times 10^{12}/L)}$$

   a. **Increased** in macrocytic anemias
   b. **Decreased** in hypochromic and microcytic anemias

3. **MCHC: mean corpuscular hemoglobin concentration**. Normal range is 32–36%, and is a measure of the average concentration of hemoglobin in grams per deciliter of RBCs. Calculate using the hemoglobin and HCT counts:

$$MCHC\ (g/dL) = \frac{Hemoglobin\ (g/dL)}{Hct} \times 100$$

   a. 31–37g/dL MCHC indicates **normochromic** RBCs.
   b. < 31 g/dL MCHC indicates **hypochromic** RBCs seen in iron deficiencies and thalassemias.
   c. > 37 g/dL MCHC indicates **hyperchromic** RBCs. May indicate spherocytosis and should be confirmed.

4. **RDW: RBC distribution width.** Normal range is 8.5–14.5 percent.
   a. Will be increased or decreased according to the degree of aniso-cytosis; coefficient of variation of red cell volume.
   b. Normal RDW: Indicates anemia of chronic disorders, aplastic anemia, and thalassemia minor.
   c. High RDW: Indicates sideroblastic and iron deficiency anemia, various hemoglobinopathies, and folate/vitamin B_{12} deficiency.

5. **MPV: mean platelet volume.** Normal range is 7.0–10.0 fL.

key concepts

Discuss RBC indices, know the formulas, and describe conditions that are associated with various values.

6. **HCT (hematocrit):** Volume of packed RBCs. Ratio of RBCs in whole blood. Is measured in percentages. Normal range is 40–52 percent.
   a. **The spun hematocrit** is the reference manual method.
   b. The buffy coat layer of leukocytes and platelets can be seen between plasma (upper) and RBC (lower) layers.

E. Relative and Absolute Blood Cell Counts

1. **Relative count** is an increase of a cell type in relation to other blood components. **Relative lymphocytosis** is an increase in the **percentage** of lymphocytes frequently associated with neutropenia. In **relative polycythemia**, RBCs appear increased due to a decreased plasma volume.
2. **Absolute count** is an increase in the total actual number of cells without respect to other blood components. **Absolute lymphocytosis** is a true increase in the **number** of lymphocytes. **Absolute polycythemia** is a true increase in the number of RBCs.

F. Basic Homeostasis

1. **Homeostasis** is the body's tendency to move toward physiological stability. In vitro testing of blood and other body fluids must replicate exact environmental body conditions. These conditions should include:
   a. **Osmotic concentration** is the body/cellular water concentration, composed of 0.85 percent sodium chloride. Normal osmotic concentration is termed **isotonic**. In a hypotonic solution ($> H_2O$ and $<$ solutes), the cells swell and may burst— **spherocytes** would form. A hypertonic ($< H_2O$, $>$ solutes) solution will cause cells to constrict—**crenated** cells will form.
   b. **pH:** Normal range: venous blood—7.36 to 7.41; arterial blood—7.38 to 7.44. Factors that affect blood pH are respiratory problems, kidney problems, and diabetes.
   c. **Temperature:** Normal body temperature is 37.0°C. Blood specimens should be analyzed as soon as possible to prevent cellular breakdown (see specimen collection for times). Cells will lyse below 4.0°C, and will lyse or be destroyed above 56°C.
   d. **Nutrients:** Blood contains sufficient nutrients to provide for adequate testing for up to 4 hours. Erythrocytes break down glucose at a rate of about 5 percent per hour, but heparin fluoride, a preservative, will inhibit glycolysis.

G. Hematology Stains

1. **Nonvital Polychrome Stain (Romanowsky)**
   a. Most commonly used routine peripheral bloodstain.
   b. Contains **methylene blue,** which stains basic cellular components blue (DNA and RNA), and **eosin,** which stains acid components red-orange (eosinophilic cytoplasmic granules). RBCs will stain pink.
   c. A **methanol fixative** is used in the staining process to prevent the plasma background on the glass slide from staining blue.

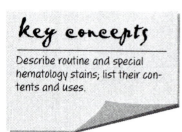

key concepts

Describe routine and special hematology stains; list their contents and uses.

   d. A phosphate buffer with a pH between 6.4 and 6.7 neutralizes
      the staining process.
   e. Examples of polychrome stains include the **Wright, Giemsa,
      Leishman, Jenner, May-Grünwald,** and various combinations
      of each.
2. **Nonvital monochrome stain**
   a. Stains specific cellular components.
   b. **Prussian Blue** stain is an example.
      1) Contains potassium ferrocyanide, HCL, and a safranin
         counterstain.
      2) Used to show **iron granules** in RBCs (siderocytic iron gran-
         ules), histocytes, and urine epithelial cells.
3. **Vital monochrome stains**
   a. Used to stain specific cellular components.
   b. No fixatives are used in the staining process.
   c. Include:
      1) **Reticulocyte** stains: methylene blue which precipitates RNA
         reticulum in early RBCs
      2) **Heinz Body** stains: brilliant cresyl green to show **denatured
         hemoglobin** associated with G-6-PD deficiency
4. **Staining problems**
   a. **Too red:** buffer/stain below 6.4 pH, excess buffer, decreased
      staining time, increased washing time, thin smear, and expired
      stains
   b. **Too blue:** Buffer/stain above 6.7 pH, too little buffer, increased
      staining time, poor washing, thick smear, increased protein, low
      HCT, heparin blood samples, and immature WBCs.

H. Special Stains (Cytochemistry)

1. **Peroxidase stain**
   a. Peroxidases are enzymes that catalyze the oxidation of sub-
      stances by hydrogen peroxide. Stain only **azurophilic** granules.
   b. Perioxidase positive **neutrophilic granules** determine the
      granulocytic component in **acute leukemias.**
   c. A positive peroxidase stain shows **dark brown granules** in granu-
      locytic cytoplasm. **Eosinophils** are also positive for peroxidase.
   d. Monocytes may be very weakly positive.
   e. Basophils and lymphocytes are **negative** for peroxidase activity.
2. **Cyanide-resistant peroxidase stain**
   a. **Eosinophilic** component of **acute myeloid** and **acute
      myelomonocytic leukemias.**
   b. Causes eosinophilic granules to become **intensely brown.**
   c. Neutrophils and all other leukocytes are negative.
3. **Acid phosphatase (AP) leukocyte stain**
   a. Shows acid phosphatase activity—useful in **differentiating T-
      lymphocyte leukemia from B-lymphocyte leukemia.**
   b. Positive for most leukocytes with lymphocytes showing less ac-
      tivity. (T-lymphocytes are positive; B-lymphocytes are negative.)
   c. A positive stain will show purple to dark red granules.

4. **Tartrate-resistant acid phosphatase stain**
   a. Used to diagnose **hairy cell leukemia.**
   b. Hairy cell leukemic cell granules stain purple to red.

5. **Leukocyte alkaline phosphatase (LAP)**
   a. Only **neutrophils** contain alkaline phosphatase.
   b. A positive stain will show deposits of blue or violet color where alkaline phosphatase activity is present.
   c. Used to separate **granulocytic leukemias** from **leukemoid reactions.**
   d. A **LAP score** is determined based on:
      1) Stain intensity.
      2) Size of granules.
      3) Percentage of cells that are stained.
      4) Results are rated from 0 to 4+ and are derived from a Kaplow count (100 neutrophils are counted as scored using LAP score criteria).
      5) Normal LAP score range is between 25–225.
   e. Examples of LAP Scores
      1) **Increased LAP score:** leukemoid reactions, late trimester pregnancy
      2) **Normal LAP score:** chronic granulocytic leukemia with remission or infection, and viral infections such as mononucleolosis and hepatitis
      3) **Decreased LAP score:** chronic granulocytic leukemias

6. **Periodic acid-Schiff (PAS)**
   a. PAS will stain leukocyte **glycogen** a bright pink.
   b. Used to diagnose erythroleukemia, Gaucher's disease, and acute lymphocytic leukemia.

7. **Sudan black B**
   a. Stains phospholipids and lipoproteins.
   b. Granulocytes stain positive (blue-black granulation), and lymphocytes are negative for Sudan Black B.
   c. Separates **lymphocytic leukemias** from **myeloid/monocytic leukemias**

8. **Alpha-naphthyl acetate esterase stain**
   a. Used to distinguish **granulocytic leukemias** (negative) from **monocytic leukemias** (positive with black granulation).

9. **Naphthol AS-D chloroacetate esterase stain**
   a. Used to distinguish **granulocytic leukemias** (positive with red granulation) from **monocytic leukemias** (negative).

10. **Prussian blue stain**
    a. Precipitates free iron into small blue/green granules in erythrocytes.
    b. **Siderocytes** are RBCs that contain free iron.
    c. Ringed sideroblasts are RBCs that contain circular iron granules.
    d. The following formula is used to determine the siderocyte percentage:

$$\% \text{ siderocytes} = \frac{\# \text{ of RBCs containing granules}}{100 \text{ RBCS}} \quad (0\text{--}1\% \text{ is normal})$$

e. **Increased percentage of siderocytes** are seen in thalassemias and following splenectomy, and ringed sideroblasts are seen in alcoholism and lead poisoning.

11. **Heinz Body**
   a. Used to stain **unstable hemoglobin.**
   b. Used in the diagnosis of **G-6-PD deficiency** and other hemolytic disorders.

I. Histograms (impedance technology)

1. **WBC histogram**
   a. 45–450 fL is the normal range for **WBCs.**
   b. 1st peak: 45–90 fL is the normal range for **lymphocytes.**
   c. 2nd peak: 90–160 fL is the normal range for **monocytes** and **immature WBCs.**
   d. 3rd peak: 160–450 fL is the normal range for **granulocytes.**

2. **Abnormal WBC histogram**
   a. Less than 50 fL may indicate nucleated RBCs **(nRBCs), sickled erythrocytes, giant** or **clumped platelets.**
   b. Peak overlap at 90 fL may indicate an **increase** in **bands** and **immature cells.**
   c. Greater than 450 fL indicates a **high granulocyte** count.

3. **RBC histogram**
   a. Normal RBC cell range is 36–360 fL.
   b. A normal RBC histogram will show a single peak between 70 and 110 fL, and will correlate with the MCV.

4. **Abnormal RBC histogram**
   a. Two peaks will indicate a microcytic and macrocytic erythrocyte population.
   b. An increased curve width will correlate with an increased RDW.
   c. Shift to the right indicates an increased MCV.
   d. Shift to the left indicates a decreased MCV.

5. **Platelet histogram**
   a. Normal range is 2–20 fL.
   b. Abnormal ranges indicate abnormal platelet morphology.

J. Automated Cell Count Errors

1. WBC counts over 50,000 result in increased cell turbidity and may increase the MCV, HCT, and hemoglobin levels.

2. Glucose over 400mg/dL (hyperosmolality) may increase the MCV, HCT, and decrease the MCHC.

3. Repeat analysis if:
   a. Rule of three does not agree.
   b. Indices are out of range.
   c. WBC/RBC are grossly out of range.
   d. Carry over from low to high WBC counts in preceding patient samples.

4. Increased cold agglutinins titer may increase the MCV and MCHC, and decrease the RBC count.

5. Lipemic samples may increase the hemoglobin, MCH, and MCHC.

II. HEMATOPOIESIS

A. *Hematopoiesis* is the production and differentiation of blood cells.

1. The **yolk sac** is located external to the developing embryo and is the first hematopoietic organ. This type of blood cell production (non–bone marrow) is called **external hematopoiesis.** The first cell to be produced is a **primitive erythroblast.**

2. At six weeks of age, the **liver** becomes a major hematopoietic organ, producing granulocytes, megakaryocytes, and nucleated erythroblasts. Activity lasts for 7 months.

3. The **spleen** has minimal hematopoietic activity during fetal development. Its primary function is filtration and the elimination of RBC inclusions and damaged and aged RBCs. The spleen also is a reservoir for platelets.

   a. The spleen is divided into **white** and **red pulp.**
   1) White pulp is concentrated with lymphocytes and macrophages.
   2) Red pulp is the area of the spleen comprised of small porous membranes, which filter erythrocytes and clears old or damaged erythrocytes.

4. After seven months of fetal life, the **bone marrow** becomes the major hematopoietic organ, with minimal lymph node support.

5. At birth, 90 percent of the bone marrow shows **red marrow,** which indicates very active blood cell production. Over time this red marrow becomes **white marrow,** indicating less cell production and more adipose tissue. Under physiological stress, white marrow may revert back to red marrow.

B. Pediatric and Adult Hematopoiesis

1. **Lymphatic tissue**
   a. **Primary lymphatic tissue** includes:
   1) **Bone marrow:** the major hematopoeitic organ after birth
   2) **Thymus:** functions in T-lymphocyte maturation
   b. **Secondary lymphatic tissue** includes:
   1) **Lymph nodes:** contain B-lymphocytes and macrophages
   2) **Spleen:** functions in blood filtration and is concentrated with lymphocytes and platelets
   3) **Gut-associated lymphatic tissue:** a reservoir for lymphocytes.

2. **Bone marrow**
   a. Newborn: 80–90 percent of bone marrow is active in producing nucleated RBCs, lymphocytes, and hemoglobin.
   b. Young adult (age 20): 60 percent of bone marrow is active and found at the proximal ends of large flat bones, pelvis, and sternum.
   c. Older adult (age 55): bone marrow is 40 percent red and 60 percent white marrow.
   d. Bone marrow function
   1) Hematopoiesis involves the production of **stem cells, progenitor cells,** and **precursor cells.**
      a) **Stem cells:** pluripotential cells that differentiate into specific cell lines. Stem cells differentiate into colony-

forming units (CFU), which further differentiate into B/T-lymphocytes, granulocytes, thrombocytes, monocytes, and erythrocytes.

    b) **Progenitor cells:** committed cells that only develop into a single cell line. These cells develop into BFU-E (erythrocytes), CFU-E (erythrocytes), CFU-MEG (thrombocytes), and CFU-GM (granulocytes).

    c) **Precursor cells:** these cells mature into blast forms.

C. Blood Cell Growth and Differentiation

1. **Pluripotent stem cell (PPSC)**
   a. Origin of all blood cells.
   b. Up to 10 percent of newborn umbilical cord cells.
   c. Less than 1 percent of adult blood cells.
   d. Differentiation of PPSC is determined by protein factors.

2. **Cell proliferation and differentiation**
   a. **Protein factors** can stimulate or inhibit blood cell production.
   b. **Cell adhesion molecules (CAMs)** are located on various cells and will influence and direct blood cells through maturation and function.
   c. **Growth factors** are factors that influence cell differentiation.
      1) Growth factors are regulatory glycoprotein hormones, including erythropoietin, interleukin, and colony-stimulating factors.

D. The Origin of Blood Cells

1. In the **bone marrow (myeloid),** the precursor of all cells is the **pluripotent stem cell (PPSC),** which develops into the **hematopoietic stem cell (HSC).**

2. Process is directed by two factors known as the **stem cell factor (SCF)** and the **myeloid stem factor (MSF).**

3. Hematopoietic stem cells develop into colony-forming units that give rise to granulocytes, erythrocytes, monocytes, and megakaryocytes—CFU-GEMM.

4. The CFU-GEMM differentiates into the following in the peripheral blood:

      BFU-E————CFU-E————Erythrocytes
      CFU-MEG————————Thrombocytes
      CFU-GM——CFEU-M——Monocytes
      ***CFU-GM——CFU-G————Segmented Neutrophils**
      ***CFU-EO————————————Eosinophils**

5. Basophils probably develop from a separate committed progenitor cell.

6. In the **tissue,** the following cells further differentiate: monocytes become macrophages, eosinophils become tissue eosinophils, and basophils become mast cells.

7. In the **lymph system,** hematopoietic stem cells under the influence of **SCF** and **LSF (lymphoid stem factor)** become **lymphoid stem cells (LSC)** that become **B-lymphocytes** (develop in the Bursa equivalent) and **T-lymphocytes** (develop in the thymus).

8. In the **tissue**, B-lymphocytes also develop into **plasma cells.**

9. Lymphoid cells are the result of extramedullary hematopoiesis, and myeloid cells result from intramedullary hematopoiesis.

E. Introduction to Progenitor and WBCs

1. CFU-GEMM are myeloid progenitor cells and are self-replicating.
2. LSCs are lymphoid progenitor cells.
3. Nonprogenitor cells include BFU-E, CFU-Mega, CFU-GM, CFU-EO, and CFU-BA.
4. Segmented neutrophils (major purpose) destroy (engulf) bacteria.
5. Monocytes destroy bacteria and relay information about the organisms to other cells.
6. Eosinophils are involved in hypersensitive reactions associated with allergies, colds, and parasitic infections.
7. Basophils probably develop from a separate committed progenitor cell.
8. Basophils mediate hypersensitivity reactions such as allergies and colds in the tissue, but not in the blood.
9. T cells develop in the thymus and produce an immune response against disease.
10. B cells produce antibodies in an immune response, can also develop into plasma cells in the tissue, and are very efficient antibody producers.
11. NK cells destroy target cells that are recognized as foreign.
12. K or lymphocyte-activated killer (LAK) cells are antibody dependent cell-mediated cytotoxic cells that destroy invading cells that have been coated with antibody.

F. Hematopoietic Terminology

1. **Medullary hematopoiesis:** Blood cell production within the bone marrow
   a. Myelopoiesis: granulocyte production
   b. Erythropoiesis: RBC production
   c. Monopoiesis: monocyte production
   d. Thrombopoiesis: platelet production
2. **Extramedullary hematopoiesis:** Blood cell production outside the bone marrow
   a. Lymphopoiesis—lymphocyte production that occurs in the bone marrow, lymph system, spleen, and peripheral blood
   b. Can refer to prenatal or abnormal blood production outside the bone marrow

G. Bone Marrow Cell Production

1. The bone marrow is responsible for producing myeloid blood cells. A bone marrow evaluation is reported as a **M:E ratio** or myeloid/erythrocyte ratio. The normal M:E ratio is **3 to 4:1**.
2. Stem cell pool is found in bone marrow and contains a supply (6–10 day lifespan) of these myeloid blood cells.
3. Most cell production in the bone marrow is myelocytic and is mostly granulocytic.
4. The myelocytic pool of cells takes 3 days to develop into mature/functioning cells. After the last stage of mitosis, they enter the storage pool until needed outside the bone marrow.

5. Myeloid pool cells can enter the peripheral blood as mature cells and are found in two places:
   a. **Marginating granulocyte pool (MGP)** is found along the blood vessel endothelial wall.
   b. **Circulating granulocyte pool (CSP)** is found in the peripheral blood.

H. Basic Cell Morphology

1. **Nucleus (N)**
   a. Contains **heterochromatin** that does **not** undergo cell division. Is dark and clumped.
   b. Also contains **euchromatin**, which undergoes cell division. Is light, loose, and contains nucleoli.
2. **Cytoplasm (C)**
   a. Contains cellular organelles that stain according to their contents.
      1) A blue color indicates components rich in RNA (a regulatory protein) and protein synthesis.
3. **Golgi apparatus**
   a. Prepares protein for secretions.
   b. Increased protein amounts within the cell will show clear areas around or near the nucleus.

I. Immature and Mature Cell Characteristics — Immature cells are very large and become smaller as they mature.

Immature Cells	Mature Cells
high N:C ratio	low N:C ratio
nucleoli present	contain no nucleoli
chromatin is loose and light	chromatin is dark and clumped
cells are **not** segmented	cells become segmented
cytoplasm is intensely blue	cytoplasm is moderately blue
organelles are **not** defined	organelles are defined

III. GRANULOCYTES

A. Basic Review

1. Granulocytes are also known as leukocytes, which are white blood cells named as such because they form pus or settle in the test tube as a white color. **Granulocytes** include **neutrophils, eosinophils,** and **basophils.** Granulocytes normally contain cytoplasmic granules.

B. Maturation and Morphology of Immature Granulocytes

1. **Myeloblast:** the first and earliest granulocyte
   a. Is a large cell (15μm).
   b. High N:C ratio (4:1).
   c. Round nucleus with loose light staining euchromatin.
   d. 1–2 nucleoli.
   e. Has minimal light blue cytoplasm.
   f. Contains **no cytoplasmic granules**.
   g. Begins to produce myeloperoxidase granules (MPO).
   h. Comprises 1 percent of the nucleated cells in the bone marrow.
   i. Takes 18 hours to mature.

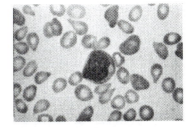

> key concepts
>
> Describe maturation and morphology of granulocytes and include characteristics of each stage.

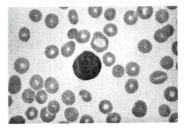

Myeloblast

Myeloblast

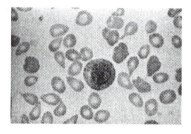

Promyelocyte

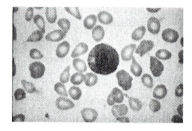

Promyelocyte

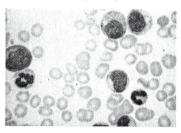

Myelocyte

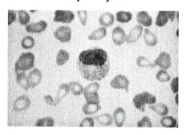

Myelocyte, band

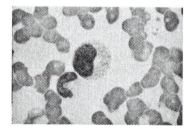

Metamyelocyte, band

2. **Promyelocyte:** larger than a myeloblast (20μm)
   a. High N:C ratio (3:1).
   b. Loose chromatin with nucleoli.
   c. Dark blue cytoplasm.
   d. Contains **large nonspecific cytoplasmic granules** containing MPO.
   e. Comprises 3 to 4 percent of nucleated bone marrow cells.
   f. Takes 24 hours to mature.
3. **Myelocyte:** medium cell size (12μm)
   a. **Round nucleus** with darker blue heterochromatin.
   b. Last stage of cell division.
   c. Has active RNA, therefore, the cytoplasm is blue.
   d. Contains MPO and secondary granules containing leukocyte alkaline phosphatase.
   e. Comprises 11.9 percent of bone marrow nucleated cells. Takes 100 hours to mature.
4. **Metamyelocyte:** last mononuclear stage, no mitosis
   a. Nucleus is **kidney** or **horseshoe** shaped, and has condensed heterochromatin.
   b. Has a prominent Golgi apparatus—**clear area** located at the indentation site of the nucleus.
   c. Cytoplasm is similar to the mature cell.
   d. Comprises 18 percent of bone marrow cells.
5. **Band**
   a. Same size as a mature neutrophil (10–12μm).
   b. N:C ratio has reversed (1:2).
   c. Nucleus is **band-** or **sausage-shaped** without segmentation.
   d. Cytoplasm is filled with small neutrophilic granules.
   e. Last immature stage.
   f. Comprises 11 percent of bone marrow cells and 0–3 percent of peripheral WBCs.
   g. Stored in the bone marrow and released when there is an increased demand for neutrophils.
   h. **Shift to the left** is an increase indicating demand for WBCs.
   i. Matures in 2 days.

C. Morphology of Mature Granulocytes
   1. **Neutrophils**
      a. Also known as segmented neutrophils, segs, polymorphonuclear cells, polys, and PMNs.
      b. N:C ratio is 1:3, and the size is 10–12μm.
      c. Average nucleus contains 3–5 segments connected by narrow filaments.
      d. **Hyposegmented** is less than 3 segments, and may indicate a shift to the left or an anomaly.
      e. **Hypersegmented** is more than 5 segments, and may indicate infection or megaloblastic anemia.
      f. Cytoplasm contains very small nuclear granules.
         1) Can become larger upon bacterial infection producing **toxic granulation**, which are numerous, large, basophilic granules.

g. Makes up 60–80 percent of all peripheral WBCs.

h. Average time spent in the blood is 10 hours; time over 10 hours may cause the neutrophil to become hypersegmented.

2. **Eosinophils**

a. Average size is 13μm.

b. Nucleus is generally bilobed.

c. Cytoplasm is **bright red** to **orange** which is due to large secretory granules containing histamines that are basic and stain with the acidic eosin stain.

d. Makes up 3 percent of WBCs the peripheral blood.

3. **Basophils**

a. Is the smallest granulocyte at 10μm.

b. The nucleus is **difficult to see** due to heavy granulation.

c. Cytoplasm contains specific secondary basophilic granules that are basic and stain purple; the granules contain **heparin** and **histamines.**

d. Makes up 0.5 percent of peripheral WBCs.

e. *Note:* **Tissue mast cells** are similar to basophils but are larger and have no developmental relationship with basophils. Mast cells have a **mesenchymal** (connective tissue) origin and have granules containing **serotonin** (basophilic granules contain no serotonin).

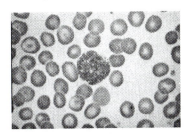

Eosinophils

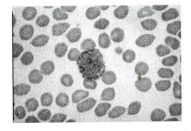

Basophils

D. Granulocyte Physiology and Function

1. **Neutrophils**

a. Neutrophils become part of circulating granulocyte pool (CGP).

b. The marginating granulocyte pool (MGP) is located along the blood vessel endothelial wall waiting to be activated by **chemotaxic substances** such as lipids, sugars, bacterial antigenic fragments, hormones, tissue injury, or cytokines.

c. When activated, neutrophils accumulate at a specific site where **phagocytosis** begins.

d. After phagocytizing bacteria, neutrophil cytoplasmic granules release their digestive enzymes (**hydrogen peroxide**) which fuse with bacteria for bactericidal action.

e. In massive infections, the supply of mature neutrophils may be exhausted, and bands will appear as demand continues.

2. **Visible response to infection by neutrophils**

a. **Toxic granulation**

1) Accumulation of dense **azurophilic,** peroxidase positive granules (may also appear as basophilic granules).

2) May not be found in all neutrophils.

3) A **response to infection** or it may indicate a genetic anomaly or (caution) stain artifacts.

b. **Cytoplasmic vacuolation**

1) Associated with infection.

2) Neutrophilic cytoplasm is normally not vacuolated.

c. **Döhle bodies**

1) Segments of endoplasmic reticulum (RNA).

2) Small oval inclusions located at the edges of the cytoplasm, stain light blue.

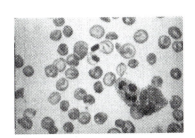

Toxic granulation

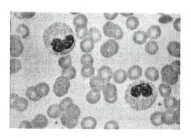

Pelger-Huët

3) Periodic acid-Schiff (PAS) positive.

4) Associated with scarlet fever, burns, infections, and aplastic anemia.

d. **Shift to the left (bands)**

1) Increased number of bands entering the peripheral blood.

2) Indicates an increased demand for neutrophils as seen in infection, and other physiological or pathological conditions requiring neutrophils.

3. **Nuclear Inherited Abnormalities of Neutrophils**

a. **Pelger-Huët**

1) Characterized by hyposegmentation of the nucleus.

2) Nucleus shows an increased chromatin density.

3) **True Pelger-Huët** is an autosomal dominant inherited trait.

4) **False Pelger-Huët** is an acquired abnormality associated with malignancies.

5) Nucleus may be referred to as "pince-nez" (bilobed).

b. **Hypersegmentation**

1) Associated with infection and macrocytic anemias.

2) Neutrophils show five or more lobes.

4. **Cytoplasmic inherited abnormalities of neutrophils**

a. **May-Hegglin anomaly**

1) Appears as Döhle-like inclusions—on Wright stain the anomalies appear as gray-blue, spindle-shaped (cigar-shaped) inclusions.

2) Associated with giant platelets and thrombocytopenia.

3) Abnormal genetic condition.

b. **Alder-Reilly anomaly**

1) Resembles toxic granulation; however, the granules are much larger and azurophilic in appearance.

2) Seen in mucopolysaccharide storage diseases.

3) Caused by an inherited autosomal recessive trait.

5. **Eosinophils**

a. Release granules in response to **parasitic infections** and **Type I hypersensitivity** reactions (allergies, hay fever, bronchial asthma).

b. Granules contain **histaminase,** eosinophil peroxidase, and lysophospholipase.

c. Eosinophils secrete tumor necrosis factor, and transforming growth factor B; both are involved in inflammation and **tissue repair**.

d. Adrenal corticosteroid hormones stimulate eosinophils to leave the peripheral blood.

6. **Basophils**

a. Basophilic granules **mediate** type 1 hypersensitivity reactions.

b. Granules release **histamine,** which results in watery eyes, runny nose, and sneezing.

c. Basophils are usually not seen in the tissue and appear in small numbers in the bone marrow and peripheral blood.

E. Nonmalignant Granulocytic Disorders

1. **Neutrophilia**
   a. **Increase** in the neutrophil count.
   b. Neutrophilia is caused by bacterial infections.
   c. Nonbacterial causes include inflammation, exercise, hormones, and leukemias.

2. **Neutropenia**
   a. **Decrease** in the neutrophil count.
   b. Also known as **agranulocytosis**.
   c. Can be caused by the following disorders:
      1) Infections that can deplete available neutrophil reserves. Prolonged neutropenia is seen in chronic or severe infections.
      2) Damaged spleen (the spleen holds large reserves of neutrophils).
      3) Aplasia and myeloid hypoplasia, when the bone marrow fails to produce cells, including neutrophils.
      4) Vitamin B_{12} deficiency, cyanocobalamin, pernicious anemia, or folate deficiency.
      5) Preleukemic states such as myelodysplastic syndromes.

3. **Abnormal neutrophil function**
   a. **Chronic granulomatous disease (CGD)**
      1) The inability of granules to release their contents, resulting in inhibited bactericidal function
   b. **Chédiak-Higashi syndrome**
      1) A genetic disorder, resulting in neutrophils containing large granules with impaired function.
      2) Patients will present with CNS disorders, abnormal skin pigmentation, and frequent infections.

4. **Eosinophilia**
   a. **Increase** associated with the following conditions:
      1) Bronchial asthma, hay fever, hives, and atopic dermatitis
      2) Parasitic infections
      3) Scarlet fever, especially the rash stage
      4) Removal of the spleen
      5) Chronic myelocytic leukemia (CML)

5. **Eosinopenia**
   a. **Decrease** seen in stressful situations, resulting in the release of adrenal corticoids, epinephrine, and acute inflammation

6. **Basophilia**
   a. **Increase** in the number of basophils associated with the following conditions:
      1) Hypersensitivity reactions.
      2) Myeloproliferative disorders, including CML, polycythemia vera, hypothyroidism, and chronic hemolytic anemia.
      3) **Relative transient basophilia** can be caused by irradiation or patients on hematopoietic growth factors.

7. **Basopenia**
   a. **Decrease** associated with acute infection and hyperthroidism.
   b. Difficult to diagnose because of their normally low normal range.

IV. MONOCYTES AND MACROPHAGES

A. Monocytes

1. Monocytes are part of the macrophage system called the **reticuloendothelial system (RES).** Macrophages are named according to their location in the body:
   a. **Histiocytes**—bone marrow
   b. **Kupffer cells**—liver
   c. **Microglial cells**—brain
   d. **Osteoclasts**—bone
   e. **Langerhans' cells**—skin
   f. **Monocytes**—peripheral blood

B. Monocyte Characteristics

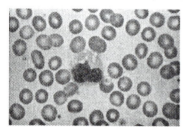

Monocyte characteristics

Monocyte characteristics

1. Largest peripheral WBC (14–20μm), normal range is 3–8 percent.
2. Peripheral blood monocytes are found between the **margination monocyte pool (MMP)** and the **circulating monocyte pool (CMP).**
3. Large population of monocytes is found in the spleen.
4. Nucleus is large and indented with **lacy chromatin.**
5. Cytoplasm is gray-blue to pink and has a **foamy appearance.**
6. Cytoplasm contains **primary granules** that are slightly peroxidase positive and **secondary granules** that are strongly alkaline phosphase positive.
7. Cytoplasm is often **vacuolated.**

C. Monocyte Function

1. Monocytes are very efficient **phagocytic** cells that are less antigen selective.
2. Unlike neutrophils, the phagocytic process does not kill the monocyte.
3. Monocytes are known as **"scavenger cells"** due to their ability to ingest foreign material, including abnormal or old RBCs where contents will be recycled. **Iron** from RBC breakdown is stored in macrophages which can be stained with the **Prussian blue** stain.
4. Monocytes process ingested material and also **process antigenic information,** which is given to the **T-helper (CD4)** lymphocyte. The T-helper lymphocyte coordinates the immune response to foreign antigens.
5. Monocytes produce and respond to **interleukins (IL)** and **cytokines (regulatory proteins).**

D. Nonmalignant Monocytic Disorders

1. **Monocytosis**
   a. **Increase** in the number of monocytes.
   b. Can be caused by the following conditions:
      1) Recovery phase of acute infections
      2) Mycobacterial infections
      3) Syphilis and brucellosis
      4) Malaria and Rocky Mountain spotted fever
      5) Arthritis and lupus
      6) Liver and spleen disorders
      7) Granulomatous disease such as Crohn's disease, colitis, and sarcoidosis

2. **Lipid storage disorders**
   a. **Gaucher's disease** is the most common lipid storage disorder, characterized by pancytopenia, hepatosplenomegaly. Gaucher cells are large cells with pale blue cytoplasm showing a fibrillar pattern.
   b. Most often diagnosed during childhood, and most common in Baltic Sea Jews.
   c. Caused by a deficiency in betaglucocerebrosidase.
   d. The peripheral blood film shows a **normocytic/normochromic** anemia, leukopenia, thrombocytopenia, and **Gaucher cells** (rarely found in peripheral blood).
   e. The identification of Gaucher cells confirms the diagnosis.
3. **Other lipid storage diseases**
   a. **Tay-Sachs**—a deficiency in hexosaminidase A
   b. **Sandhoff's**—a deficiency in hexosaminidase A and B
   c. **Niemann-Pick**—a deficiency in sphingomyelinase
   d. **Sea-blue histiocytosis**—causes an unknown deficiency, categorized as a lipid storage disease
   e. **Fabry's disease**—a deficiency in ceramide trihexosidase/alpha galactosidase
4. **Histiocytic diseases**
   a. **Histiocytes** are bone marrow macrophages, and are also called antigen-processing cells (APCs).
   b. Histiocytes are not found in the peripheral blood but are only found in the bone marrow and body tissue.
   c. Associated with rare histiocyte disorders.

V. LYMPHOCYTES AND PLASMA CELLS

A. Lymphocytes contain the following cells—T-cells, B-cells, plasma cells, K-cells (killer), NK-cells (nonkiller)
1. T- and B-lymphocytes migrate and circulate in the blood and lymphoid tissue, including spleen, lymph nodes, and intestines, in addition to circulating in the associated lymphoid tissue (Peyer's patch and tonsils). Lymphocytes can live for a number of years.

B. Lymphocyte Morphology
1. Round nucleus with uniform chromatin.
2. Light blue cytoplasm with no granules.
3. High N/C ratio.
4. Atypical lymphocytes are also called **reactive lymphs, Turk** and **Downey cells,** which become stimulated by **viral infections** such as mononucleosis or hepatitis.
5. Atypical lymphocytes show the following characteristics:
   a. Generally larger.
   b. Less mature nucleus with visible nucleoli.
   c. Smaller N/C ratio.
   d. Increased amount of cytoplasm.
   e. Cytoplasm becomes dark blue due to increased RNA production.
   f. Golgi apparatus is enlarged and visible as a clear area near the nucleus, and is called a perinuclear halo or **Hof area.**

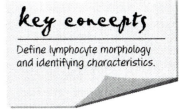

key concepts

Define lymphocyte morphology and identifying characteristics.

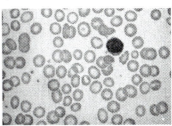

Lymphocyte morphology

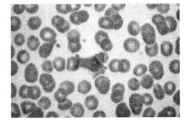

Atypical lymphocytes

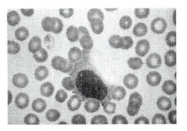

Atypical lymphocytes

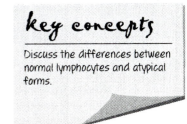

key concepts

Discuss the differences between normal lymphocytes and atypical forms.

C. T-lymphocytes (T-cells)

1. Produced in the thymus; make up 80 percent of the peripheral blood lymphocytes.
2. In the thymus, T-cells can be identified by membrane marker and nuclear enzyme analysis.
3. T-cell membrane proteins make up the histocompatibility complex antigens (MHC-1, MHC-II) which are also called histocompatible leukocyte antigens (**HLA-I, HLA-II**).
4. HLA-I is associated with organ and graft rejections, and HLA-II is associated with the **T-helper** recognition of foreign antigens.
5. **T-lymph function**
   a. Act in cell-mediated immunity (CMI). Examples of CMI are graft rejections, lysis of neoplastic cells, attack, and the destruction of intracellular organisms.
   b. Obtain antigenic information from monocytes, which is passed to other T-cells and B-cells.
   c. Destroy foreign/abnormal cells.
   d. Produce cytokines, which activate and destroy neoplastic cells.
6. **T-cell subsets** are differentiated by cluster differentiation (**CD**) markers.
   a. **T-helper cell (T-h)**
      1) Identified by **CD4** membrane proteins.
      2) T-h cells receive antigenic information from monocytes and macrophages, which passes this information to other cells.
   b. **T-suppressor cell (T-s)**
      1) Identified by **CD8** membrane markers.
      2) T-s cells keep the immune response controlled by three different T-s cells: inducer, mediator, and effector
   c. **Cytotoxic T cell (T-c)**
      1) Function in viral infections and organ rejections.
   d. **T memory cells (T-m)**
      1) Have a long life and can respond quickly to a prior antigenic exposure.
   e. Healthy people have a **T-h/T-s ratio of 2:1,** this ratio is used to monitor HIV patients. T-h (CD4) cells are destroyed by the HIV virus, which increases the ratio as the infection spreads.

D. B-lymphocytes (B-cells)

1. Make up 20 percent of peripheral blood lymphocytes and are identified by surface antibodies, receptors, and protein markers.
   a. Major producers of antibodies.
   b. When stimulated become **plasma cells,** which are the most efficient producers of antibodies.
   c. **Plasma Cells**
      1) Larger than normal lymphocytes.
      2) Contain abundant blue cytoplasm.
      3) Have an **eccentric nucleus** with a **wheel chromatin pattern.**
      4) Contain a prominent Golgi apparatus with a perinuclear halo.

Plasma cells

5) Makes up less than 5 percent of nucleated cells in the bone marrow.
6) Not usually found in the peripheral blood.

2. B-lymphocyte function

a. B-cells are stimulated to produce antibodies (humoral immunity) by contact with foreign antigens.
b. The stimulated B-lymphocyte becomes a **reactive lymphocyte** with the characteristic morphology associated with reactivity.

E. Large Granular Lymphocytes

1. Large cells with low N/C ratios.
2. Lack B-cell or T-cell membrane markers.
   a. All large granular lymphocytes are positive for **CD16.**
3. Function in the production of interferons, colony-stimulating factors, and IL-2.
4. Large granular lymphocytes include the following subsets:
   a. **Killer cells (K-cells)**
      1) Activated by antibody bound to cells, also called **antibody-dependent cytotoxic cells (ADCC).**
   b. **Natural killer cells (NK)**
      1) Not antibody dependent.
      2) Survey cells for surface alterations such as cells infected with viruses or cancer cells.
      3) Important in **monitoring** tumor development.
   c. **Lymphokine-activated killer cells (LAK)**
      1) Activated by IL-2. Destroy tumor cells not previously destroyed by NK-cells.

F. Nonmalignant Lymphocytosis Associated with Viral Infections

1. **Infectious mononucleosis**
   a. Caused by the **Epstein-Barr** virus (EBV).
   b. Common in the 17–25 age group with symptoms ranging from malaise and fever to pharyngitis, lymphadenopathy, and splenomegaly.
   c. Lymphocytes can account for 90 percent of the WBCs with 20 percent being atypical lymphs. **Not associated with monocytes.**
   d. Can cause a **normocytic, normochromic hemolytic anemia.** Diagnosed by serological testing.

2. **Cytomegalovirus (CMV)**
   a. Characteristics similar to mononucleosis.
   b. Transmission is by blood transfusions and saliva exchange.
   c. 90 percent of lymphocytes can be atypical.
   d. Transfused blood products are often tested for CMV.

3. **Infectious lymphocytosis**
   a. Contagious disease mostly affecting young children.
   b. After a 12–21 day incubation period, symptoms appear, including vomiting, fever, rash, diarrhea, and possible CNS involvement.

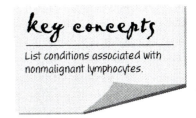

key concepts

List conditions associated with nonmalignant lymphocytes.

G. Additional Examples of Viral and Bacterial Lymphocytosis
1. Hepatitis, influenza, mumps, measles, rubella, and varicella.
2. **Examples of bacterial lymphocytosis**
   a. Pertussis, mycobacteria, cat-scratch disease, and mycoplasma pneumoniae.

VI. LEUKEMIAS

A. Lymphocytic Leukemias
1. **Acute lymphocytic (lymphoblastic) leukemia (ALL) (FAB L1)**
   a. Most common childhood (less than 5 years old) cancer, also found in 20- to 40-year-old adults.
   b. Clinical: fever, bone/joint pain, bleeding, hepatosplenomegaly.
   c. Leukemic blasts are pre–B-cell immunophenotype.
   d. **Protein marker characteristics of L1 (pre–B-cell origin)**
      1) ALL antigen (CALLA) negative
      2) CD7 negative, CD10 and CD19 positive
      3) HLA-DR positive
      4) TDT (terminyl dexoynucleotidyl transferase) positive
   e. Common genetic translocations include **t(4,11), 11q23–25, 9p21–22.**
   f. Laboratory: **normocytic/normochromic** anemia with **nRBCs, thrombocytopenia,** varied WBC count, and **small lymphocytes** with a high N/C ratio. Predominant cells are **lymphoblasts.**
   g. Patients respond with a greater than 50 percent cure rate.
2. **Acute lymphocytic leukemia (FAB L2)**
   a. Also called Adult T-cell leukemia (ATL).
   b. More common in adults, with higher incidence in Japan.
   c. Larger irregular lymphocytes (the morphology can vary from case to case). Indented nuclei are often present in lymphoblasts.
   d. **Protein marker characteristics of L2 (T-cell origin)**
      1) ALL antigen (CALLA) negative
      2) CD7 positive and CD19 negative
      3) HLA-DR negative
      4) TDT positive
   e. Very close association with **HTLV-I.**
   f. Characterized by the development of **t(9,22)** translocation; also called the **Ph1 chromosome (Philadelphia chromosome).**
   g. Patients show a poor prognosis.
3. **Acute Lymphocytic Leukemia (FAB L3)**
   a. Also known as acute lymphoblastic leukemia or the leukemic phase of Burkitt's lymphoma.
   b. Lymphocytes are large and uniform with prominent nucleoli; cytoplasm stains deeply basophilic and may show vacuoles.
   c. Lymphocytes are mature B-cells.
   d. Common translocations **t(8;14)** and **(q24;q32)** with a rearrangement of the **c-myc** oncogene.
   e. **Protein Marker Characteristics (B-Cell Origin)**
      1) ALL antigen (CALLA) negative
      2) CD7 negative, CD19, CD20, and CD24 positive

key concepts

Define and describe the various leukemias.

    3) HLA-DR positive

    4) TDT negative

  f. Shows a very poor prognosis.

  g. **Burkitt's lymphoma** of the L3 leukemic phase

    1) Endemic in East Africa.

    2) Detected in 96 percent of patients with Epstein-Barr viral (EBV) infections.

    3) Children present with jaw tumors.

    4) A rare, aggressive disease.

4. **Chronic lymphocytic leukemia (CLL)**

  a. Found in over 60 year olds, rare before the age of 40, with survival rate of approximately 6 years.

  b. Has a B-cell phenotype. (CD19, CD20, CD24 positive).

  c. Patients present with enlarged lymph nodes, hepatosplenomegaly, anorexia, and fatigue.

  d. Diagnosed secondary to other diseases.

  e. Laboratory: **homogeneous small lymphocytes.** Anemia is not generally present but if present will be an **autoimmune hemolytic anemia** characterized by **thrombocytopenia** and **smudge cells.**

  f. **Cytogenetics of CLL**

    1) Greater than 50 percent of CLL patients show an extra chromosome 12.

    2) Chromosomes 8 and 14 translocation.

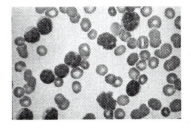

Cytogenics of CLL

  g. **CLL Variants**

    1) **Lymphosarcoma leukemia (LSL)**

      a) Small lymphocytes with **deep clefts** in the nuclei with condensed chromatin

      b) Associated with poorly differentiated lymphocytic lymphoma

      c) Diagnosed by observing nodules of poorly differentiated cells in enlarged lymph nodes

    2) **Prolymphocytic leukemia (PL)**

      a) Characterized by lymphocytosis ($>100 \times 10^9$/L) with many prolymphocytes.

      b) Less responsive to treatment (refractory).

      c) Poorer prognosis than regular CLL, especially the T-cell type.

      d) Results in splenomegaly, anemia, and thrombocytopenia. Occurs more frequently in males.

      e) Can be B-cell (most common) or T-cell type.

    3) **Hairy cell leukemia (HCL)**

      a) A rare B-cell disease characterized by lymphocytopenia.

      b) Seen in patients over 50 years of age; causes severe spleen problems.

      c) Laboratory: lymphocytes show a **notched** or **dumbbell-** shaped nucleus. Cytoplasm shows **hairlike** projections. Lymphocytes stain with **tartrate-resistant acid phosphatase.**

    4) Etiology associated with irradiation and **HTLV-1.**

5. **Waldenström's macroglobulinemia** (plasma cell malignancy)
   a. Involvement of a **B-cell** or **plasma cell** malignancy, which produces excessive **IgM (monoclonal gammopathy).**
   b. Identified by protein electrophoresis.
   c. Affects older patients (60–70 years of age).
   d. Excessive IgM production causes hyperviscous blood.
   e. Abnormal protein binds to platelets, which alters coagulation factors, resulting in prolonged bleeding.
   f. **Differential:** Normocytic, chronic, or hemolytic anemia, lymphocytosis, thrombocytopenia, and **rouleaux** formation of RBCs.
   g. Erythrocyte sedimentation rate (ESR) is increased.
6. **Multiple myeloma** (plasma cell malignancy)
   a. Monoclonal gammopathy producing excessive **IgG.**
   b. Average age is 62 years with a greater incidence in males.
   c. Neoplasic cell, the plasma cell, is called a **myeloma** cell. The myeloma cell is larger than the normal plasma cell and contains multiple nuclei.
   d. Myeloma cells produce large amount of **M protein**, which causes:
      1) An inhibition of normal antibody production.
      2) M proteins bind to RBCs, platelets, and coagulation proteins, resulting in bleeding and anemia.
   e. **Laboratory: normocytic/normochromic anemia,** variable WBC count, **marked rouleaux,** and an **increased ESR.**
   f. **Bence Jones** proteins are found in the urine, and seen as a **M spot** on protein electrophoresis.
   g. Three-year survival rate, and can progress into sideroblastic anemia and acute leukemia.

B. Malignant Lymphomas
   1. **Hodgkin's lymphoma**
      a. **Reed-Sternberg** cells found in lymph node biopsy are large multinucleated cells with large nucleoli.
      b. **Differential: normochromic/normocytic** anemia. WBC count is variable, monocytosis, and lymphocytopenia.
      c. Seen in patients between 15–35 and over 50 years of age. Seen more frequently in males.
      d. Rye classification
         1) Lymphocytic predominant group
         2) Lymphocyte depleted group
         3) Mixed cell group
         4) Nodular sclerosis group
   2. **Non-Hodgkin's lymphoma**
      a. No Reed-Sternberg cells are present.
      b. Graded as to cell type and size.
      c. National Cancer Institute classification: low- middle- and high-grade malignancies.
   3. **Mycosis Fungoides and Sézary syndrome**
      a. Cutaneous T-cell lymphoma (CTCL).
      b. Seen in patients over 45 years of age.
      c. Characterized by dermatitis.

d. Spreads to organs, and leads to death within 2 years due to infection.

e. Leukemia phase of mycosis fungoides is called Sézary syndrome.

f. CD2, CD3, and CD4 positive.

g. Laboratory: Sézary cells (neoplastic cells) in the peripheral blood show characteristic monocytic nucleus.

C. FAB Classification of Acute Leukemias (Myeloproliferative Disorders) — Characterized by spontaneous proliferation of platelet, erythroid, granulocyte, and monocyte precursors. Clonal in origin.

1. **Acute myelogenous leukemia (AML, M1-M2)**

   a. Seen during the first few months of life and during the mid–late years. Prognosis after diagnosis is several months.

   b. Clinical characteristics include fever, malaise, and mouth/throat ulcers.

   c. Types of AML

      1) **M1** (AML without maturation) shows **90 percent myeloblast**

         a) Laboratory: anemia, increased WBCs, decreased platelets, and myeloblasts

         b) Positive for Sudan black B and myeloperoxidase

      2) **M2** (AML with maturation) shows **< 90 percent myeloblast** with **Auer rods.**

         a) Seen more in midlife.

         b) Laboratory: anemia, increased WBCs, decreased platelets. M2 will show more granulocytes than M1.

         c) Positive for Sudan black B, myeloperoxidase, and naphthol AS-D chloroacetate esterase.

2. **Acute promyelocytic leukemia (APL, M3)**

   a. Characterized by **hypergranular promyelocytes** (hypergranular M3) with azurophilic granules.

   b. Laboratory: multiple **Auer rods** are present (can occur in bundles known as **faggot cells**), slightly increased WBC count, hypergranular promyelocytes, blasts, and thrombocytopenia.

   c. Survival time is approximately two years.

   d. Clinical characteristics include severe bleeding, hepatomegaly, and disseminated intravascular coagulation (DIC).

   e. **Microgranular M3 variant**

      1) Laboratory: markedly increased WBC, promyelocytes with nongranulated cytoplasm, rare faggot cells, and Auer rods

3. **Acute myelomonocytic leukemia (AMML, M4)**

   a. Shows a **monocytosis,** 30 percent myeloblast in the bone marrow (1% is normal) and Auer rods.

   b. Can see both monocytic and granulocytic cells.

   c. Positive for urine/serum lysozyme, alpha-naphthyl acetate esterase stain, and CD14 markers.

   d. **M4E** is a subclass of AMML with eosinophilia.

      1) Occurs in midlife.

      2) Laboratory: eosinophils show very large basophilic granules that stain with ASD chloroacetate esterase.

3) Normal eosinophils will not stain with ASD chloroacetate esterase.

4) Characterized by an inversion or deletion of **chromosome 16.**

4. **Acute monocytic leukemia (AMOL, M5)**

a. Rare form of leukemia accounting for less than 10% of all leukemias.

b. Characterized by showing large numbers of monocytic cells in the bone marrow.

c. Complications include DIC and renal insufficiency.

d. Cells stains positive for fluoride-inhibited nonspecific esterase and alpha-naphthyl acetate esterase.

e. **CD14, CD4** positive.

f. Contains two subclasses

1) **M5A** is seen in younger patients, characterized by poorly differentiated cells, with 80% monoblasts in the bone marrow.

2) **M5B** shows well-differentiated cells, an increase in promonocytes and monocytes in the peripheral blood, and less than 80% blasts in the bone marrow. Occurs in middle age adults.

5. **Chronic myelomonocytic leukemia (CMML)**

a. Classified as a myelodysplastic syndrome.

b. Seen in patients over 50.

c. Characterized by monocytosis and refractory anemia.

d. Hypercellular bone marrow with an increased number of blasts.

e. Is a preleukemia/dysplastic syndrome with a high percentage of cases progressing to overt leukemia.

f. Shows a very poor prognosis.

6. **Acute erythroleukemia (AEL, M6)**

a. Also called **Di Guglielmo's disease.**

b. Characterized by a proliferation of malignant erythrocytes.

c. Greater than 50 percent dysplastic erythrocytes in the bone marrow with normoblasts containing dense cytoplasmic glycogen.

d. Stains positive with periodic acid-Schiff (PAS).

e. Howell-Jolly bodies and ringed sideroblasts.

f. Positive for anticarbonic anhydrase I, **CAI, FA6-152.**

g. Seen in middle-age adults.

7. **Acute megakaryocytic leukemia (AMeqL, M7)**

a. Very rare type of leukemia.

b. Characterized by a proliferation of megakaryoblast.

c. Cells are identified by flow cytometry.

D. Chronic Myelocytic Leukemia (CML) — also known as chronic granulocytic leukemia (CGL)

1. Seen in older adults and is diagnosed secondary to other conditions such as pneumonia or anemia.

2. **Normocytic/normochromic** anemia resulting from excessive neutrophil production.

3. WBC > 50×10^9/L with mostly mature segmented neutrophils, bands, metamyelocytes, and myelocytes

4. CML can appear like a bacterial infection (leukemoid reaction) with a decreased LAP.

5. Hypercellular bone marrow inhibits aspiration (dry tap).

6. **Philadelphia (Ph1) chromosome** may be present in over 90 percent of CML patients.

7. Clinical characteristics include weight loss, enlarged spleen, fever, night sweats, and malaise.

E. Miscellaneous Myeloproliferative Disorders

1. **Essential thrombocythemia (ET)**
   a. Characterized by uncontrolled proliferation of megakaryocytic stem cells.
   b. Rare disorder affecting individuals from 20 to 60 years of age.
   c. Laboratory: marked thrombocytosis with giant forms, leukocytosis, and decreased RBC indices if anemia is present.
   d. More than 50 percent of patients with ET survive 5 years after diagnosis and treatment.

2. **Polycythemia vera (PV)**
   a. Increase in erythrocytes (**erythrocytosis**) and all cell lines (**polycythemia**). Produces a thick, viscous blood.
   b. Can cause high blood pressure, stroke, and heart attack. Often leads to leukemia. Occurs in patients in the early to mid 60s.
   c. Caused by excessive erythropoiesis and can be hereditary.
   d. Laboratory: increased Hct (> 60%) and increased hemoglobin (> 20%) indicate polycythemia, in addition to an increase in marrow iron reserves. WBC and RBC counts are increased.
   e. **Polycythemia vera** results from a multipotential stem cell failure. A clonal disorder that can progress into acute myelogenous leukemia (AML).
   f. Erythropoietin (**EPO**) is decreased.
   g. Treatment is therapeutic phlebotomy, splenectomy, and chemotherapy. A chronic disease with a prognosis after diagnosis of up to 20 years.
   h. **Other forms of polycythemia**
      1) **Stress polycythemia or relative polycythemia**
         a) Due to normal physiologic fluid movement caused by unrelated problems such as dehydration or IV fluid administration.
         b) Dehydration can result from diarrhea, diuretics, or burns.
         c) Increased Hct, normal total RBC mass, normal WBC and platelet count.
      2) **Absolute benign polycythemia**
         a) Increase in erythrocytes in response to increased EPO and decreased tissue oxygen.
         b) Can be caused by smoking (sometimes known as spurious polycythemia), emphysema, and high altitudes
      3) **Absolute malignant polycythemia** is excessive erythropoiesis due to renal tumors.

3. **Myelofibrosis with myeloid metaplasia (MMM)**
   a. Caused by a stem cell disorder resulting in proliferation of erythrocytes, granulocytes, and thrombocytes.
   b. Fibrosis is secondary to the primary proliferation event and is seen in the liver, spleen, and kidneys.
   c. MMM affects individuals past 50 years of age.
   d. Individuals with MMM often show bleeding, splenomegaly, and hepatomegaly in addition to extremity pain.
   e. Laboratory: moderate to severe normocytic/normochromic anemia, marked anisocytosis and poikilocytosis. Hypochromic anemia can be present if bleeding occurs. Reticulocytosis and a variable platelet/WBC count.
   f. Prognosis after diagnosis and treatment up to 5 years.

4. **Myelodysplastic syndromes (MDS)**
   a. Group of disorders that are generally benign stem cell disorders that can progress into leukemia "type" diseases.
   b. Possibly caused by oncogenes, resulting in maturation inhibitions. MDS development can be stimulated by chemotherapy, radiation, and toxic substances.
   c. MDS is most common in elderly individuals but can occur in children.
   d. Laboratory: moderate to severe anemia, neutropenia and thrombocytopenia. Erythrocytes can be macrocytic (with oval macrocytes) or microcytic and hypochromic. Other findings include marked anisocytoisis and poikilocytosis, Howell-Jolly bodies, basophilic stippling, and nucleated RBCs.
   e. FAB classification of myelodysplastic syndromes
      1) **Refractory anemia (RA)**
         a) Moderate to severe anemia that is refractory (not responsive) to therapy.
         b) Laboratory: macrocytic RBCs, decreased reticulocytes, rare blasts, and a normal WBC and platelet count.
      2) **Refractory anemia with ringed sideroblasts (RARS)**
         a) Ringed sideroblasts comprise 20 percent of bone marrow nucleated cells.
         b) Laboratory is similar to RA.
      3) **Refractory anemia with excess blasts (RAEB)**
         a) Two or more cell lines showing cytopenia.
         b) Laboratory: anemia is normocytic, increased reticulocytes, blasts range from 5 percent to 20 percent of the WBC count.
         c) Survival rate correlates to the number of blasts present.
      4) **Refractory anemia with excess blasts in transformation (RAEB-T)**
         a) Very similar to acute leukemia.
         b) Poor survival rate which may be as short as 10 months.

VII. HEMOGLOBIN — an oxygen-transporting protein contained within erythrocytes. The heme portion of hemoglobin gives erythrocytes their characteristic red color. Hemoglobin types are determined by amino acid sequence. This sequence determines function and hemoglobin electrophoresis pattern.

A. Hemoglobin Structure
1. The amino acid sequence of the globin chain determines type of hemoglobin.
2. Four globin (polypeptide) chains.
3. Four heme (protoporphyrin) groups.
4. Four iron (Fe^{2+}) molecules and must be in the ferous state.

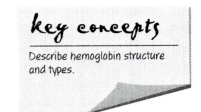

key concepts

Describe hemoglobin structure and types.

B. Hemoglobin Synthesis
1. 65 percent hemoglobin synthesis occurs in immature nRBCs.
2. 35 percent hemoglobin synthesis occurs in reticulocytes.
3. Heme synthesis occurs in the mitochondria of normoblasts, and is dependent on vitamin B6.
4. Globin synthesis occurs in the ribosomes where glycine/succinyl co-A condenses. Limited by amino levulinic acid (ALA), resulting in the protoporphyrin ring combining with iron to form heme. Heme then combines with the globin chains.
5. Globin-chain synthesis is coded on **chromosome 16** (alpha-chains) and **chromosome 11** for all other chains.

C. Hemoglobin/Erythrocyte Breakdown
1. **Intravascular hemolysis**
   a. Occurs when hemoglobin breaks down in the blood and free hemoglobin is released into plasma (red color).
   b. Free hemoglobin binds to **haptoglobin** (major free hemoglobin transport protein), **hemopexin,** and **albumin,** which will be phagocytized by macrophages.
2. **Extravascular hemolysis**
   a. Occurs when altered RBCs are phagocytized by macrophages in the liver or spleen.
   b. **Bilirubin** is product of heme catabolism.
   c. Bilirubin is excreted in urine and feces.
   d. Globin chains are recycled back to the amino acid pool.
   e. Heme releases **iron** that binds to **transferrin.** This goes to bone marrow for new RBC production or is stored for future use.
      1) **Ferritin** in macrophages
      2) **Hemosiderin** in organs

D. Hemoglobin and Iron
1. Most iron in the body is in hemoglobin and must be in the ferrous state (Fe^{++}) to be used. Fe^{++} binds to oxygen for transport to lungs and body tissues. Fe^{+++} (ferric state) is not able to bind to hemoglobin. Iron is an **essential** mineral and cannot be produced by the body.

E. Types of Hemoglobin
1. **Fetal hemoglobin**
   a. **Hb F** contains 2 alpha and 2 gamma globin chains. Hb F functions in a reduced oxygen environment. Hb F switches to hemoglobin A shortly before birth and is complete in 6 months.
      1) Is resistant to acid and alkaline elutions.

    2) Laboratory: Alkaline denaturation test—add KOH to the hemoglobin solution, read the absorbance, report as part of fetal hemoglobin.

    3) Hb F can be increased in most hemolobinopathies.

  b. **Hb Bart's:** contains four gamma chains, is seen in the fetus and in newborn infants (no alpha chains).

    1) Hydrops fetalis—fetal or neonatal death with severe anemia. Usually found in Southeast Asians and Filipinos. Hb Bart's > 80 percent

    2) Hb H disease—chronic hemolytic anemia; Hb Bart's 20–40 percent

    3) Seen in patients with thalassemia, Hb Bart's 2–20 percent

2. **Adult**

  a. **Hb A:** polypeptide chains in globin are composed of two alpha and two beta chains. Major adult hemoglobin.

  b. **Hb A$_2$:** two alpha and two delta chains. The delta chains differ from the beta chains on Hb A.

  c. Hb A is subdivided into glycosylated fractions. **A$_{1C}$** fraction reflects sugar levels in the blood and is very sensitive in monitoring diabetics. A$_{1C}$ is a stable hemoglobin.

    1) Normal range of A$_{1C}$ is 3 to 6 percent.

    2) Diabetic range of A$_{1C}$ is 6 to 15 percent.

  d. Adult erythrocytes contain **96–98% Hb A, 0.5–0.8% Hb F, and 1.5–3.2% Hb A$_2$.**

F. Different Forms of Normal Hemoglobin

1. **Oxyhemoglobin:** hemoglobin + O_2 = HbO_2, seen in arterial circulation.

2. **Deoxyhemoglobin:** hemoglobin with no O_2 = hemoglobin.

3. **Carboxyhemoglobin:** hemoglobin + CO = HBCO, CO has 210X greater affinity for hemoglobin. HbCO carries no O_2 and will result in death, but is reversible if given pure O_2. Is cherry pink.

4. **Sulfhemoglobin:** hemoglobin + S = SHb; cannot transport O_2; seldom reaches fatal levels.

5. **Methemoglobin (Hi):** increased Hi levels will cause cyanosis and anemia. A manual hemoglobin determination uses Hi+ cyanide for color production that can be measured.

VIII. TYPES OF HEMOGLOBINOPATHIES

A. Sickle Cell Trait (Hb AS)

1. Caused by genetic substitution of **glutamic acid** by **valine** at the sixth beta-hemoglobin chain position.

2. Contains **Hb AS** where one of two hemoglobin genes is the S gene, and the other is a normal hemoglobin gene. Hemoglobin S makes up about 40 percent of hemoglobin in sickle cell trait individuals.

3. A **heterozygous trait** affecting about 8 percent of the black population. Most common hemoglobinopathy in the United States.

4. Anemia is rare but if present will be **normochromic/normocytic,** and sickling will occur during rare crisis states (same as in Hb S); otherwise **sickle cell trait generally produces no clinical symptoms.**

5. Sickle cell trait is diagnosed by sickle cell screening tests and confirmed by hemoglobin electrophoresis.

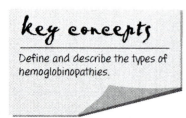

key concepts

Define and describe the types of hemoglobinopathies.

6. Hb S containing erythrocytes cannot be infected with **malaria,** *Plasmodium falciparum.*

B. Sickle Cell Disease (Hb S)

1. Caused when **valine** replaces **glutamic acid,** and results in a decrease in hemoglobin solubility and function. Sickle cell gene must be inherited from **both parents.**
2. **Homozygous** trait of both S genes which produces a chronic hemolytic anemia.
3. Hemoglobin insolubility results when deoxyhemoglobin is formed. This causes hemoglobin to crystallize within erythrocytes. Characterized by the classic sickled shape of erythrocytes.
4. Clinical characteristics
   a. Erythrocytes become rigid and become trapped in the bodies' capillaries, this restricts blood flow and will cause tissue necrosis from the lack of oxygen.
   b. All organs are affected with **kidney failure** being a common outcome, joint swelling and leg ulcers also occur.
   c. **Crisis** occurs with increased RBC production. Crisis can be initiated by many physiological factors including surgery, trauma, pregnancy, high altitudes, etc.
   d. Immunity to *P. falciparum.*
5. Occurs in **0.2 percent** of the black population. Also affects Arabs, South/Central Americans, and peoples in the Mediterranean region.
6. Diagnosis is made during childhood with fatalities historically within 30 years. Death usually results from infection or congestive heart failure. Maternal and fetal mortality in sickle cell disease patients approaches 25 percent.
7. **Laboratory**
   a. **Normochromic/normocytic** anemia and polychromasia resulting from premature release of reticulocytes.
   b. Also present are **sickle cells, target cells, nucleated RBCs,** and **Howell-Jolly bodies.**
   c. Neutrophilia and increased platelets. Osmotic fragility test will be decreased.
   d. There are various screening tests for insoluble hemoglobins in addition to alkali denaturation and acid elution tests.
   e. Sickle cell anemia is confirmed by hemoglobin electrophoresis.
   f. Can be diagnosed by DNA analysis.

C. Miscellaneous Sickle Cell Hemoglobinopathies

1. **Sickle-β thalassemia**
   a. Caused by the inheritance of the β-thalassemia gene from one parent and the sickle cell gene from the other parent.
   b. Symptoms include hemolytic anemia and splenomegaly.
   c. Laboratory: hypochromic, microcytic erythrocytes, marked polychromasia, target cells, and rare sickled cells.
   d. Diagnosis is based on hemoglobin electrophoresis, which shows 80 percent hemoglobin S and 20 percent hemoglobin F (ratios may differ slightly in patients).

S7791

2. **Sickle-C disease**
   a. Causes moderate hemolytic anemia.
   b. Peripheral blood film shows target cells and sickle cells.
   c. Clinical symptoms vary with patients.

D. **Rare hemoglobinopathies** involve a sequence change in amino acids in the globin chain position, and most show **target cells.**
   1. **Hb C disease**
      a. Inherited **homozygous** disorder caused when glutamic acid is replaced by **lysine** (different amino acid than sickle cell disease) at the sixth amino acid of the beta chain.
      b. Affects mostly blacks and generally produces no symptoms.
      c. Laboratory: **normochromic/normocytic** anemia, **spherocytes,** and **target cells.**
      d. Characterized by **tetragonal red crystals** within the erythrocyte caused by deoxyhemoglobin C, resulting in decreased solubility.
      e. Hb C becomes **cathodal** on electrophoresis.
   2. **Hb D disease**
      a. Caused by an amino acid substitution in the beta chain at position 121 of the glutamate with a glutamine amino acid.
      b. Inherited **heterozygous** trait found more commonly in Asians and Indians.
      c. Hb D migrates with Hb S on hemoglobin electrophoresis.
      d. Sickle cell screening tests are negative.
   3. **Hb E disease**
      a. Inherited **homozygous** trait found mostly in Asians.
      b. Results in a mild form of anemia.
      c. Caused by the substitution of lysine for glutamic acid in the beta chain.
      d. Laboratory analysis: target cells, increased reticulocyte count, hypochromic/microcytic anemia.
   4. **Hb SC disease**
      a. Double **heterozygous** trait where a different abnormal beta chain is inherited from each parent (hemoglobin S and hemoglobin C).
      b. Seen in blacks with symptoms similar to sickle cell anemia but in milder form.
      c. Laboratory: **target cells, sickle cells** (rare), and **Hb CC crystals.**
      d. Sickle cell screening tests are positive.
      e. Hb SC patients lack hemoglobin A and will have increased hemoglobin F levels.

E. **Thalassemias**
   1. Caused by a **decrease** synthesis of one or more globin chains.
   2. Mostly seen in **Mediterranean** and **Southeast Asian** populations.
   3. The old name for β-thalassemias was **Cooley's anemia.**
   4. There are no thalassemia screening tests.
   5. Diagnosis is confirmed when hemoglobin electrophoresis shows **Hb A_2** increased over 2 percent, and increased levels of **Hb F.**

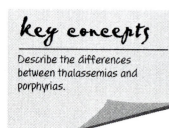

key concepts

Describe the differences between thalassemias and porphyrias.

6. Laboratory
   a. **Microcytic/hypochromia** anemia with moderate number of **target cells**
   b. **Nucleated RBCs, schistocytes,** and **spherocytes**
   c. **Howell-Jolly bodies, siderocytes,** and **Cabot rings**
7. Thalassemia types are based on the globin chain affected. **Thalassemia major** has a **total lack** of alpha or beta globin production whereas **thalassemia minor** has **decreased** chain production.
8. Clinical picture
   a. Prominent facial bones, especially the cheek and jaw.
   b. Growth and maturity are stunted and prolonged.
   c. Liver and spleen disorders, especially in young children.
9. **Types of α-thalassemias**
   a. **α-thalassemia**
      1) **Alpha** chains are missing, which causes decreased hemoglobin to be formed. Different forms of α-thalassemia result from a decrease in α-chain production.
      2) Excess unused β chains form inclusions that are phagocytized by macrophages.
   b. **α-thalassemia 2 (α + -thalassemia)**
      1) Characterized by showing no clinical symptoms.
      2) At birth there is 2 percent Hb-Bart's; the adult will show normal Hb A.
      3) Lacks **one** pair of α-globin genes.
   c. **α-thalassemia 1 (α° - thalassemia)**
      1) Generally no clinical symptoms; at birth there is 5–10 percent Hb Bart's. Adults will show normal Hb A.
      2) Caused by a deletion on chromosome 16 of both linked α-globin genes, resulting in no α-chains being produced.
   d. **α-thalassemia minor**
      1) Generally a less severe form resulting from a decrease in α-chain synthesis.
      2) More common in Filipinos, Chinese, and other Asians.
   e. **Hb C̄S̄ Disease**
      1) Characterized by splenomegaly.
      2) Caused by a deletion of three genes.
      3) Heinz bodies are usually present.
      4) At birth there is less than 5 percent Hb Bart's; adults will show 70 percent Hb A.
      5) Most common in Southeast Asia, the Middle East, and Greece. Rare in African Americans.
   f. **Hb CS Constant Spring Disease**
      1) Caused by the addition of amino acids to globin chains resulting from α-globin mutations.
      2) Found in Asian and Mediterranean populations.
10. **Types of β-thalassemias**
    a. **β-thalassemia major**
       1) Caused by a reduction in the production of β-chains, resulting from two thalassemia β alleles on chromosome 11.
       2) Most severe form of β-thalassemia.

3) Often associated with severe hemolytic anemia. Requires frequent blood transfusions.

4) Children will develop characteristic features (without transfusion therapy): prominent facial bones in addition to cardiomegaly, ulcers, and growth and sexual development deficiencies.

b. **Thalassemia intermedia**

1) Classification term (not genetic) used to describe clinically a condition less severe than β-thalassemia major but more severe than β-thalassemia minor.

c. **Thalassemia minor**

1) Caused by a single β-thalassemia allele.

2) Usually produces no clinical symptoms.

d. **Thalassemia minima**

1) The "silent" form that produces no clinical symptoms.

F. Porphyrias

1. Caused by genetic enzyme deficiencies resulting in a decreased production of heme.

2. Characterized by photosensitivity, abdominal pain, and CNS disorders.

3. Laboratory: **microcytic/hypochromia** anemia and ineffective hematopoiesis. **Heinz bodies** and **basophilic stippling** is often present.

4. MCV, MCHC, and MCH are decreased.

5. Porphyrins are precursors of alpha aminolevulinic acid and can be found in urine, feces, and blood.

6. Porphyrias can be inherited or acquired.

a. **Inherited**

1) **Acute intermittent porphyria** produces a leukocytosis. Caused by decreased levels of porphyrinogen I and III synthetase.

2) **Hereditary coproporphyria** is caused by a deficiency in coproporphyrinogen decarboxylase activity. Patients have very light-sensitive skin.

3) **Varigate porphyria** produces cutaneous lesions due to light sensitive skin. Caused by a deficiency in protoporphyrinogen oxidase.

4) **Congenital erythropoietic porphyria** is an often fatal disorder caused by a deficiency in uroporphyrinogen III cosynthetase.

5) **Erythrohepatic protoporphyria** is caused by inhibited activity of heme synthetase.

b. **Acquired**

1) **Porphyria cutanea tarda** results from liver disease, estrogen therapy, or alcoholism. Uroporphyrinogen III decarboxylase is inhibited.

2) **Lead intoxication:** lead inhibits ALA dehydrase activity.

G. Hemoglobin Measurement

1. Blood oxygen capacity: measures functional hemoglobin.

$$\frac{\text{Oxygen capacity in mL/dL blood}}{1.34 \text{ (hemoglobin oxygen capacity)}} = \text{grams of hemoglobin/dL blood}$$

2. Blood iron content: measures total iron content of blood that is bound to hemoglobin.

$$\frac{\text{Blood iron content in mg/dL}}{3.47 \text{ (hemoglobin iron content)}} = \text{grams of hemoglobin/dL blood}$$

3. Oxyhemoglobin method: does not measure sulfhemoglobin or methemoglobin; read patient's sample at 540nm.
4. Cyanmethemoglobin method: the **reference method** for all hemoglobins except for sulfhemoglobin. Uses **Drabkin** solution (potassium ferricyanide and NaCN) that is added to blood; read at 540nm.

IX. ERYTHROCYTES

A. General Characteristics

1. Transport oxygen, removal of metabolic waste.
2. Loss of nucleus is required for function.
3. Cytoplasmic granules not required for function.
4. Only one cell line population.
5. 120 day lifespan.

B. Erythropoietin

1. Produced mainly by the kidneys with minimal production by the liver.
2. Stimulates erythrocyte production by influencing colony-forming unit-erythrocytes (CFU-Es) to differentiate into erythroblasts.
3. Influences the production of platelet precursors.

C. Erythrocyte Maturation

1. **Pronormoblast (rubriblast)**
   a. Earliest RBC, large cell (20μm), with a 5:1 N/C ratio.
   b. 0–5 nucleoli, nucleus has dark areas of DNA.
   c. Deep blue cytoplasm.
   d. Chromatin is fine and uniform, which stains intensely.
   e. Contain no granules.

2. **Basophilic normoblast (prorubricyte)**
   a. Decreased N:C ratio of 4:1. Size is up to 18μm.
   b. Centrally located nucleus with no nucleoli.
   c. Cytoplasm is less blue but intensely basophilic (RNA activity).
   d. Chromatin is coarse with a bicycle pattern and is more clumped.

3. **Polychromatophilic normoblast (rubricyte)**
   a. 1:1 N/C ratio. Size is up to 16μm.
   b. Begins to produce hemoglobin, resulting in grayish cytoplasm.
   c. Chromatin shows more clumping.

4. **Orthochromic normoblast (metarubricyte)**
   a. Final nucleated stage.
   b. 10–12μm in size.
   c. Chromatin is pyknotic or compact.
   d. Pale acidophilic cytoplasm.

key concepts

List the stages of erythrocyte maturation.

5. **Reticulocyte**
    a. Last immature stage.
    b. Contains no nucleus but has a mitochondria and ribosomes.
    c. Last stage in bone marrow before release to the blood.
    d. Normal ranges are 0.5–1.5 percent for adults and 2.5–6.5 percent for newborns. Slightly increased in females and higher altitudes.
    e. Wright stain appearance is slightly macrocytic and polychromatic.
    f. Reticulocyte stain (a supra vital stain) is used to show reticulocytes
    g. **Reticulocyte counts** are used to determine bone marrow erythropoeitic activity. Generally increased in anemias, blood loss, and leukemias.
    h. Reticulocytes are one of the best indicators of bone marrow function
    i. **Stress reticulocytes** are large bluish cells released from bone marrow under erythrocyte stress such as anemia, and occurs when all mature RBCs and mature reticulocytes have been released.
    j. Hemoglobin continues to be produced by reticulocytes for approximately 24 hours after exiting the bone marrow.
6. **Mature erythrocyte**
    a. Small cell 6–8μm in size.
    b. Round and biconcave.
    c. Red with clearing in the center (central pallor) that results from uneven hemoglobin distribution.
        1) Normal cells will show a one-third area of central pallor.
        2) Decreased central pallor is seen in spherocytosis, including burns and liver disorders.
        3) Increased central pallor is seen in anemias and other disorders.
    d. Reference value is $4.2–5.4 \times 10^3/\mu L$ for females and $4.6–6.2 \times 10^3/\mu L$ for males
    e. Erythropoiesis is regulated by **erythropoietin** produced in the kidney. Additional regulation includes:
        1) Any changes in production or usage.
        2) Hypoxia due to high altitudes, heart and lung pathology, and anemia.
        3) Androgens (male hormones that appear to enhance the activity of erythropoietin) and hemolytic anemias (increased erythrocyte destruction).
    f. Erythrocytes do not have a nucleus or mitochondria.

D. Erythrocyte physiology

1. Early RBCs get energy from oxidative phosphorylation. During maturation, the mitochondria is lost, and energy is derived from glycolysis.
2. Erythrocytes need proper volume ratio for exchange of blood gases and flexibility to travel through capillaries. This is accomplished by the Na/K pump mechanism.
3. Erythrocyte membrane is 50–60 percent lipid (phospholipids, cholesterol, and glycolipids) and 40–50 percent protein.

E. Substances Needed for Erythropoiesis
1. **Iron:** needed for maturation.
2. **Folic acid/Vitamin B$_{12}$:** needed for DNA replication/cell division.
3. **Hormones:** erythropoietin, thyroxine, androgens.
4. **Other substances:** manganese, cobalt, zink, vitamins C, E, B$_6$, thiamine, riboflavin, and pantothenic acid.

F. Erythrocytic Morphology and Associated Disease (Size and Shape)
1. **Normocytes (discocytes)** are normal erythrocytes
2. **Macrocytes**
   a. Erythrocytes that have an MCV greater than 100 fL.
   b. Seen in megaloblastic anemias, such as B$_{12}$/folate deficiency.
   c. Occurs in anemia of liver disease.
3. **Microcytes**
   a. Are small RBCs less than 6μm in diameter.
   b. Shows an MCV less than 80 fL.
   c. Seen in iron deficiency anemia, thalassemias, hemolytic anemias, sideroblastic anemia, and chronic disorder anemias.
4. **Echinocytes (crenated RBCs)**
   a. Show uniform round bumps or spikes on the RBC surface.
   b. Usually indicate artifact of staining or increased platelets.
   c. No pathology is indicated.
   d. Caused by changes in cellular osmotic pressure.
5. **Burr cell (keratocytes)**
   a. Irregular in size with spiny projections.
   b. Seen in renal insufficiency, liver disease, ulcers, and heparin therapy.
   c. Caused by cell membrane breakup due to cytoplasmic vacuoles.
   d. Can be confused with crenated erythrocytes.
6. **Acanthocytes**
   a. Appear as small, densely stained RBCs with multiple irregularly spaced spikes or clublike projections.
   b. Associated with liver disease (hepatitis, especially neonatal) and abetalipoproteinemia.
   c. Caused by excessive cholesterol in the membrane.
7. **Target cells (codocytes or Mexican hat cells)**
   a. Show a central area of hemoglobin surrounded by a colorless ring and a peripheral ring of hemoglobin.
   b. Considered artifacts if appear in only one section of the smear.

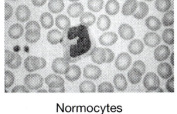

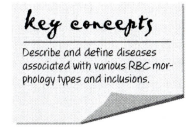

Normocytes (discocytes)

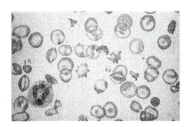

key concepts

Describe and define diseases associated with various RBC morphology types and inclusions.

Echinocytes (crerated RBCs)

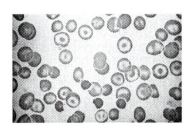

Target cells

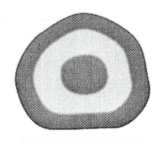

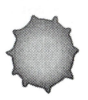

FIGURE 2.1
Crenated cell

FIGURE 2.2
Burr cell

FIGURE 2.3
Leptocyte

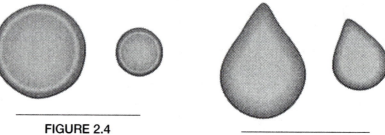

FIGURE 2.4
Spherocytes

FIGURE 2.5
Teardrops (dacrocytes)

c. Seen in liver disease, hemoglobinopathies, iron deficiency anemia, hemolytic anemia, and liver disease.

d. Caused by excessive cholesterol in the membrane or a hemoglobin distribution imbalance.

e. **Leptocytes** are similar in appearance to target cells but fail to show a complete detachment between the inner and outer membrane. Seen in iron deficiency anemia, thalassemia, and liver disease.

8. **Spherocytes**
    a. Slightly smaller (6.2–7.0μL) than normal erythrocytes.
    b. Shows no central pallor.
    c. Increased MCHC and increased osmotic fragility.
    d. Seen in hereditary spherocytosis, burns, and extravascular hemolytic processes.
    e. **Microspherocytes** are frequently seen in severe burn cases.
    f. Spherocytes and microspherocytes result when the erythrocyte surface area decreases due to a decrease in cell volume.

9. **Teardrops (dacryocytes)**
    a. Show a tapered and round end. Slightly smaller than normocytes.
    b. Seen in pernicious anemia (megaloblastic), myelofibrosis, acquired hemolytic anemia, and extramedullary hematopoiesis.

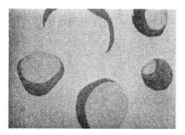

Sickle cells
(drepanocytes)

10. **Sickle cells (drepanocytes)**
    a. Shapes vary but show thin, elongated pointed ends, and will appear crescent shaped.
    b. Contain hemoglobin S.
    c. Seen in sickle cell anemia.
    d. Cell shape is caused by cell membrane alterations due to hemoglobin S.

11. **Helmet cells**
    a. Interior portion of cell is hollow, resembling a helmet.
    b. Caused by hemolytic processes.
    c. Seen in hemolytic anemia, and other conditions resulting from intravascular hemolysis.

12. **Schistocytes (RBC fragments)**
    a. Erythrocyte fragmentation results from passage through damaged or altered blood vessels.
    b. Seen in DIC, burns, renal transplant rejection and hemolytic processes.

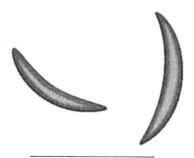

FIGURE 2.6
Sickle cell
(depranocytes)

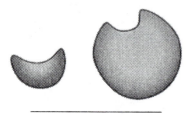

FIGURE 2.7
Schistocytes

13. **Stomatocytes (mouth cells)**
    a. Characterized by an elongated or slitlike area of central pallor.
    b. May indicate liver disease, also seen in hereditary stomatocytosis.
    c. Caused by an increase in sodium (cytoplasmic) and a decrease in potassium.

14. **Elliptocytes (ovalocytes)**
    a. Cigar to pencil shaped. Function normally.
    b. Caused by a membrane integrity defect.
    c. Seen in hereditary elliptocytosis, iron deficiency anemia, megaloblastic anemia, thalassemia major, and sickle cell anemia.

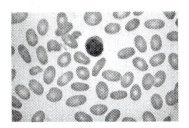

Elliptocytes

15. **Nucleated RBCs (nRBCs)**
    a. Most are orthochromic normoblasts but can appear in any erythrocytic stage of maturation.
    b. Indicate some type of bone marrow stimulation or increased erythropoiesis.
    c. Normally found in newborns.
    d. Seen in acute blood loss, leukemias, hypoxia, megaloblastic anemias, heart disease, and myelofibrosis.
    e. As few as one nRBC should be reported when seen on adult peripheral blood films.

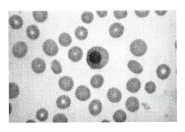

NRBCs

16. **Blister cells**
    a. Show cellular vacuoles.
    b. Seen in burns, damaged blood vessels, and sickle cell anemia.
    c. Caused by damaged cellular membranes.

G. Erythrocyte Inclusions and Associated Disease

1. **Howell-Jolly bodies**
    a. Appear as small, round fragments (1 to 2μm in diameter) of nuclear material (DNA) that may be **single** or **multiple.**
    b. Caused by nuclear disintegration.
    c. Fragments stain reddish/blue to purple.
    d. Positive for the Feulgen stain, which stains DNA.
    e. Not seen in normal erythrocytes.
    f. Seen in sickle cell anemia, megaloblastic anemia, alcoholism, splenectomy, hemolysis, and hemoglobinopathies.

2. **Basophilic stippling**
    a. **Multiple,** tiny, fine, or coarse inclusions (ribosomal RNA remnants) throughout the cell.
    b. Stain dark blue to purple.

FIGURE 2.8
Stomatocyte

FIGURE 2.9
Howell-Jolly bodies

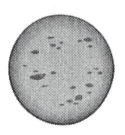

FIGURE 2.10
Basophilic stippling

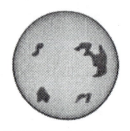

FIGURE 2.11
Pappenheimer bodies

    c. Will not stain with Prussian blue stain.

    d. Seen in thalassemias, megaloblastic anemias, **lead poisoning,** alcoholism, and disorders that increase erythropoiesis.

    e. Larger more coarse granules hold greater pathological importance.

    f. Smaller than Howell-Jolly bodies—avoid misidentification.

3. **Pappenheimer bodies**

    a. Small irregular, dark-staining granules (iron granules) **clumped together at one end or region.**

    b. Stain with the Prussian blue stain and appear dark violet with Wright's stain (although difficult to see with Wright's stain).

    c. Caused by an accumulation of ribosome, mitochondria, and iron fragments.

    d. Seen in sideroblastic anemia, thalassemia, hemosiderosis, and megaloblastic anemia.

4. **Cabot rings**

    a. Thin, blue to reddish-purple, single to multiple **ringlike** structures that may appear in loop or figure-eight shapes.

    b. Seen in megaloblastic anemia, **lead poisoning,** and dyserythropoiesis.

    c. Caused by fragments of nuclear material.

5. **Hemoglobin H inclusions**

    a. Small greenish/blue bodies that stain with cresyl blue.

    b. Seen in hemoglobin H disease and α-thalassemia.

6. **Hemoglobin CC crystals**

    a. Hexagonal with blunt ends.

    b. May appear after splenectomy.

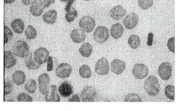

Hemoglobin
CC crystals

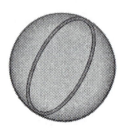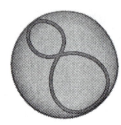

FIGURE 2.12 Cabot rings

7. **Hemoglobin SC crystals**
    a. Blunt-pointed projections extending from the cell membrane.
    b. Seen in hemoglobin SC disease.
8. **Heinz bodies**
    a. Multiple inclusions ranging in size from 0.3 to 2.0μm.
    b. Must stain with crystal violet or cresyl blue stain.
    c. Seen in **G6PD deficiency.**
    d. Results from denatured hemoglobin.
9. **Parasites** (covered in more detail in Chapter 8)

H. Erythrocyte Hemoglobin Content and Associated Diseases

1. **Normochromasia:** cells have the normal one-third clear central pallor area.
2. **Hypochromasia**
    a. Increased central pallor area.
    b. MCH and MCHC usually decreased.
    c. Often associated with microcytosis.
    d. Seen in iron deficiency anemia, thalassemia, and sideroblastic anemia.
    e. Normocytic hypochromasia is seen in rheumatoid arthritis, chronic infections, and inflammation.

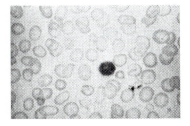

Hypochromasia

3. **Polychromasia**
    a. Variation in hemoglobin content showing a slight blue-orange color.
    b. Indicates an increase in reticulocytes.
    c. Erythrocytes are usually slightly larger than normocytic RBCs.
4. **Hyperchromasia (term no longer used)**

I. Erythrocyte Size/Shape Variations and Associated Disease

1. **Anisocytosis**
    a. Variation in RBC size and diameter.
    b. Quantitated from 1+ through 4+.
    c. RDW will correlate with anisocytosis, especially when the RDW exceeds 15.0.
    d. Often associated with anemias.
2. **Poikilocytosis**
    a. Variation in shape.
    b. Quantitated from 1+ to 4+.
    c. Associated with a variety of pathological conditions.

J. Abnormal Erythrocyte Distributions and Associated Disease

1. **Rouleaux**
    a. Characterized by erythrocytes appearing in short or long stacks of overlapping cells.
    b. Seen in hyperproteinemia, multiple myeloma, macroblobuline-mia, and conditions that produce increased fibrinogen (infec-tions, tissue necrosis, and pregnancy).
    c. May result from staining artifacts and normally exists in the thick area of a peripheral smear.
    d. True rouleaux is determined in the thin area of a peripheral smear.

2. **Agglutination**
   a. Characterized by erythrocytes appearing in clusters and groups.
   b. Produced when erythrocytes are exposed to erythrocyte antibodies.
   c. Seen in hemolytic anemias, DIC, and atypical pneumonia.

X. ANEMIAS

A. Anemias—caused by a decrease in erythrocytes and hemoglobin. They are classified as normocytic, normochromic, microcytic, hypochromic, or macrocytic. Each anemia has a specific etiology. Anemias are suspected when the hemoglobin is **<12 g/dL in men** or **< 11 g/dL in women.**

key concepts

Define and describe the various types of anemias.

1. **Relative anemias**
   a. RBC count is normal, but a shift in fluid levels give the clinical picture of anemia.
   b. Secondary to an unrelated condition and can be transient in nature.
   c. Causes include pregnancy, cirrhosis of the liver, nephritis, congestive heart failure, multiple myeloma, and IV fluid administration.
   d. **Reticulocyte** count is **normal.**
   e. **Normocytic/normochromic** anemia.

2. **Absolute anemias**
   a. Indicated by a true decrease in erythrocytes and hemoglobin.
   b. Caused by **aplasia** (lack of bone marrow production), **dyserythropoiesis** (abnormal RBC production), **hemolysis** (increased rate of RBC destruction), and **DNA/heme** disorders.

3. **Anemia classification**
   a. Blood loss anemia, including acute and chronic
   b. Defective or impaired production
      1) Aplastic
      2) Iron deficiency
      3) Sideroblastic anemia
      4) Megaloblastic (vitamin B_{12} and folic acid deficiency)
   c. Anemia of chronic disease
   d. Hemolytic anemia
   e. Genetic anemia
   f. Anemia of systemic disorders

B. Blood Loss Anemia
   1. **Acute blood loss anemia**
      a. Characterized by a sudden loss of blood resulting from trauma or other severe forms of injury.
      b. Clinical symptoms include hypovolemia, rapid pulse, low blood pressure, and pallor.
      c. Laboratory: Normal **reticulocyte** count; **Hct/Hgb** is normal when immediately drawn; increase in **platelet** count followed by a drop in platelets; **neutrophilic leukocytosis** with a shift to the left; **normocytic/normochromic** anemia.
   2. **Chronic blood loss anemia**
      a. Characterized by a gradual, long term loss of blood. Caused by a wide variety of diseases such as bleeding ulcers, GI bleeds, etc.

b. Laboratory: increased **recticulocytes,** the anemia is **normocytic/normochromic.** The anemia overtime causes a decrease in **Hct/Hgb,** and the loss of **iron** results in a **microcytic/hypochromic** anemia.

C. Defective or Impaired Production Anemia

1. **Aplastic anemia**
   a. Anemia of decreased cell production.
   b. Laboratory: decrease in **Hct/Hgb, normochromic** and **normocytic** anemia, no response to **erythropoietin, pancytopenia** including **neutropenia** and **thrombocytopenia.**
   c. Affects people around the age of 50, and is more common in Asians. Can rarely occur in children.
   d. Special tests for diagnosis: increased **hemoglobin F** and increased **LAP** score.
   e. Patients have a poor prognosis with a variety of complication, including bleeding, infections, and iron overload.
   f. Treatment includes bone marrow transplants and chemotherapy.
   g. **Aplastic anemia has two types of etiology** (genetic and acquired)
      1) **Genetic aplastic anemia**
         a) **Diamond-Blackfan syndrome**
            (i) Causes a decreased production of RBCs. A hypoplastic anemia.
            (ii) Defective stem cell disorder is probable cause.
            (iii) Laboratory: normochromic/normocytic anema, decreased reticulocytes.
         b) **Fanconi's anemia**
            (i) Caused by an autosomal recessive trait more common in males.
            (ii) Disease results in skeletal disorders (short stature), renal disease, and mental retardation.
            (iii) Laboratory: progressive pancytopenia with decreased hemoglobin.
            (iv) Strong association with malignancy development, especially acute leukemia.
      2) **Acquired aplastic anemia (acquired pure red cell aplasia)** caused by the following:
         a) Antibiotics: chloramphenicol and tetracyclines.
         b) Chemicals: benzene, alcohol, and herbicides.
         c) Viruses: B19 parvovirus secondary to hepatitis, measles, CMV, and Epstein-Barr virus.
         d) Radiation and chemotherapy.
         e) Thymus gland tumors and malnutrition.
         f) Laboratory: severe **normocytic** anemia, decreased **reticulocyte** count; **WBC and platelets counts** are normal.

2. **Myelophthisic anemia**
   a. Hypoproliferative anemia common in patients with cancer and chronic infections.
   b. Caused by bone metastasizing cancers such as breast, prostate, lung, and melanoma.

3. **Lead intoxication**
   a. Result in decreased RBC production leading to anemia.
   b. Seen mostly in children when lead-based paint is present.
   c. Clinical: abdominal pain, muscle weakness, and a **gum lead line** which are blue/black deposits of lead sulfate.
   d. Laboratory: **normocytic/normochromic** anemia with characteristic basophilic stippling.

4. **Iron deficiency anemia**
   a. Most common form of anemia in the United States.
   b. Prevalent in young women not eating a proper diet during pregnancy, excessive menstural flow, and in the elderly with poor diets.
   c. Any long-term blood loss will progress into iron deficiency anemia.
   d. Laboratory: **hypochromic/microcytic** anemia. Total iron-binding capacity **(TIBC)** is increased; all other **iron tests** are decreased. Most **RBC indices** and **Hct/Hgb** will be decreased. **WBCs** and **reticulocytes** are normal, and **platelet count** is increased.
   e. Clinical: most patients show fatigue, dizziness, stomatitis (cracks in the corners of the mouth), glossitis (sore tongue), and koilonychia (spooning of the nails).

5. **Sideroblastic anemia**
   a. Not as common in the United States.
   b. Caused by abnormal iron metabolism.
   c. Excess iron accumulates in the mitochondrial region of the erythrocyte and these cells are called siderocytes or sideroblasts.
   d. **Siderocytes** shown best by **Prussian blue stain.** Typed according to their **ferritin aggregate** content. **Type I** has four aggregates of ferritin, **Type II** has six aggregates of ferritin, and **Type III** has ringed ferritin and are called **ringed sideroblasts**.
   e. Siderocytes can accumulate in body tissue in a disease state called **hemochromatosis**, which is characterized by iron deposits in body tissue, resulting in the skin taking on a bronze color.
   f. Siderocytes will stain with the Wright stain but appear as Pappenheimer bodies.
   g. Considered a **myelodysplastic syndrome.**
   h. Laboratory: **microcytic/hypochromic** anemia. With increased **transferrin** and **serum iron**, the **TIBC** is decreased.

6. **Vitamin B$_{12}$ deficiency (cyanocobalamin)**
   a. Caused by a failure of the gastric mucosa to produce intrinsic factor necessary in the absorption of B$_{12}$ which is required for DNA synthesis. A **megaloblastic anemia**.
   b. Causes of vitamin B$_{12}$ deficiency are celiac disease, tapeworms, bacterial and parasitic infections, and poor diet. *Note*: Strict vegetarians run the risk of developing B$_{12}$ deficiency anemia.
   c. Clinical: jaundice, sore tongue, and gastrointestinal (GI) CNS problems.

    d. Laboratory: **macrocytosis (oval macrocytes), hyperseg-mented neutrophils,** and **macrocytic/normochromic** anemia.

    e. The **Schilling Test** measures B_{12} levels, which will be decreased in B_{12} anemia.

    f. **Pernicious anemia** is a nutritional deficiency of B_{12}, resulting from a lack of intrinsic factor (IF) secreted by gastric mucosa.

       1) Pernicious anemia can be inherited or acquired (gastrectomy).

7. **Folic acid deficiency** is an anemia similar to B_{12} anemia, and is associated with poor diet and pregnancy. A **megaloblastic anemia.**

8. **Macrocytic anemias not associated with megaloblastic nuclei** include alcoholism, liver disease, and lead poisoning.

D. Hemolytic Anemias

1. **Intravascular hemolysis** is trauma to erythrocytes that produces schistocytes.

2. **Paroxysmal nocturnal hemoglobinuria**: autoimmune intravascular hemolysis where sensitivity of erythrocytes to complement causes hemolysis to occur in an acid pH during sleep. The first morning void is red urine containing free hemoglobin.

3. **Paroxysmal cold hemoglobinuria (PCH)** results from activation of cold antibodies, e.g., anti-P, that activate complement.

E. Genetic Anemias

1. **Abetalipoproteinemia** is a rare genetic anemia resulting in abnormal formation of the erythrocyte membrane. Differential: poikilocytosis and **acanthocytes.**

2. **Spherocytosis** is caused by defective Na/K pump mechanisms. MCV is below 80 fL, and the MCHC is above 36 percent.

F. Anemia of Systemic Disorders

1. **Anemia of chronic renal disease** is a hypoproliferative anemia due to decreased erythropoietin production.

2. **Anemia of endocrine disorders** is caused by hypothyroidism which results in a decrease in hemopoiesis and erythropoiesis. Presents as a **macrocytic** anemia.

3. **Anemia of pregnancy** usually results from an increase in fluid levels and loss increased iron use. Hemoglobin rarely falls under 10g/dL.

XI. HEMATOLOGY TESTS
A. Blood Cell Enumeration

1. **WBC count** manual counts use a hemacytometer.

    a. Use a white cell diluting pipet or Unopette^{TM} with a dilution factor of 20. Reagent lyses RBCs.

    b. Count the 4-corner 1mm large squares.

    c. **Formula**

$$\text{WBC/mm}^3 = \frac{\text{WBCs} \times \text{depth} \times \text{dilution}}{\text{area counted (mm}^2)}$$

    d. **Nucleated RBC correction formula**

$$\text{WBCs counted} = \text{\# of nRBCs} / + 100$$

2. **Platelet count**
   a. Dilution is 1:100. Hemacytomter is filled, covered with a Petri dish for 15 minutes to allow platelets to settle in one optical plane.
      1) Count the central large square (1mm); the 25 smaller squares within the large square are 0.2mm each.
      2) **Formula**

      # of platelets = total PLTs counted $\times$ 100 $\times$ 10

3. Sources of error involving manual cell counts
   a. Specimen contains small clots due to insufficient mixing with anticoagulant, not maintained at proper temperature, or exceeds allowable time limit.
   b. Sample inadequately mixed before diluting.
   c. Equipment that is not thoroughtly cleaned and dried (hemacytometer and pipettes) or does not meet U.S. Bureau of Standards.
   d. Technical due to inaccuracies in diluting samples, following steps of procedure, counting of cells, and calculating results; failure to consider abnormalities, additional calculations, i.e., WBC counts when nRBCs are present or correct reporting of results.

B. Blood Cell Enumeration—Automated Methods
1. Electrical impedance
   a. Cells pass through an aperture with an electrical current flowing through simultaneously. Cells change electrical resistance which is then counted as voltage pulses.
   b. Sample is diluted in isotonic conductive solution that preserves cell shape.
      1) RBCs are diluted 1:50,000
      2) Platelets are counted simultaneously with RBCs in triplicate.
      3) Sample for counting WBCs is mixed with reagent to lyse RBCs, i.e., 3 percent saponin. A commercially available reagent which both lyses RBCs and converts Hgb to HiCN can be used to determine Hgb and WBCs in one dilution. Dilution for WBCs is 1:500.
2. Light scattering optical method
   a. Uses a light-sensitive detector that measures light scattering.
   b. Detects size of pulse that is proportional to size of particle (cell)
   c. Sample is diluted similar to electrical impedance.

C. Additional Blood Cell Information—Automated Methods
1. Platelet distribution is determined and the **mean platelet volume (MPV)** is mathematically determined from the histogram.
   a. MPV ranges 6.5–12 fL.
   b. Platelet size normally varies inversely with the platelet count.
   c. There is no standard to determine this value so it is of questionable use.
2. RBC anisocytosis is estimated by the **red cell distribution width (RDW)**
   a. RDW is the coefficient of variation (CV) of the distribution of individual red cell volumes.
   b. Helpful in diagnosis and treatment of anemias.

3. MCV is determined by sizing of individual red cell volumes.
4. HCT is calculated: MCV × RBC count.
   a. No automated instrument incorporates the Hct reference-spun method in its system at this time.
5. **Histograms** display cell size distributions by *plotting cell volume versus relative number*—WBCs, RBCs, and platelets.
   a. Suspect **"flags"** indicate problems: linearity, lack of agreement among aperatures, unacceptable distribution caused by unusual cell populations.
      1) Identifies erythrocytic, i.e., "ANISO+++, MICRO, MACRO++" or "3+ Anisocytosis, 3+ Macrocytosis, Anemia."
      2) Identifies leukocytic abnormalities, i.e., "L shift, atyp, blasts, other" or "Leukocytosis."
   b. Interpretative reports give percentages and absolute counts for 5 leukocyte cell types (most instruments).
   c. Provide an interpretative **"differential"** of leukocyte cell types.
6. Scattergram plots of WBCs are displayed on a cathode ray tube (monitor) (CRT), color-coded for different population densities.
   a. Scattergrams plot leukocyte volume (determined by impedance) versus laser light scatter (DF1).
   b. Correlation between cells plotted in specified areas and suspect flags is considered excellent; reports indicate 6 percent false-negative and 3 percent false-positives.

D. Hemoglobin Measurement

1. Blood oxygen capacity: measures functional hemoglobin.

$$\frac{\text{Oxygen capacity in ml/dL blood}}{1.34 \text{ (hgb oxygen capacity)}} = \text{grams of Hgb/dL blood}$$

2. Blood iron content: measures total iron content of blood that is bound to hemoglobin.

$$\frac{\text{Blood iron content in mg/dL}}{3.47 \text{ (Hgb iron content)}} = \text{grams of Hgb/dL blood}$$

3. Oxyhemoglobin method does not measure sulfhemoglobin or methemoglobin. Read patients sample at 40 nm.
4. Cyanmethemoglobin method is the **reference method** for all hemoglobins except for sulfhemoglobin. Uses **Drabkin** solution (potassium ferricyanide and NaCN) that is added to blood. Read at 540 nm.

E. Reticulocyte Counts

1. Supravital stains are used to demonstrate reticulum in reticulocytes.
2. Formula:

$$\text{Retics (\%)} = \frac{\text{\# of Retics}}{1,000 \text{ RBCs observed}} \times 100$$

3. Corrected reticulocyte counts **(CRC)** are calculated to account of degree of anemia by using a standard normal Hct of 0.45 L/L.
   a. Formula

$$\text{CRC-Retics (\%)} \times \frac{\text{Hct (l/L)}}{0.45 \text{ L/L}}$$

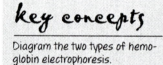

key concepts

Identify various hematology tests; explain the principal and major reagent(s) for each procedure. Compare and contrast reference and automated methods.

F. Erythrocyte sedimentation rate (ESR) — measures degree of settling of RBCs in plasma in an anticoagulated specimen during a specific time, usually 1 hour. Setting dependent on RBC mass and plasma viscosity.

1. Normal range is 0–20 mm/hr
2. **Increased:** inflammatory conditions resulting from increased plasma proteins.
    a. Includes arthritis, tuberculosis, hepatitis, heart disease, and tissue damage.
    b. Also increased in menstruation, pregnancy, and multiple myeloma.
    c. Nondisease increase includes tilting the tube and hemolysis.
3. **Normal to decreased:** polycythemia, sickle cell anemia, and spherocytosis (all produce an increased number of cells).
4. **Modified Westergren** method
    a. Ethylenediamine tetraacetic acid (EDTA) blood specimen diluted with sodium citrate or sodium chloride.
    b. Not affected by anemia. Anemia affects older **Wintrobe**/Westergren methods.
    c. Must test within 2 hours of blood collection if not refrigerated.
    d. Used to monitor inflammatory processes.
    e. Must test at room temperature with tube in a vertical position.

G. Hemoglobin F (Kleihauer-Betke method) — count HgbF cells (dense-staining cells) and the number of ghost cells. Normal is 1 percent, infants 70–90 percent.

H. Hemoglobin Electrophoresis

1. Procedure for the identification of normal and abnormal hemoglobins.
2. Methodology based on net negative charges, which cause hemoglobins to migrate from the negative **(cathode)** region toward the positive **(anode)** region. Different hgbs migrate at different rates.
3. Two types of electrophoresis: **cellulose acetate pH 8.4** and **citrate agar pH 6.2**
4. Migration of hemoglobin is dependent on the isoelectric point, and buffer pH.

key concepts

Diagram the two types of hemoglobin electrophoresis.

5. Cellulose Acetate (pH 8.4) Hemoglobin Electrophoresis

Cathode (−)					Anode (+)
(x) origin	**A₂**	**S**	**F**	**A**	
		C	**D**		
		E	**G**		
		O			

6. Citrate Aagar (pH 6.2) Hemoglobin Electrophoresis

Cathode (−)					Anode (+)
C	**S**	(x) origin	**A**	**F**	
			D		
			G		
			E		

   a. At pH 8.4, HbA migrates the fastest, and HbC migrates the slowest.
   b. At pH 6.2, HbS is separated from HbD and HbG.
   c. HbC is differentiated from HbO, HbS, and HbG.
   d. There is a large separation between HbF and HbA₂.

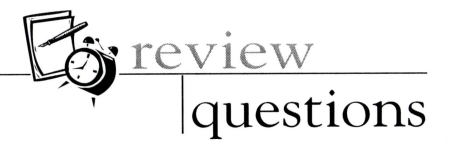

review questions

DIRECTIONS Each of the questions or incomplete statements below is followed by suggested answers or completions. Select the **one answer** that is best in each case.

1. Which of the following can produce an increased buffy coat?
   a. Erythrocytosis
   b. Neutrophilia
   c. Thrombocytopenia
   d. Monocytopenia

2. Which of the following would indicate an immature cell?
   a. Low N:C ratio, clumped chromatin, no nucleoli
   b. No nuclear segmentation, high N:C ratio, clumped chromatin
   c. Light to loose chromatin, high N:C ratio, nucleoli are present
   d. Poorly defined organelles, nuclear segmentation, high N:C ratio

3. A medium-size immature cell with a round nucleus showing heterochromatin, cytoplasm indicating active RNA synthesis, and containing both nonspecific and specific granules would be:
   a. Metamyleocyte.
   b. Promyelocyte.
   c. Myelocyte.
   d. Myeloblast.

4. The two types of acute myelogenous leukemia (M1 and M2) can be differentiated on the basis of:
   a. Percentage of myeloblasts.
   b. Presence or absence of Auer rods.

   c. Type of granulation.
   d. Clinical symptoms.

5. Macrophages found in the brain are called:
   a. Monocytes.
   b. Langerhans' cells.
   c. Kupffer cells.
   d. Microglial cells.

6. What is the average ratio of T-lymphocytes to B-lymphocytes?
   a. 50/50
   b. 80/20
   c. 20/80
   d. 40/60

7. In the most common childhood cancer, the differential shows a normocytic-nocyrochromic anemia with nRBCs, thrombocytopenia, varied WBC, and small homogenous lymphocytes with a high N/C ratio, which are called:
   a. CLL.
   b. L1.
   c. L2.
   d. L3.

8. Which of the following is B-cell malignancy, considered a monoclonal gammopathy, which results in the excessive production of IgM?
   a. Prolymphocytic leukemia
   b. Multiple myeloma
   c. Waldenström's macroglobulinemia
   d. Hodgkin's lymphoma

9. Acquired aplastic anemia can be caused by all the following EXCEPT:
   a. Chloramphenicol.
   b. Diamond-Blackfan syndrome.
   c. Alcohol.
   d. B19 parvovirus secondary to hepatitis.

10. Which of the following is an erythrocyte morphology found in most hemoglobinopathies?
   a. Target cells
   b. Schistocytes
   c. Dacryocytes
   d. Drepanocytes

11. Which of the following is a major diagnostic characteristic of plasma cells?
   a. Eccentric nucleus with clumped chromatin
   b. Round nucleus with blue cytoplasm
   c. Found in the peripheral blood
   d. None of the above

12. Which of the following is a rare subtype B-cell disease characterized by lymphocytopenia and is positive for tartrate-resistant acid phosphatase?
   a. Waldenström's macroglobulinemia
   b. Prolymphocytic leukemia
   c. Hairy cell leukemia
   d. Multiple myeloma

13. Which of the following is characterized by an inversion or deletion of chromosome 16?
   a. M4E
   b. M5
   c. M5A
   d. M5B

14. M2 has which of the following characteristics?
   a. Less than 90 percent myeloblast with Auer rods
   b. Promyelocytic granules are very small and sparse
   c. Positive for serum lysozyme
   d. CD14 and CD4 positive

15. Which of the following is characterized by monocytosis and refractory anemia?
   a. M7
   b. L1
   c. APL
   d. CMML

16. Identify the correct statement regarding hemoglobin synthesis.
   a. Thirty-five percent hemoglobin synthesis occurs in immature nRBCs and 65 percent in reticulocytes.
   b. Heme synthesis occurs in the ribosomes of normoblasts.
   c. Globin synthesis occurs in the mitochondia of normoblasts.
   d. Sixty-five percent hemoglobin synthesis occurs in immature nRBCs and 35 percent in reticulocytes.

17. Thalassemias will show which of the following laboratory characteristics?
   a. Macrocytic/hypochromic anemia, target cells, nRBCs
   b. Howell-Jolly bodies, siderocytes, spherocytes
   c. Microcytic/hypochromia anemia, target cells, nRBCs
   d. Both b and c

18. Which hemoglobins are used to diagnose thalassemia on hemoglobin electrophoresis?
   a. HbA and HbF
   b. HbA2 and Hb-H
   c. HbA2 and HbF
   d. HbA and Hb-Barts

19. All of the following are associated with the diagnosis of multiple myeloma EXCEPT:
   a. Chloramphenicol.
   b. Diamond-Blackfan syndrome
   c. Alcohol.
   d. B19 parvovirus secondary to hepatitis.

20. Iron deficiency anemia will show which of the following laboratory characteristics?
   a. Hyperchromic/microcytic anemia, increased TIBC, increased iron
   b. Hypochromic/microcytic anemia, increased TIBC, decreased iron
   c. Hypochromic/macrocytic, increased TIBC, increased iron
   d. Increased WBC count, reticulocytosis, increased platelets

3

Coagulation

contents

➤ COMPREHENSIVE KEY CONCEPTS

1. Analyze and explain the steps and components needed in the formation of a clot, including primary hemostasis, secondary hemostasis, and the intrinsic, extrinsic, and common coagulation pathways. Include in the analysis various diseases and conditions that can affect coagulation.

2. Define the function of the fibrinolytic system, including the necessary components, steps, and inhibitors, in addition to the conditions and diseases that affect fibrinolysis.

3. Outline the various intrinsic and extrinsic pathway disorders including their laboratory (focus on prothrombin time [PT] and activated partial thromboplastin time [PTT] testing) and clinical characteristics.

I. INTRODUCTION TO THROMBOCYTES (PLATELETS)
A. Thrombocyte Characteristics
1. **Platelets** range in size from 1 to 4μm.
2. The reference range for healthy individuals is **150–400 × 10⁹/L** or 9 to 20 per high power field.
3. Life span averages 5 to 10 days but can be shorter in certain disease states.
4. Mature **platelets** have **no nucleus.** The cytoplasm contains inclusions: lysosomes, mitochondria, glycogen, granules, and peroxisomes.
5. Platelets are found in the bone marrow, tissue, and blood vessels where they function in hemostasis.
6. Unlike erythrocytes and leukocytes, platelets originate from only one cell population group.
7. Mature platelets are released from the bone marrow and enter the peripheral blood as cytoplasmic fragments.
   a. Platelet cytoplasm stains gray-blue with purple granules with Wright's stain.
   b. Platelets contain two types of **functional granules:**
      1) **Alpha granules** contain fibrinogen, von Willebrand's factor, platelet-derived growth factor (PDGF), PF4 (platelet factor), and other proteins.
      2) **Dense core granules** contain ADP, ATP (energy molecules), 5-HT, and calcium.
8. Larger platelets indicate premature release from the bone marrow resulting from demand due to disease, anemia, etc.
9. Immature platelets are usually not found in the peripheral blood except in certain diseases such as **megakaryocytic leukemia.**

B. Thrombocyte Maturation
1. **Megakaryoblast**
   a. Earliest thrombocyte stage where the nucleus undergoes nuclear division without cytoplasmic division (process know as **endomitosis**).
   b. Endomitosis results in the formation of giant multinucleated cells.
   c. Nucleus contains nucleoli, but chromatin is not yet visible.

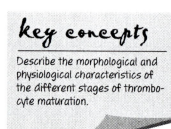

key concepts

Describe the morphological and physiological characteristics of the different stages of thrombocyte maturation.

    d. Megakaryoblasts range in size from 20 to 50µm.

    e. Cytoplasm contains **no granules,** stains blue, and is irregularly shaped with **cytoplasmic tags** (blunt extensions of cytoplasm).

2. **Promegakaryocyte**

    a. **Increases** in size to 20–80µm.

    b. Contains a double nucleus.

    c. **Cytoplasmic granules** begin to appear, and cytoplasmic tags continue to be present.

    d. **Demarcating membrane system (DMS)** begins to form.

       1) DMS is an invagination of the plasma membrane that becomes the future site of platelet fragmentation.

3. **Megakaryocyte**

    a. **Increases** in size to 30–100µm.

    b. Contains multiple nuclei with many small granules, which are reddish to blue in color.

    c. Nuclear chromatin is coarse.

    d. **Last stage** of development where no platelets are produced.

    e. Represents 1 percent of nucleated bone marrow cells.

    f. Seen in peripheral blood on rare occurrences due to increased demand for platelets; acute bleeding episodes.

4. **Metamegakaryocyte**

    a. Largest cell in the body.

    b. Begins to show a **decreased N/C ratio.**

    c. The nucleus is multilobed and **ploidy** (refers to the number of 23 chromosome sets in the cell).

    d. Stage where platelets break away from the cytoplasm in the DMS region.

5. **Mature platelets**

    a. 1–4µm in size, appearing as dense blue particles with azurophilic granules.

    b. Comprised of **four** major areas:

       1) **Peripheral zone:** outer membrane and related structures.

       2) **Submembrane area:** links the platelet membrane together with the internal cell structure.

       3) **Sol-gel zone:** matrix or skeletal portion of the platelet.

       4) **Organelle zone:** contains granules, lysosomes, and the mitochondria. Controls platelet function in response to coagulation, viruses, and other foreign bodies.

C. Identifying Maturation Stages

1. Cytoplasmic appearance is important in early stage identification.

2. The number of nuclei can be misleading as they are not well defined.

3. **Size** is diagnostic.

4. Other large cells may be similar in appearance: osteoblasts, plasma, Reed-Sternberg, and neoplastic cells.

D. Thrombocyte Function

1. Platelet function is dependent on **platelet secreted proteins, ATP, ADP, calcium, and platelet factors.**

2. **Platelet secreted protein**
   a. Stimulates blood vessels to constrict when injured.
   b. Activates other platelets and coagulation factors.
   c. Contracts the thrombus at the end of the coagulation process.
3. **Platelet factors**
   a. **PF4** neutralizes heparin.
   b. **PF3** is a platelet phospholipid needed for proper platelet function and coagulation.
      1) PF3 is needed in the production of **thromboxane A2** (aggregating substance and vasoconstrictor).
      2) Provides a surface for fibrin formation.
4. Proper platelet function involves **adhesion, release of granules, aggregation, and clot compaction.**
   a. **Adhesion**
      1) Platelets alter their shape and adhere to vascular surfaces.
      2) Is a response to subendothelial surface exposure caused by vascular injury.
      3) Dependent on **platelet and plasma vWF** and **VIII:vWF.**
      4) Can also be activated by thrombin.
   b. **Platelet granule release**
      1) Platelet granule release is regulated by:
         a) **Collagen**
         b) **Thrombin**
         c) **Epinephrine**
         d) **Thromboxane A2**
      2) The degree of granule release is regulated by the response intensity.
         a) A strong response causes more **dense core granules** to be released.
         b) A weak stimuli causes more **alpha granules** to be released.
   c. **Aggregation**
      1) Platelets clump together to form the initial plug.
      2) Platelets release **ADP** (energy source), **serotonin** (constricts blood vessels), and **PF4** (neutralizes heparin).
      3) During aggregation, **PF3** is released to provide the surface for fibrin formation.
   d. **Clot compaction**
      1) Successful clot formation depends on clot compaction.
      2) Dependent on **thrombasthenin** and **glycoprotein IIa** and **IIIb.**

E. **Laboratory Analysis of Platelets**
   1. Platelet numbers: blood smear estimates, hemocytometer and automated counts.
   2. Platelet adhesion: bleeding time.
   3. Clot retraction: time required for a clot to retract.
   4. Aggregating agents such as ADP, epinephrine, collagen, thrombin, and ristocetin: increased platelet aggregation.
   5. VIIIvWB factor: antigen and functional activity assays.

II. DISEASES AND CONDITIONS ASSOCIATED WITH PLATELETS

A. Genetic Disorders (Adhesion Defects)

1. **Bernard-Soulier syndrome**
   a. Seen with larger platelets that lack glycoprotein Ib, which prevents the binding of the platelet to von Willebrand's factor.
   b. Deficiency in glycoprotein Ib results in defective adhesion.
   c. Laboratory: mid to moderate thrombocytopenia, marked platelet anisocytosis, and an increased bleeding time.

2. **von Willebrand's disease (platelet type)**
   a. Lacks a plasma protein needed for platelets to adhere to damaged vessels.
   b. Results in decreased platelet adhesion and mild bleeding.
   c. Laboratory: normal to decreased platelet count, prolonged bleeding time, and a decreased aggregation response to ristocetin.

B. Genetic defects (aggregation defect)

1. **Glanzmann's thrombasthenia**
   a. Hemorrhagic disorder seen in ethnic populations where consanguinity is prevalent.
   b. Decreased surface membrane glycoproteins IIa and IIb.
   c. Results in the inability of platelets to bind to fibrinogen and fibrin.
   clot retraction (diagnostic), normal
   ased PF3.

eficiency of one or more types of storage

characterized by large platelets void of
les resulting in defective aggregation due

ne: characterized by a lack of stored or
s are prone to hemorrhage and infection.
rome: dense core granules are not pro-
cteristic oculocutaneous albinism.
y: patients may exhibit (partial) albinism,
and hemorrhage. Platelets produce giant
ontain giant inclusion granules.

ation Defects)

1. **Drugs**
   a. Common: aspirin, nonsteroidal anti-inflammatory drugs, antimicrobials, penicillin, cardiovascular, anticoagulants, psychotropics, chemotherapeutics, anesthetics, and alcohol will inhibit **thromboxane A2** synthesis.

2. **Diet**
   a. Fish containing C19 or C21 chain fatty acids found in fish oil replaces arachidonic acid which is a prostaglandin needed for platelet aggregation.
   b. Onions and garlic contain substances that affect aggregation. Herbs in Szechuan foods are said to have aggregation inhibitory properties.

key concepts

Be able to categorize platelet disorders such as adhesion, aggregation, genetic, or acquired defects.

key concepts

List and discuss the diseases associated with platelet disorders.

3. **Diseases** such as **myeloproliferative disorders, uremia,** and **disseminated intravascular coagulopathies (DIC)** will affect aggregation.

E. Quantitative Platelet Disorders

1. **Primary (essential) thrombocytosis**

   a. Uncontrolled proliferation of platelets which can be caused by **polycythemia vera, essential thrombocythemia,** and **chronic granulocytic leukemia.**

2. **Secondary (reactive) thrombocytosis**

   a. Increase in platelet production, which is not as pronounced as primary thrombocytosis. Can result from the following:

      1) **Malignant disease**

      2) **Chronic and acute inflammatory disease,** i.e., tuberculosis, cirrhosis.

      3) **Iron deficiency:** iron regulates thrombopoiesis by inhibiting thrombopoietin.

      4) **Rapid blood regeneration:** due to hemolytic anemia and acute blood loss.

      5) **Exercise, prematurity, and response to drugs.**

      6) **Other conditions:** alcohol and cytotoxic drug withdrawal, postoperative state from tissue damage, and splenectomy.

3. **Thrombocytopenia**

   a. Decrease in the production of platelets which can result from the following diseases:

      1) **Megakaryocyte hypoproliferation:** caused by aplastic anemia, drug and alcohol abuse, and viral infections.

      2) **Ineffective thrombopoiesis:** caused by megaloblastic anemia, thrombopoietic deficiency, or iron deficiency anemia.

      3) **Increased loss/destruction**

         a) **Nonimmune** loss due to severe hemorrhages, extensive transfusion (dilution loss), and increased consumption seen in DIC, hemolytic uremic syndrome, and chronic bleeding.

         b) **Immune** loss can be due to neonatal purpura, posttransfusion purpura, immune thrombocytopenic purpura, and idiopathic thrombocytopenic purpura.

      4) **Splenic sequestration**

         a) Can result in thrombocytopenia due to increased phagocytosis.

         b) Increased destruction of damaged platelets and normal platelets.

         c) Gaucher's disease and sarcoidosis.

      5) **Satellitism syndrome:** platelets adhere to neutrophils when exposed to EDTA resulting in falsely decreased platelet counts.

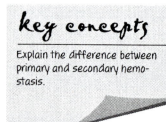

key concepts

Explain the difference between primary and secondary hemostasis.

III. INTRODUCTION TO HEMOSTASIS

A. Primary Hemostasis

1. Starts when platelets come in contact with exposed collagen, microfilaments, and the basement membrane of endothelial tissue.

2. Small blood vessels constrict, which allows platelets to adhere to exposed tissue causing **ADP/ATP** (promotes platelet aggregation, energy source) and **thromboxane A2** to be released.

3. Platelets begin to aggregate, which causes the release of additional ADP, ATP, and **serotonin** (substance that promotes vaso-constriction).

B. Secondary Hemostasis

1. Results in the formation of a fibrin clot in association with the intrinsic and extrinsic coagulation pathways.

2. **Fibrin clot** includes fibrin formed in secondary hemostasis and the platelet plug formed in primary hemostasis.

3. **Intrinsic pathway** is activated when specific coagulation proteins come in contact with subendothelial tissue.

4. **Extrinsic pathway** starts with the release of tissue factor from injured blood vessel endothelial cells and subendothelium. Tissue factor is found in most organs and large blood vessels.

5. **Common pathway** begins with **factor X** activation by either the intrinsic or extrinsic pathway.

6. **Alternative pathways** link the extrinsic, intrinsic, and common pathways.

C. Coagulation Proteins (Coagulation Factors)

1. Coagulation factors are also known as **enzyme precursors** or **zymogens,** which are found in the plasma, along with nonenzymatic cofactors and calcium.

2. **Zymogens** are substrates having no biologic activity until converted by enzymes to active enzymes, which are then called **serine proteases.**
   a. These factors include **II, VII, IX, X, XI, XII,** and **prekallikrein.**

3. **Cofactors** assist in the activation of zymogens and include **V, VIII, tissue factor,** and **high molecular weight kininogen (HMWK).**

D. The Coagulation Groups

1. **Contact group**
   a. Includes **prekallikrein, HMWK, XI,** and **XII.**
   b. Not vitamin K dependent.
   c. Present in BaSO₄ absorbed plasma.
   d. Produced in the liver.
   e. Functions of the contact group:
      1) XII and HMWK activate XI and convert prekallikrein to kallikrein.
      2) Kallikrein and HMWK play roles in intrinsic coagulation activation, activation of fibrinoysis, kinin formation, and activation of the complement system.

2. **Prothrombin group**
   a. Includes **II, VII, IX,** and **X.**
   b. Vitamin K dependent.
   c. Not present in BaSO₄ absorbed plasma.
   d. Produced in the liver.

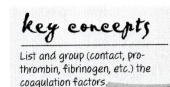

key concepts

List and group (contact, prothrombin, fibrinogen, etc.) the coagulation factors.

e. Functions of the prothrombin group:
1) Vitamin K reactions are inhibited by vitamin K deficiencies and antibiotics that kill intestinal bacterial flora where vitamin K is synthesized.
2) Oral anticoagulant therapy (warfarin) inhibits the activity of the prothrombin group.

3. **Fibrinogen group**
a. Includes **I, V, VIII,** and **XIII.**
b. Serve as substrates for the fibrinolytic enzyme plasmin.
c. All fibrinogen group factors are found in platelets except for VIII
d. Not vitamin K dependent.
e. Found in $BaSO_4$ absorbed plasma.
f. Functions of the fibrinogen group:
1) Factor VIII is composed of two fractions.
a) **VIII:C** (antihemophilic factor) is the coagulation portion that acts as a cofactor in the intrinsic coagulation pathway.
b) **VIII:vWF** (von Willebrand's portion) is important in normal platelet function.
2) Other factor VIII components:
a) **vW AgII** (von Willebrand antigen II) is released by endothelial cells and platelets.
b) **vWF B:Co** is detected by botrocetin (snake venom) by causing vWF to bind to platelets.
c) **vWF** is the carrier protein for VIII:C, also the component that binds to endothelium.

E. Complement System and Coagulation

1. The complement system is activated during coagulation and fibrinolysis.
2. Contains more than 30 circulating blood proteins, primarily to mediate inflammatory response, and immune and allergic reactions.
3. Complement functions in lysing antibody-coated cells.
4. **Plasmin** (in association with antibody-antigen complexes) activates **C1** and causes cleavage of C3 to C3a and C3b. **C3a** increases vascular permeability, and **C3b** causes immune adherence of erythrocytes to neutrophils, which enhances phagocytosis.
5. Complement activation is regulated by **C1 inactivator,** which also inhibits several coagulation factors.

F. Kinin System in Coagulation

1. The **kinin system** contains four plasma proteins: Hageman factor, clotting factor, XI, prekallikrein (Fletcher factor), and HMWK (Fitzgerald factor).
2. Generates bradykinin, an active peptide, and kallikrein, a proteolytic enzyme.
3. Involved in chemotaxis and pain sensation.
4. Function: mediate inflammatory responses, vasodilatation, and activates intrinsic coagulation and complement.

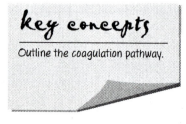

key concepts

Outline the coagulation pathway.

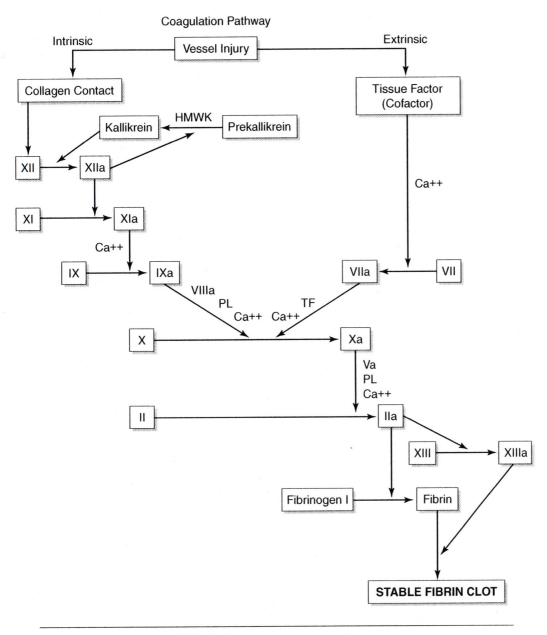

FIGURE 3-1. Coagulation pathway

IV. THE FIBRINOGEN SYSTEM

A. Thrombin Feedback

1. Thrombin activates coagulation (low thrombin levels); activates factors **V, VIII,** and **XIII;** and induces platelet aggregation.
2. Thrombin inhibits coagulation (high thrombin levels) by inhibiting the activation of factors V and VIII.
3. Starts fibrinolysis by converting plasminogen to plasmin, and activates **protein C** (potent anticoagulant).

B. Fibrin Clot Formation and Stabilization

1. Thrombin activity on fibrinogen starts the final phases of coagulation.

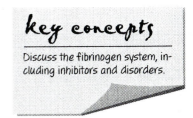

key concepts

Discuss the fibrinogen system, including inhibitors and disorders.

2. Conversion of fibrinogen to fibrin is a three-step process:
   a. Fibrinogen alpha and beta ends are cleaved by thrombin, which is then called a soluble fibrin monomer.
   b. Fibrin monomers aggregate together.
   c. Clot stabilization occurs requiring **XIII, calcium,** and **thrombin.**

C. Fibrinolytic System Function

1. Keeps blood vessels clear. Is important in clot dissolution. During this process, **plasminogen** is activated to **plasmin.**
2. **Plasminogen**
   a. A zymogen (inactive or inert form), found in the plasma.
   b. Converted to plasmin by plasminogen activators.
   c. A glycoprotein produced in the liver.
   d. Stored and transported by **eosinophils.**
3. **Plasmin**
   a. Not found in the blood in the active form.
   b. Degrades fibrin clots (fibrinolysis) and native fibrinogen (fibrinogenolysis).
   c. Promotes coagulation and activates the complement system.

D. Inhibitors of Fibrinolysis and Coagulation

1. **Antithrombin III** (AT-III)
   a. Produced in the liver.
   b. Inhibits thrombin, IX, X, XI, XII, kallikrein, and plasmin.
   c. **Heparin enhances** the action of antithrombin III.
2. **Alpha 2-macroglobulin**
   a. Inhibits the development and function of plasmins.
   b. Not enhanced by heparin.
3. **Alpha 1-antitrypsin**
   a. Inhibits factor XI, and inactivates plasmin.
   b. Heparin has no effect.
4. **C1 Inactivator**
   a. Inhibits XI, XII, and plasmin.
   b. Heparin has no effect.
5. **Alpha 2-antiplasmin**
   a. **Principle inhibitor** of fibrinolysis.
   b. Neutralizes plasmin.
   c. Heparin has no effect.

E. Thrombosis Disorders

1. **Primary thrombosis disorders**
   a. **Antithrombin III deficiency**
      1) Occurs about 1:2,000 in the general population.
      2) Can cause lower extremity thrombophlebitis and pulmonary embolism.
      3) Laboratory: quantitative AT-III levels.
      4) Treatment is **heparin** for the acute stage and **warfarin** (Coumadin) for long-term management.
   b. **Protein C deficiency**
      1) Vitamin K dependent.
      2) Inactivates factors **V** and **VIII.**

3) More common at an early age.

4) Can cause superficial and deep vein thrombophlebitis with frequent pulmonary emboli.

  c. **Protein S deficiency**

    1) Cofactor that promotes the inactivation of **factor V** by **protein C.**

    2) Characterized by frequent venous thromboses.

    3) Laboratory: protein S assay.

    4) Treatment is warfarin/Coumadin.

2. **Secondary thrombosis disorders**

  a. **Lupus anticoagulant**

    1) The body develops autoantibodies against platelet phospholipids, increasing the risk of thrombosis.

  b. **Postoperative status**

    1) Thrombotic event starts after blood is exposed to activating tissue substances exposed during surgery.

  c. **Malignancy:** risk of malignancy increases due to release of coagulation factors by neoplastic cells.

  d. **Pregnancy:** the placenta is rich in tissue thromboplastin, which may enhance thrombosis during pregnancy, especially high-risk patients having caesarian section surgery.

  e. **Estrogen/oral contraceptives:** increases risk of venous thrombosis and renal artery thrombosis.

  f. **Morbid obesity:** results in decreased AT-III levels and thrombosis.

F. Disorders of Coagulation and Fibrinolysis

1. **Inherited** disorders generally affect only one hemostatic component.

2. **Acquired** disorders involve multiple hemostatic components or pathways.

G. Inherited Intrinsic Pathway Disorders

1. **Factor XII (Hageman factor) deficiency**

  a. Autosomal recessive trait.

  b. Clinical: excessive clotting, no bleeding.

  c. Laboratory: **prolonged aPTT;** factor XII assay confirms.

2. **Prekallikrein (Fletcher factor) deficiency**

  a. Autosomal recessive trait.

  b. Clinical: possible excessive clotting and no clinical bleeding.

  c. Laboratory: **normal aPTT,** decreased aPTT in patient plasma incubated with **kadin.**

    1) Kadin is a low molecular weight substance made up of amino acids.

3. **HMWK (Fitzgerald factor) deficiency**

  a. Autosomal recessive trait.

  b. Characterized by **poor contact-phase reactions,** resulting in defective fibrinolysis.

  c. Laboratory: **aPTT** is slightly prolonged.

4. **Factor XI (hemophilia C) deficiency**

  a. Mainly seen in the Jewish population.

key concepts

Describe disorders of coagulation and fibrinolysis as related to clinical and laboratory analysis.

   b. Characterized by clinical bleeding that is asymptomatic until surgery or trauma.

   c. Laboratory: **prolonged aPTT, normal bleeding time,** and is confirmed by XI analysis.

  5. **Factor X activation phase disorders**

   a. Caused by **decreased VIII: C** and **IX** levels.

   b. Causes a serious bleeding disorder.

  6. **Factor VIII: C deficiency (hemophilia A or classic hemophilia)**

   a. Predominant congenital bleeding disorder in the United States.

   b. Sex-linked disorder transmitted on the **X chromosome** by carrier women to their sons.

   c. Many new cases of hemophilia A result from spontaneous mutations.

   d. Clinical: severity of bleeding is related to the percent of VIII:C deficiency. Bleeding occurs often and is especially bad in joint regions.

   e. Laboratory: **prolonged aPTT,** confirm diagnosis by VIII:C assay.

   f. Treatment: replacement of factor VIII:C, or in mild cases medication can be used to stimulate the release of VIII:C from stored reserves.

   g. A small percentage of hemophiliacs develop antibody to VIII:C; associated with a poor prognosis.

  7. **Factor IX (hemophilia B, Christmas disease) deficiency**

   a. Sex-linked recessive trait.

   b. Less severe form of hemophilia.

   c. Clinicals: generally not prone to bleeding.

   d. Types of the disease are based on their antigenic reactivity of Factor IX, and include **CRM+, CRM−,** and **CRM-R.** The three variants are termed cross-reactive material +, −, or R.

    1) CRM+: the antigen reacts with specific antibody.

    2) CRM−: antigen is not detected.

    3) CRM-R: antigen reactivity detected in decreased form.

   e. Laboratory: **prolonged aPTT,** definitive diagnosis—XI assay.

  8. **von Willebrand's disease**

   a. Autosomal dominant trait.

   b. Most frequently inherited coagulopathy.

   c. Caused by a deficiency or defect in VIII:C and VIII vWF.

   d. Clinical: severe bleeding in children that decreases in severity with age.

   e. Laboratory: **prolonged aPTT** and **bleeding times;** decreased VIII:C activity.

H. Inherited Extrinsic and Common Pathway Disorders

  1. **VII deficiency**

   a. Autosomal recessive trait.

   b. Contains the **CRM+** and **CRM-R** variants.

   c. Clinical: soft tissue bleeding.

   d. Laboratory: **prolonged PT.**

2. **X (Stuart-Prower) deficiency**
   a. Autosomal recessive trait.
   b. Clinical: soft-tissue bleeding and chronic bruising.
   c. Laboratory: **prolonged PT** and **aPTT.**
3. **V deficiency (Owren's disease, labile factor deficiency)**
   a. Autosomal recessive trait.
   b. Patients with the acquired form of V deficiency will develop autoantibodies of IgG and IgM to factor V.
   c. Clinical: mild to moderate hemophilia.
   d. Laboratory: **prolonged PT** and **aPTT.**
4. **II (prothrombin) deficiency**
   a. Autosomal recessive trait.
   b. Clinical: mild hemophilia.
   c. Laboratory: **prolonged PT and aPTT** rule out vitamin K deficiency and liver disease.
5. **I (fibrinogen) deficiency**
   a. Results from the following inherited disorders:
      1) **Afibrinogenemia:** inherited lack of fibrinogen
      2) **Hypofibrinogenemia:** inherited deficiency of fibrinogen
      3) **Dysfibrinogenemia:** inherited production of abnormal fibrinogen
   b. Clinical: spontaneous bleeding of mucosa, intestines, and intracranial sites.
   c. Laboratory: **increased reptilase;** however, the **PT** and **aPTT** may be **decreased** or **prolonged.**
6. **XIII (fibrin-stabilizing factor) deficiency**
   a. Autosomal recessive trait.
   b. Clinical: spontaneous bleeding, poor wound healing, and unusual scar formation.
   c. **Is incompatible with pregnancy.**
   d. Laboratory: XIII and immunological studies.

I. Acquired Disorders of Coagulation and Fibrinolysis

1. **Hepatic disease**
   a. The liver is the major site of factor synthesis.
   b. Problems can result from a decreased synthesis of coagulation factors or the impaired clearance of activated hemostatic components.
   c. Laboratory: **prolonged PT, aPTT, bleeding times,** and **increased platelet counts.**
2. **Vitamin K deficiency**
   a. Vitamin K is produced by normal intestinal flora.
   b. Deficiencies in vitamin K can result from oral antibiotics, vitamin K antagonists (coumarin), or decreased absorption resulting from obstructive jaundice.
   c. Breast-fed babies are more prone to vitamin K deficiency because breast milk is sterile, which allows no bacterial intestinal colonization to occur.
   d. Laboratory: **prolonged PT.**

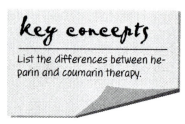

V. INTRINSIC AND EXTRINSIC PATHWAY TESTING

A. Activated Clotting Time (ACT)

1. **Whole** blood is placed in a glass tube, activator is added. Determine time it takes the clot to form, keep blood at 37°C.
2. Reference range: 75–120 seconds
3. Prolonged **ACT** results indicate intrinsic or common pathway factor defects or the presence of heparin.

B. Activated Partial Thromboplastin Time (aPTT)

1. Common test of the **intrinsic/common** pathways and for **heparin monitoring.**
2. Reagents include:
   a. **Platelet substitute** (brain or plant phospholipids)
   b. **Activator** (kaolin, celite, silica, or ellagic acid)
   c. **Calcium choride**
3. Principle: add reagents to citrated patient plasma sample. Calculate the time required for clot formation.
4. Include high and low controls (essential for quality control).
5. Reference range: 20–45 seconds (round result to the nearest tenth).
6. **Prolonged aPTT** can indicate the following:
   a. Factor deficiency (intrinsic pathway)
   b. Acquired circulating anticoagulant, lupus inhibitor, or antibody to a specific factor
   c. Heparin therapy
7. **Sources of error**
   a. Improper sample collection and preparation: short sample, hemolysis (< aPTT), plasma containing platelets (< aPTT), or heparin contamination.
   b. Incorrect reagent preparation: incorrect dilution, water impurities, or improper storage.
   c. Instrumentation: problems with temperature or light source.

C. Prothrombin Time (PT)

1. Screening test for factors **I, II, V, VII, X (extrinsic pathway).**
2. Monitors anticoagulation therapy by vitamin K antagonists (warfarin, coumarin).
3. Reagents: **thromboplastin.**
4. Reference range: 10–14 seconds.
5. **INR:** international normalized ratio:
   a. Standardized PT value not dependent on type of thromboplastin used.
   b. INR values are only used to monitor coumarin therapy.
   c. Formula

$$INR = \frac{\text{Patient PT (ISI)}}{\text{Normal PT}}$$

   d. ISI is the International Sensitivity Index for thromboplastin; this number may vary as to the manufacturer.
6. **Prolonged PT:** extrinsic/common factor abnormalities or factor inhibitors.

7. **Sources of error**
   a. Improper sample collection and preparation: short sample, hemolysis (< aPTT), plasma containing platelets (< aPTT), or heparin contamination.
   b. Incorrect reagent preparation: incorrect dilution, water impurities, or improper storage.
   c. Instrumentation: problems with temperature or light source.

D. **Factor V Leiden (Activated Protein C Resistance PCR Assay)**
   1. Specific test for activated protein C (APC) resistance due to single point mutation in the gene for factor V.
   2. DNA-based analysis is recommended, using PCR technology.

VI. EVALUATION TESTS FOR FIBRINOLYSIS

A. **Fibrinogen Modified Thrombin Clotting Time**
   1. Also known as fibrinogen assay (functional assay).
   2. Concentrated thrombin is added to diluted platelet-poor plasma (PPP) to convert fibrinogen to fibrin.
   3. Clotting time is inversely proportional to the fibrinogen concentration.

B. **Latex Fibrin Degradation Products (FDP)** — Latex particles are coated with antibody against fibrinogen and are mixed with patient serum. Macroscopic agglutination indicates degradation products. Highly specific to measure degradation of fibrin and fibrinogen.

C. **Latex D-Dimer Assay** — measures fibrinolysis or the presence of D-dimers. Highly specific degradation measurement of fibrin, *not* fibrinogen.

VII. COAGULOPATHY CAUSED BY FACTOR DEFICIENCIES OR INHIBITOR PROBLEMS

A. **Factor deficiencies** — may be **inherited,** i.e., hemophilia A, or **acquired** as shown by development of inhibitors, i.e., to factor VIII (specific), or **lupuslike anticoagulant (nonspecific).**

B. **Laboratory Analysis**
   1. Factor assays: identify deficiency of a specific factor.
   2. Mixing studies: mixing patient plasma with normal plasma for **PT** and **aPTT** testing.
      a. Factor deficiencies will be corrected (from prolonged) to normal times.
      b. Inhibitors will *not* be corrected; times will remain prolonged.

VIII. SAMPLE COLLECTION, HANDLING, AND PROCESSING FOR COAGULATION TESTING

A. **Nontraumatic venipuncture is *essential*** — Trauma may introduce tissue thromboplastin that would activate coagulation.

B. **Use plastic or silicone-coated glass tubes** — Plain glass tubes will activate the alternative pathway, including the activation of prekallikrein, XI, and XII.

C. **Ratio of blood to anticoagulant in collection tubes is critical** — inadequate amount of blood renders specimen unacceptable.

D. **Specimens must be processed as soon as possible** — within 2 hours. Centrifuge and remove plasma or freeze plasma at $-20°C$.

E. **Testing must be performed at 37°C** — Labile factors V and VIII will break down at room temperature. Factors VII and XI will be activated at cold temperatures.

IX. COAGULATION THERAPY

A. **Heparin therapy**

1. Treatment of choice for venous thrombosis, pulmonary emboli, thrombophlebitis, and arterial thrombosis.
2. Inhibits factors XII, XI, X, IX, II.
3. Inhibits the conversion of fibrinogen to fibrin.
4. Inhibits platelet aggregation.
5. Inhibits the activation of fibrin-stabilizing enzymes.
6. Requires AT-III to be present for heparin to work.

B. **Heparin activity can be immediately reversed by protamine sulfate.**

C. **Drugs that inhibit heparin activity** — antihistamines, digitalis, nicotine, penicillin, and tetracycline.

D. **Laboratory monitoring** — aPTT therapeutic range is 1.0–1.5 times the normal aPTT control range.

E. **Coumadin (Warfarin) therapy**

1. Oral anticoagulant prescribed for venous thrombosis.
2. Mode of action is the inference with vitamin K metabolism
3. Inhibits factors II, VII, IX, X.
4. Administered after heparin therapeutic level achieved, usually for several months.
5. **PT** is used to monitor the effects of coumarin.

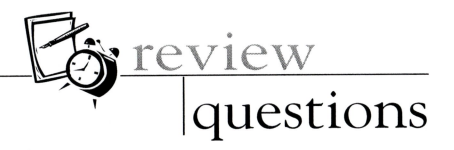

review questions

DIRECTIONS Each of the questions or incomplete statements below is followed by suggested answers or completions. Select the **one answer** that is best in each case.

1. The common pathway begins with the activation of factor:
   a. II.
   b. III.
   c. X.
   d. XI.

2. In primary hemostasis, which substance promotes vasoconstriction?
   a. Serotonin
   b. Fibrin split products
   c. ADP
   d. ATP

3. Which of the following is the best test to monitor heparin therapy?
   a. PT
   b. ACT
   c. Reptilase
   d. aPTT

4. Which *two* of the following can result from excessive aspirin ingestion?
   a. Deficient aggregation
   b. Inhibition of thromboxane A2
   c. Inhibition of glycoprotein IIa
   d. Decreased platelet adhesion
   e. Increased platelet adhesion
   f. Increased platelet count

5. Secondary thrombosis disorders can be caused by which of the following?
   a. Iron deficiency
   b. Protein C deficiency

   c. Oral contraceptives
   d. Splenectomy

6. Jean Doe is being worked up by a coagulation specialist for diagnosis. The following information is obtained from Jean's medical chart: 21-year-old Jewish female. Lab tests show a PTT of 71 seconds and a bleeding time of 5 minutes. Jean presents with morbid obesity and is currently on estrogen therapy for mood swings. From the list, choose TWO possible conditions that are causing Jean's problems.
   a. Hemophilia A
   b. Hemophilia C
   c. Hageman Factor deficiency
   d. HMWK deficiency
   e. Secondary thrombosis
   f. Protein S deficiency
   g. Primary thrombosis
   h. Protein C deficiency

7. PT is the only coagulation test that is increased in which of the following disorders of the extrinsic pathway?
   a. Factor X deficiency
   b. Factor VII deficiency
   c. Factor V deficiency
   d. Factor I deficiency

8. An extrinsic disorder, the acquired form develops from IgG or IgM autoantibodies:
   a. Factor IX deficiency
   b. Factor XI deficiency

c. Factor V deficiency
d. Factor X activation phase disorder

9. Platelet dense granules release:
   a. ADP.
   b. FGN.
   c. PDGF.
   d. PF3.

10. John Doe is being treated for a gastrointestinal infection with antibiotics that act against gram-negative bacilli (enterics). The resulting vitamin deficiency would be:
    a. Vitamin C.
    b. Vitamin A.
    c. Vitamin D.
    d. Vitamin K.

4

Clinical Chemistry

contents

➤ COMPREHENSIVE KEY CONCEPTS

1. Analyze the diseases of the body that alter the values of specific chemicals in the body.
2. Analyze instrument function to facilitate instrument selection and troubleshooting.

---

key concepts

List the different types of glassware, parts of a centrifuge, calculation of solution concentrations, preanalytic variation, sample storage, and transportation.

I. GENERAL LABORATORY PRINCIPLES
A. Chemicals and Related Substances
1. **Reagent grade chemicals** are used in analytical work. **Reagent grade** is an unofficial classification of chemicals.
2. **National Bureau of Standards** (NBS) sells standard reference materials.
3. **Reagent grade water** consists of three types: I, II, III.
   a. **Type I** is the highest quality. Used in test methodologies where minimum interference and maximum precision and accuracy are needed. Must be used quickly after production. Type I water resistance is less than 10Ω.
   b. **Type II** is used for general laboratory use. Storage time should be short because chemical and bacterial contamination can occur while stored.

    c. **Type III** is used for initial rinsing of laboratory glassware.

    d. **Preparing reagent grade water:** filters are used to purify water.

       1) **Prefilters** are glass or cotton microfibers that remove 98 percent of the particulate matter.

       2) **Activated carbon** removes organic matter and chlorine.

       3) **A submicron** removes all particles or microorganisms larger than the membrane pore size.

       4) **Reverse osmosis** is a process that removes 95–99 percent of bacteria and organic and other particulate matter.

4. **Primary standards** are ultra pure chemicals that are weighed or measured to produce a solution with an exact concentration.

5. **Secondary standards** are solutions whose value is determined by repeated analyses, using a reference method.

6. **Standard reference materials** are produced by the NBS. Exact chemical or physical properties are known.

7. **Dessicant** drying agent: chemical that absorbs water.

8. **Laboratory supplies**

    a. **Types of glass**

       1) **Disposable glass** is made of borosilicate.

       2) **Pyrex** and **Kimax** are glasses that can withstand high temperatures. Made of borosilicate with a low alkali content.

       3) **Corex:** extra hard glassware used to make high temperature thermometers.

       4) **Vycor** glass can be heated to 900°C and is used for extremely high temperatures.

    b. **Types of plasticware**

       1) **Polyolefins** (polyethylene): chemically inert resins.

       2) **Fluorocarbin resins** (Teflon): chemically inert and used for temperatures from −270° C to 255°C.

    c. **Pipettes and calibration**

       1) **Pipettes:** common types are transfer and measuring

          a) Transfer pipettes are **volumetric** and **Ostwald-Folin**

            (i) **Volumetric pipettes** accurately deliver a fixed volume of aqueous solution. They drain by gravity.

            (ii) **Ostwald-Folin pipettes** have the bulb closer to the delivery tip because they deliver viscous fluids. These pipettes contain an accurate volume and are to be "blown out."

          b) Measuring pipettes are **serologic** and **Mohr.**

            (i) **Serologic pipettes** are calibrated to the tip and can be "blown out."

            (ii) **Mohr pipettes** are calibrated between marks and cannot be "blown out." They are "to deliver."

          c) Automatic pipettes are **handheld** and **automated.**

            (i) **Handheld pipettes** use disposable tips, and the technician performs aspiration and dispensing.

            (ii) **Automated pipettes** are electronic, and usually do not require tips. Many use a glass syringe that aspirates and dispenses through the same tube.

2) **Verification of pipette calibration**
   a) **Gravimetric pipette calibration:** This method verifies the amount of liquid dispensed by a pipette. All equipment and water must be at room temperature before beginning. A specific amount of water is pipetted into a container and the water is weighed. The weight of the water is proportional to the volume of water pipetted. The volume of water pipetted is noted on the pipette.
   b) **Volumetric pipette calibration:** Uses a dye of known concentration and water. A specific amount of dye is pipetted into a specific volume of water. Depending on the volume of the pipette, the absorbance of the solution will read a predetermined number. The pipette can then be adjusted, and the calibration repeated.

d. **Centrifuges**
   1) **Centrifuges** accelerate gravitational separation of substances differing in their masses. They are used to separate blood cells from serum or plasma, separate particulate matter in urine, and separate two liquid phases of different densities.
   2) Types of centrifuges
      a) **Horizontal centrifuges or swinging buckets** allow the tubes to attain a horizontal position in the centrifuge when spinning and a vertical position when the head is not moving.
      b) **Fixed angle or angle-head** have angled compartments for the tubes and allow small particles to sediment more rapidly.
      c) **Ultracentrifuges** are high-speed centrifuges used to separate layers of different specific gravities. Commonly used to separate lipoproteins. Separation may require many hours or days, so the chamber must be refrigerated.

e. **Balances and weighing**
   1) **Mass** is a physical property of matter. A balance compares the mass of an unknown against a known mass. Balances work on three principles
      a) **Direct comparison:** weights are added to one side of the beam to counterbalance the weight of the object.
      b) **Substitution:** weights are removed to restore equilibrium
      c) **Electromagnetic force** uses an electromagnetic force to balance the weight of the object.
   2) Types of balances
      a) **Double pan:** a single beam with arms of equal length. Standard weights are added manually to the right side to counterbalance the weight of the object.
      b) **Single pan:** arms are unequal in length. The object is placed on a pan attached to the shorter arm. A restoring force is applied mechanically to the other arm until the indicator is balanced.
      c) **Electronic single pan:** the electromagnetic force replaces the weights as the counterbalance.

B. Solute and Solvent

1. **Solute:** substance dissolved in a solution
2. **Solvent:** substance in which the solute is dissolved
3. **Solution:** homogenous mixture of solutes and solvent
4. **Saturated solution:** dissolves as much of a solute as possible at a given temperature.
5. **Miscible:** two liquids dissolve in one another.
6. **Immiscible:** two liquids that cannot be mixed, e.g. oil and water.
7. **Solution Concentrations**
   a. **Molarity:** one mole of solute is dissolved in 1 liter of solution.
      M = moles/liter of solution
   b. **Normality:** one gram equivalent weight of solute is dissolved in 1 liter of solution
      N = gram equivalent weight/liter of solution
      1 gram equivalent = 1 mole/valence
   c. **Molality:** one mole of solute is dissolved in 1 kg of solvent.
      m = moles/kg of solvent
   d. **Percent solutions:** 100 mg of solute is dissolved in 1 dL of solution
      % = 100 mg solute/1 deciliter of solution

C. Sources and Control of Preanalytical Error

1. **Preanalytical variation** includes
   a. **Cyclic variation:** changes in analyte concentration occur at different times during the day, week, or month.
   b. **Diurnal variation:** variation according to sleeping and waking times.
   c. **Circadian variation:** occurs during a 24-hour period.
   d. **Circannual variation:** occurs twice a year (elevated in the summer, decreased in the winter).
   e. **Physical variables**
      1) **Exercise:** potassium, phosphate, creatinine, and protein values are altered.
      2) **Eating:** increased glucose and other analytes.
      3) **Stress** can reversibly alter cortisol (increased), total cholesterol (increased), and even decreased hormone production.
   f. **Blood collection technique errors** in **preservatives** and/or **anticoagulants** or **specimen type** or **drawing technique**.
      1) **Short draws** in coagulation tubes.
      2) **Proper anticoagulants** must be used; plain red tops or serum separator tubes must be used for the appropriate tests.
      3) **Improper drawing techniques can lead to increased electrolytes, proteins, and metabolic by-products,** as well as hemolysis of red blood cells.
      4) **Hemolysis** causes increased lactate dehydrogenase (LD), potassium, and magnesium as well as decreased sodium.
      5) **Drawing from a vein receiving IV fluid** dilutes all blood analytes, but increases the value of analytes in the fluid, e.g., sodium and chloride
   g. **Patient identification, sample identification,** and **chain of custody** are also concerns in specimen collection.

h. **Sample transportation** is important for **blood gas** and **coagulation** analyses. These specimens are usually placed on ice for transport to the lab.

i. **Sample processing** involves **logging the specimen into a computer or log** and **assigning the sample a number, sorting** and sending specimens to various departments for testing, **centrifuging** to separate serum from red blood cells, and **removing serum** from red blood cells (if not in a serum separator tube).

j. **Sample storage**

1) **EDTA tubes** can be stored at 2–8°C for 24 hours.

2) **Coagulation tubes** can be stored at 2–8°C for 8 hours.

3) **Serum** can be stored at 2–8°C for 2–3 days or indefinitely at −20°C.

II. LABORATORY SAFETY

A. Personal Safety

1. **Use fume hoods** whenever possible when dispensing or pipetting dangerous chemicals.

2. **Safety goggles/glasses with side shields should be worn** at all times in the laboratory.

3. **Fluid-resistant laboratory coats (buttoned up) will be worn at all times in the laboratory** and removed when leaving the laboratory.

4. **Gloves will be worn when contact with blood and body fluids is expected** in the laboratory and removed when leaving the laboratory.

5. **Wash hands before leaving the laboratory** and after taking off gloves.

6. **DO NOT MOUTH PIPET!**

7. **Avoid** having long hair, loose sleeves/cuffs, rings, bracelets, etc., dangling in front of your eyes or outside of your lab coat.

8. **Do not apply cosmetics** in the laboratory.

9. **EATING AND DRINKING IS FORBIDDEN IN THE LABORATORY!**

B. Fire Prevention

1. **Be aware of ignition sources** in your laboratory area (heat sources, electrical equipment).

2. **Do not store flammable liquids in standard refrigerators.** Explosion-proof refrigerators are needed for storage of flammable liquids.

3. **Store flammable liquids** in appropriate safety cabinets/safety cans.

4. **Make sure** that all electrical cords are in good condition. All electrical outlets should be grounded and should accommodate a 3-pronged plug.

C. Housekeeping

1. **Eliminate safety hazards** by maintaining laboratory work areas in a good state of order.

2. **Keep the laboratory floor dry** at all times. Immediately attend to spills of chemicals/water.

D. Emergency Procedures

1. **In event of an emergency, dial your emergency number.** By calling this number, a variety of emergency response departments can then be alerted to your situation.

key concepts

Discuss the importance of safety.

2. **Look at** the names and phone numbers of personnel to be contacted in an emergency and contact the appropriate personnel.
3. **Be familiar** with the location and use of the following safety devices:
   a. Safety shower
   b. Fire blanket
   c. Eyewash station
   d. Fire alarm
   e. First aid kit
   f. Fume hood
   g. Spill cleanup kit
   h. Fire extinguisher
4. **Clean up** all small spills immediately.

E. Waste Collection

1. **Dispose of all biohazardous substances in BIOHAZARD bags.**
2. **Dispose of** swab wrappings, band aid wrappings, used paper towels, kit boxes, and any other nonbiohazardous waste in regular trash bags.
3. **Dispose of all used needles, pipettes, broken glass,** and **slides** in PLASTIC BIOHAZARDOUS SHARPS containers.
4. **Dispose of all used tubes** in RED BIOHAZARD bags.
5. **Dispose of all bacterial and fungal culture plates** in RED BIO-HAZARD bags.
6. **DO NOT** throw nonbiohazardous waste into red biohazard bags.

F. Personal Protective Equipment

1. **Eye protection:** goggles
2. **Protective clothing**
   a. The lab coat is designed to protect the clothing and skin from chemicals that may be spilled or splashed. It should be worn buttoned up and with the sleeves extended to the wearer's wrist.
3. **Hand protection**
4. **Foot protection**
   a. **Foot protection is designed to prevent injury from corrosive chemicals or heavy objects.** If a corrosive chemical or heavy object were to fall on the floor, the most vulnerable portion of the body would be the feet. For this reason, shoes **that COMPLETELY COVER AND PROTECT** the foot are worn in the laboratory.

G. Laboratory Safety Equipment

1. **Laboratory chemical fume hoods**
   a. **Chemical fume hoods capture, contain, and expel emissions generated by hazardous chemicals.**
2. **Chemical storage cabinets**
   a. Storage of flammables and corrosives in the lab should be limited to as small a quantity as possible. They should be stored in ventilated cabinets that meet OSHA 1910.106d and NFPA 30 specifications.

key concepts

List how to wear personal protective equipment, use safety devices, recognize biohazardous waste, use first aid procedures, identify properties of hazardous materials.

3. **Individual storage containers**
   a. Selecting the best means of storage for chemical reagents will, to a great extent, depend on that reagent's compatibility with the container. A safety can is an approved container of no more than 5-gallon capacity. It has a spring-closing lid and spout cover, and is designed to safely relieve pressure buildup within the container.

4. **Refrigerators**
   a. Domestic refrigeration units are **not appropriate for storing flammable materials. Laboratory refrigerators are not appropriate for storing food for consumption**. Separate, labeled refrigerators are used for storing food.
      1) Use and maintenance
         a) Each refrigerator and freezer must be monitored daily to ensure proper functioning.
         b) Each refrigerator and freezer must be labeled: "No Food or Beverages may be stored in this refrigerator."
         c) Containers placed in the refrigerator will be completely sealed or capped, securely placed, and permanently labeled. Use caps or parafilm to cover containers.

5. **Safety showers**
   a. Safety showers provide an effective means of treatment in the event that chemicals are spilled or splashed onto the skin or clothing.

6. Fire safety equipment
   a. **Alarms** are designed so that endangered personnel are alerted. All individuals should become familiar with the EXACT LOCATION of the fire alarm stations nearest to their laboratory.
   b. **Extinguishers**
      1) Extinguishers are classified according to a particular fire type and are given the same letter and symbol classification as that of the fire.
         a) **Type A**—combustibles: wood, cloth, paper, rubber, and plastics
         b) **Type B**—flammable liquids: oil, grease, and paint thinners
         c) **Type C**—energized electrical equipment: electrophoresis
         d) **Type D**—combustible metals: magnesium, titanium, sodium, lithium, potassium
      2) **Multipurpose extinguishers** are highly recommended because they are an effective agent against Type A, B, and C fires.
      3) **How to use an extinguisher:** Remember the "PASS" word.
         a) **Pull the pin:** place your hand on the top of the cylinder and pull the pin. This will unlock the handle and allow you to activate the unit.
         b) **Aim:** point the nozzle of the hose at the base of the fire.
         c) **Squeeze** the handle (lever) releasing the fire fighting agent.

d) **Sweep** the nozzle from side to side over the fire. Keep the nozzle/hose directed at the base of the flame. Empty the fire extinguisher onto the fire.

7. **Fire blankets**
   a. Laboratory personnel are *discouraged* from using fire safety blankets as a means to extinguish a fire.
   b. Fire safety blankets should be used as a means to keep shock victims warm.

8. **Chemical spill clean-up kits**
   a. Laboratories are equipped with clean-up kits for various types of spills. Wear the appropriate personal protective equipment (i.e., gloves, goggles) when cleaning up spills.
      1) Acid spills
         a) Apply neutralizer (or sodium bicarbonate) to perimeter of spill.
         b) Mix thoroughly until fizzing and evolution of gas ceases.
         c) Transfer the mixture to a plastic bag, tie shut, fill out a waste label, and place in a fume hood.
      2) Solvent spills
         a) Apply activated charcoal to the perimeter of the spill.
         b) Mix thoroughly until material is dry and no evidence of solvent remains.
         c) Transfer absorbed solvent to a plastic bag, tie shut, and place in fume hood.

H. Properties of Hazardous Chemicals

1. **Flammability**
   a. Flammability is a measure of how easily a gas, liquid, or solid will ignite and how quickly the flame, once started, will spread.
   b. **Flammable liquids themselves are not flammable; rather, the vapor from the liquids are combustible.** There are two physical properties of a material that indicate its flammability: flash point and volatility (boiling point).
      1) **The flash point of a material** is the temperature at which a liquid (or volatile solid) gives off vapor in quantities significant enough to form an ignitable mixture with air.
      2) **The volatility of a material** is an indication of how easily the liquid or solid will pass into the vapor stage. Volatility is measured by the boiling point of the material—the temperature at which the vapor pressure of the material is equal to the atmospheric pressure.
   c. Some materials are **pyrophoric, meaning that they can ignite spontaneously with no external source of ignition.** Potassium metal, for example, can react with the moisture in air.
   d. **Labeling and information**
      1) **Flammability information** can be found in the **Material Safety Data Sheet (MSDS)** under **Fire and Explosion Data.** Flash point and boiling point information can be found in the section entitled Physical Properties.

     e. **Storage**

       1) **Flammable materials should never be stored near acids**.

       2) **Storage areas should be cool** enough to prevent ignition in the event that vapors mix with air. Adequate ventilation should be provided to prevent vapor buildup.

       3) **Avoid storage of flammable materials in conventional** (nonexplosion-proof) **refrigerators.** Sparks generated by internal lights or thermostats may ignite flammable material inside the refrigerator, causing an extremely dangerous explosion hazard.

     f. **Handling**

       1) Use gloves and safety goggles when handling flammable liquids or vapors.

       2) Dispensing of flammable or combustible liquids should only be carried out under a fume hood or in an approved storage room.

       3) DO NOT use water to clean up flammable liquid spills.

I. Bloodborne Pathogens

1. **Bloodborne pathogens such as HIV, HBV, and HCV** are transmitted through contact with infected blood and body fluids including:

   a. Semen

   b. Vaginal secretions

   c. Cerebrospinal fluid

   d. Synovial fluid

   e. Pleural fluid

   f. Peritoneal fluid

   g. Amniotic fluid

   h. Saliva (in dental procedures)

   i. Any body fluid visibly contaminated with blood

2. **Bloodborne diseases are most commonly transmitted by** sexual contact; sharing of hypodermic needles; puncture from contaminated needles, glass, or sharps; contact between broken or damaged skin and infected body fluids; and contact between mucous membranes and infected body fluids.

3. **Personal protective equipment (PPE)** includes latex gloves, fluid resistant laboratory coats (buttoned up), face shields, protective goggles, and respirators.

4. **Always wear PPE** in exposure situations.

5. **Replace PPE** when it becomes torn, punctured, or soiled.

6. **Remove PPE** before leaving the work area and wash your hands.

7. **Use standard precautions** and treat all blood or potentially infectious body fluids as if they are contaminated. Avoid contact whenever possible, and whenever it's not, wear personal protective equipment.

8. All surfaces, tools, equipment, and other objects that come in contact with blood or potentially infectious materials **must be decontaminated** and sterilized as soon as possible. Decontamination is recommended with 5.25 percent bleach solution (1:10 dilution of household bleach).

9. **Sharps:** all sharps, including needles and broken glass, will be disposed of in labeled plastic sharps containers. Needles may be recapped only by using a mechanical device and may not be broken, cut, or bent. Sharps containers must be closable, puncture-resistant, leak-proof on sides and bottom, and labeled biohazard.

III. LABORATORY QUALITY ASSESSMENT
A. Definitions

1. **Quality assurance:** a systemic laboratory program that monitors and corrects excessive variation in personnel competencies, test methodologies, instruments, specimens, quality control, and reagents. This process is used to ensure accurate patient test results.

2. **Accuracy:** the measure of a lab test result's closeness to the true value.

3. **Precision:** when consecutive laboratory results yield the same number; reproducibility.

4. **Quality control (QC):** a process used to monitor the accuracy and precision of laboratory test results.
   a. **Internal:** performed by the lab using control materials and comparing the control values periodically. These values are analyzed using Westgard rules to detect errors.
   b. **External:** unknown specimens sent to laboratories and compared against referred values using the same specimen for analysis.

5. **Random errors** occur spontaneously, unable to predict; no known pattern.

6. **Systemic errors** are caused by a malfunction, incorrect calibration, or another part of an instrument not functioning correctly.

7. **Preanalytical variation** occurs before a sample is run on an instrument. Variables include age, sex, ethnicity, exercise, etc.

8. **Analytical variation** occurs during the diagnostic testing process and includes reagents, instruments, controls, etc.

9. **Postanalytical variation** occurs after the test is performed and refers to clerical errors.

10. **Linearity check** determines the lowest and highest values that can be accurately measured by a particular procedure.

11. **Reference ranges** are determined by each laboratory to fit their particular population. Intervals are constructed by adding and subtracting 2 standard deviations from the mean.

12. **Standard:** sample of known concentration (should be traceable to National Bureau of Standards) that are used to calibrate instruments.

13. **Control:** synthetic material that is analyzed with patient samples to determine proper instrument function.
   a. **Assayed:** values assigned by manufacturer
   b. **Unassayed:** values determined by each individual laboratory

14. **Westgard rules:** statistical "rules" applied to graphical summaries of control data to determine if an instrument is functioning correctly.

key concepts

Compare and contrast internal and external quality control and when to use each to determine the accuracy and precision of laboratory test results.

B. Specimen Quality

1. Test result quality depends on the quality of the specimen submitted. **Garbage in = garbage out.**
2. Quality specimen depends on
   a. Patient preparation
   b. Type of specimen needed for the test
   c. Special timing for specimen
   d. Transportation requirements
   e. Labeling procedures
   f. Criteria for unacceptable specimens
   g. Specimen handling
   h. Special collection instructions

C. Operating Instructions

1. Procedures should contain the following information: test name, test principle, significance of procedure, patient preparation, test specimen requirements, instrumentation, equipment and materials, reagent preparation, test procedure, calculations, quality control procedures, reference intervals, panic values, limitations of the procedure, references, signature of all techs, and date and signature of reviewers.

D. Selecting Instruments

1. Selection criteria include cost, reagent cost, technical support, training, linearity, reagent storage, and test methodologies.
2. Instruments are evaluated to determine the instrument and method's **accuracy and precision, systemic error, turnaround-time, linearity, preventive maintenance time,** and **calibration stability.**

E. Reference Intervals

1. **Reference intervals are calculated for each laboratory's menu of tests.** Each laboratory serves a unique population so the reference intervals must be calculated.
2. Use a minimum of 20 test values drawn from **"healthy" people.**
3. Calculate the **mean** and **standard deviation.**
4. Construct **confidence intervals of the mean plus or minus 3 standard deviations** and eliminate any outliers.
5. **Reference ranges are** the mean plus 2 standard deviations (high value) and the mean minus 2 standard deviations (low value) to include 95 percent of the "healthy" population.

F. Internal Quality Control

1. **Purpose:** comprehensive program involving statistical analysis of control samples, which are analyzed with a batch of patient samples to determine acceptability of the run.
2. **Controls**
   a. Commercially manufactured solutions that imitate patient specimens and evaluate the test process.
   b. **Controls are handled exactly like patient specimens:** incubation time, analysis temperature, preanalysis conditions (precipitate, protein-free filtrate), etc.

    c. Controls are selected so that values will be at **medically signifi-cant levels.**

    d. **Long (at least 1-year) shelf life.**

    e. **Low vial-to-vial variability.**

    f. Minimum reconstitution requirements (liquid or frozen is best).

    g. Available in large enough quantities to meet the laboratory's need for one year.

    h. **Unassayed controls** are preferred, but assayed controls can also be used.

    i. **Qualitative controls** use a control material that will provide positive, negative, or trace, 1+, 2+, 3+, and 4+ results. If the desired test result is not obtained, the procedure needs to be investigated.

3. **Data evaluation procedures**

    a. **Levey Jennings (L-J) charts:** constructed using the mean and 3 standard deviations to construct a graph that will allow visual detection of shifts and trends (systematic error)

       1) **Shift:** 6 or more consecutive values that are suddenly at the high end or low end of the control value ranges. This can occur without losing precision.

       2) **Trend:** a gradual consecutive decrease or increase of 6 control values.

       3) **A loss of precision** is obvious on the chart when control values are more dispersed.

    b. **Westgard Rules**

       1) 1_{2s}—1 control value exceeds 2 standard deviations

       2) 1_{3s}—1 control value exceeds 3 standard deviations

       3) 2_{2s}—2 consecutive control values exceed the same 2s limit (same side of the mean)

       4) R_{4s}—2 consecutive control values exceed a 4 standard deviation spread

       5) 4_{1s}—4 consecutive values are recorded on one side of the mean

       6) 10_{x}—10 consecutive values are recorded on one side of the mean

4. **Absurd values:** values that are not consistent with life.

5. **Delta checks:** comparing current results with results from previous runs. If the difference is greater than expected, an analytical error may be the cause.

G. External Quality Control

1. **Definition:** a program where an agency contracts with a manufacturer to send prepared specimens to clinical laboratories to analyze. The same specimens are sent to a few "reference" laboratories. These reference laboratories analyze the specimens, then the agency determines the mean and standard deviation for the samples, and laboratories receive a result sheet showing where their test result falls in comparison to other laboratories that use the same reagents and instrument.

2. **Proficiency survey:** consists of the specially prepared specimens that are sent to clinical laboratories to analyze.

3. **Standard deviation index (SDI):** a measure of the difference between the test result submitted by the clinical laboratory and the mean test result of the reference laboratories.

4. **SDI = (value − group mean)/group standard deviation.**

5. **Youden plot:** a graph used to evaluate external quality control.
   a. This graph was developed to assess precision and accuracy using paired samples.

6. **Proficiency samples**
   a. Very different from patient samples. The samples must be shipped and must maintain their integrity. The samples are usually lyophilized, with special diluent shipped with the sample. Some samples may be frozen and others may arrive in liquid form. The constitution of the sample depends on the nature of the tests to be performed.

7. **Limitations of external quality control programs**
   a. Specimens treated differently than normal patient specimens—special handling, running controls before and after each survey specimen, calibrating the test before running the survey, etc.—will not reflect the accuracy and precision of the laboratory.
   b. Specimens do not reflect collection procedures, handling procedures, instrument maintenance, etc. There could be problems in these areas that this program will not be able to address.

8. **Clinical Laboratory Improvement Amendment (CLIA) regulations**
   a. To report outpatient results for a particular analyte, laboratories must pass their proficiency surveys for that analyte with 80 percent of the samples within 2 SDI. If a laboratory goes below 80 percent for that analyte for two proficiency surveys in a row, they will be unable to report outpatient results until satisfactory performance (within 2 SDI) is achieved with proficiency testing.
   b. Laboratories reporting patient results for an analyte must participate in quarterly proficiency surveys that have 5 specimens each to be tested.

IV. SPECTROPHOTOMETRY

A. Definitions

1. **Light:** electromagnetic radiation with wavelike and particlelike properties.

2. **Wavelength (λ):** distance traveled by 1 complete wave cycle measured in **nanometers (nm).**

3. **Frequency (ν):** number of cycles occurring per second.

4. Particles of light are called **photons.** The energy of a photon is $E = h\nu$, where h = Planck's constant, 6.62×10^{-27} erg/sec.

5. Light is classified according to its wavelength: **infrared light** has very long wavelengths; **ultraviolet light** has very short wavelengths. When all visible wavelengths of light are combined, white light results.

6. **Color:** wavelength of light reflected (not absorbed) by an object.

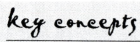

key concepts

List the parts of the spectrophotometer and how they work together to determine the concentration of an analyte in a sample.

7. When an atom absorbs a photon, the atom becomes excited in one of three ways:
   a. An electron is moved to a higher energy level,
   b. The mode of the covalent bond vibration is changed, or
   c. The rotation around its covalent bonds is changed.
8. **Near-infrared** and **visible light** produce changes in the **vibrational** energy of atoms.
9. **Visible, ultraviolet**, or **x-ray energy** is needed to boost an electron to a higher energy level.
10. **Absorption spectrum** is characteristic of a molecule and can help identify a molecule. It demonstrates all the energy transitions for the various wavelengths of light

B. Spectrophotometer

1. A spectrophotometer is used to measure the light transmitted by a solution in order to determine the concentration of the light-absorbing substance in the solution.
2. **Components of a Spectrophotometer**
   a. Power supply
   b. Light source
   c. Entrance slit
   d. Monochromator
   e. Exit slit
   f. Cuvet/sample cells
   g. Photodetector
   h. Readout Devices
   i. Recorders
3. **Power supply and exciter lamp** need electricity to operate the lamp and the spectrophotometer.
   a. Exciter lamp must produce an intense, constant beam of light and a reproducible beam of light
      1) Types of lamps
         a) **Tungsten:** most common, used invisible and near ultraviolet regions
         b) **Quartz lamp:** intense beam, used in the near ultraviolet region
         c) **Hydrogen lamp:** used in the ultraviolet region
         d) **Mercury lamp:** uneven emission spectrum, not widely used
         e) **Xenon lamp:** brilliant emission; too bright for routine work
         f) Hydrogen, mercury, and xenon are all vapor lamps
      2) **Important:** When a lamp is changed in the spectrophotometer, the instrument must be recalibrated because changing the bulb changes the angle of the light striking the monochromator. This angle change causes the color of light striking the cuvet to be different.
4. **Types of Monochromators**
   a. Glass filter–absorption filters
   b. Interference filters

    c. Prisms

    d. Diffraction gratings

5. **Band pass**

    a. The range of wavelengths passed through the monochromator and exit slit is called the **band pass**, that is, the range of wavelengths that a monochromator can isolate between two points of a spectral scan where the transmittance is one-half of the peak transmittance.

    b. Bandpass widths from widest to narrowest

      1) Prisms and diffraction gratings (< 5 nm)

      2) Interference filters (10–20 nm)

      3) Glass filters (> 50 nm)

6. **Glass filters**

    a. Simplest and least expensive: thin layers of colored glass, colored gelatin sandwiches between two glass plates.

    b. Certain metal complexes or slats are dissolved or suspended in glass that absorbs specific wavelengths, leaving the desired wavelength of light to be transmitted through the filter.

    c. Used for transmitting visible and near visible light.

7. **Interference filters**

    a. Interference filters are made of two glass pieces, each with a layer of silver on one side separated by a dielectric material (an insulating material that doesn't allow electric current to flow), usually magnesium fluoride.

    b. The thickness of the spacer determines the wavelength of energy transmitted. They are designed to be precisely half of the desired wavelength.

    c. Energies of wavelengths that are multiples of this thickness also stay in phase as they reflect back and forth between the silvered surfaces and finally pass through (constructive interference). Other wavelengths will cancel out because of phase difference (destructive interference).

    d. Only specific wavelengths or multiples—not for all wavelengths such as prisms. Spectrophotometer limited to one wavelength.

8. **Prisms**

    a. A narrow beam of light focused on a prism is reflected as it enters the more dense glass (quartz, fused silica, or sodium chloride, or other material that permits transmission of light).

    b. Shorter wavelengths are refracted (bent) more than long wavelengths (violet refracted the most, red the least), resulting in a dispersion of white light into a continuous spectrum.

    c. Glass prisms: visible region; quartz or fused silica; ultraviolet.

9. **Diffraction gratings**

    a. Most common monochromator.

    b. **Reflectance:** lines are engraved on the surface of a mirror, which may consist of either a polished metal slab or a glass plate on which a thin metallic film has been deposited.

    c. Usually a thin layer of an aluminum copper alloy on the surface of a flat glass plate that has many small parallel grooves etched on to the surface (15,000–30,000/inch) with a diamond stylus.

d. As the incident light strikes the grooves on the reflectance grating, many tiny spectra are formed, one from each groove. Wave fronts formed from these spectra that are in phase reinforce one another, and those out of phase cancel each other out. This results in a linear spectrum that is parallel.

e. The prism or grating may be tilted or rotated so that the proper wavelength will be incident on the cuvet and detector.

10. **Monochromator:** entrance slit, diffraction grating, and an exit slit.

a. Entrance slit: allows lamp light to enter. Slit if fixed in position and size.

b. Monochromator

c. Exit slit: selects the bandpass and allows light of particular wavelengths to pass through the same cuvet onto the detector.

C. Photodetectors

1. A **detector** converts the electromagnetic radiation (light) transmitted by a solution into an electrical signal. The more light that is transmitted, the more energy, the greater the electrical signal that measures light intensity going through the sample.

2. Two types of photodetectors

a. **Barrier layer cell** (photocell) made up of a film of light sensitive material (selenium or cadmium) which is a semiconductor with a silver layer on one side and an iron or copper layer on the other.

b. **Photomultiplier tubes (PM)**

1) Most commonly used. Electron tube that is capable of significantly amplifying a current. Similar to a barrier-layer cell in that it has photosensitive material that gives off electrons when light energy strikes it.

2) Different in that it requires outside voltage for operation.

3) A **cathode** is a light-sensitive metal that absorbs light and emits electrons in proportion to the radiant energy that strikes the surface of the light-sensitive material.

D. Readout Devices

1. Electrical energy from a detector is displayed on some type of meter or readout system.

E. Recorders

1. Spectrophotometers may be equipped with recorders in addition to or instead of digital display of values.

2. Recorders are synchronized to provide line traces of transmittance or absorbance as a function of either time or wavelength.

V. ATOMIC ABSORPTION

A. Principle—ground state atoms absorb light at defined wavelengths.

1. **Line spectrum:** wavelengths at which an atom absorbs light.

2. The ionic state of the element is put into a flame to allow the atom to get to the ground state.

3. Then a beam of light is passed through the flame.

4. The **atom absorbs** the same wavelengths of light as it would emit when excited.

5. A decrease in intensity is measured by a detector.

key concepts

Compare and contrast atomic absorption spectroscopy and spectrophotometry, including clinical applications.

B. **Function** measures concentration of a sample by detecting absorbance of electromagnetic radiation by atoms.

C. **Diagram**

light source → chopper → sample atoms in flame → monochromator → PM tube

D. **Hollow-cathode tube**—usual light source.
   1. **Contains** an anode, cylindrical cathode made of metal being analyzed and inert gas fillers of helium or argon.
   2. **Principle:** applied voltage causes ionization of filler gas and the excited electrodes knock off electrons on the cathode. When the metal ions of the cathode return to the ground state, characteristic energy of that metal is emitted.
   3. Vaporized metal atoms from the sample can be found in the flame. (Heat from the flame breaks chemical bonds and allows the metals to become vaporized.) **The flame serves as the sample cell in this instrument.**
   4. The light from the hollow cathode ray tube excites the metal in the sample so that it absorbs electrons and emits energy at a specific wavelength.
   5. The energy emitted from the sample will be a **steady emission.**
   6. The photomultiplier tube will read the steady emission and lead to a readout of the concentration of the metal.
   7. A graphite furnace ("flameless") can also be used to vaporize the metal.

VI. NEPHELOMETRY

A. **Definition**—measurement of light scattered in a forward direction by a particulate solution. The amount of scatter is directly proportional to the number and size of particles present in the solution.
   1. **Three types of light scatter**
      a. **Rayleigh:** small particles and light is scattered symmetrically but hardly any at 90 degrees.
      b. **Mie:** very large particles and the light is mostly scattered forward.
      c. **Rayleigh-Debye:** large particles and the light is scattered mostly forward, with a small amount in other directions.
   2. The **sensitivity of a nephelometer** depends on the absence of blank or background scatter.

B. **Turbidimetry**
   1. **Definition:** measures light scattering as a decrease in the light transmitted through the solution.
   2. **Turbidimetry uses a spectrophotometer** for measurement, and it is limited by the photometric accuracy and sensitivity of the instrument.

VII. MOLECULAR EMISSION SPECTROSCOPY

A. **Four Re-emitting Processes in Atoms**
   1. **Fluorescence:** when an atom absorbs energy, it raises electrons to higher electronic states. The electrons release excess energy by emitting energy at a longer wavelength than the exciting wavelength. This shift to a longer wavelength is called a Stokes shift. The emitted light has a very short lifetime.

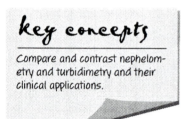

key concepts

Compare and contrast nephelometry and turbidimetry and their clinical applications.

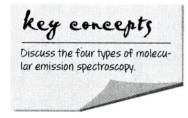

key concepts

Discuss the four types of molecular emission spectroscopy.

    a. **Variables affecting fluorescence** include Rayleigh scatter, Raman scatter, quenching, and the inner filter effect.

    b. **Advantages:** more sensitive than absorption, analytical applications requiring high sensitivity, increased specificity.

    c. **Limitations:** solvent, pH, temperature, absorbance of the solution, presence of interfering or specifically quenching compounds.

2. **Phosphorescence:** emission of light produced by certain substances after they absorb energy. Short lifetime, but longer than fluorescence.

3. **Chemiluminescence:** chemical reaction produces light. Produces more light energy for easier detection.

4. **Bioluminescence:** chemical reaction that produces light in a biological system, i.e., cellular oxidation of a substrate in the presence of an enzyme. Used as a diagnostic test, the methods use enzymes, which increases the specificity of the test.

VIII. FLOW CYTOMETRY

A. **Principle**—single cells suspended in a fluid are bombarded with a laser beam. The scattered and fluorescent light is measured, and the cell's properties are differentiated by computers. Information about the number of cells, cellular surface markers, and cell size is recorded.

B. **Major Components of the Flow Cytometer**
1. Cell transportation system
2. Light source
3. Flow chamber
4. Filters
5. Lenses
6. Mirrors
7. Photodetectors
8. Computers for data analysis

C. **Specimens Analyzed by Flow Cytometry**—lymph nodes, peripheral blood, bone marrow, tumors, and other tissues.

D. **Hydrodynamic Focusing**—uses a laminar flow to line the cells up single file.

E. **Fluorescent Dyes Used in Flow Cytometry**—include acridine orange, pyronin Y, fluorescein isothiocyanate, rhodamine isothiocyanate, and chromomycin A3.

F. **Light Is Scattered Only at 90-degrees or Forward**—the amount of forward scatter determines cell size, whereas 90-degree scatter indicates granularity of the cell.

G. **Clinical Applications**—differentiation of T- and B-cells; cell cycle analysis; diagnosing and following patients with leukemias, lymphomas, and autoimmune or deficiency diseases; karyotyping; and monitoring a patient's response to drug therapy.

IX. ELECTROCHEMISTRY

A. **Definitions**
1. **Electricity:** the flow of electrons.
2. **Conductor:** a substance whose high-energy electrons can be easily moved as free electrons.

key concepts

Discuss the principle behind flow cytometry and clinical applications.

key concepts

Discuss the principle behind ion selective electrodes and what they measure.

3. **Insulator:** high-energy electrons are held tightly in the orbits and cannot be easily moved as free electrons.
4. **Semiconductors:** electronic conductivity between conductors and insulators.
5. **Electromotive force:** the force produced in a substance when there is an excess of electrons on one end and an electron deficit on the other end.
6. **Volt:** unit of measure of electromotive force.
7. **Direct current:** produced when chemical energy is converted to electrical energy; a steady current in one direction in a circuit.
8. **Alternating current:** produced when a rotating mechanism produces mechanical energy and converts it to electrical energy by induction. A current that reverses direction in regular cycles.
9. **Conventional current flow theory:** work is performed when positive charges move to a more negative potential.
10. **Electron theory:** electrons leave the negative pole of an electrical source, travel through the circuit, then travel back to the positive pole.
11. **Circuit:** a closed loop of a conductor.
12. **Coulomb (Q):** unit for measuring charge. 1 coulomb = the charge of 6.24×10^{18} electrons
13. **Current (I):** rate at which a charge moves through a conductor. Measure in amperes (A). **1 ampere** is when 1 coulomb of charge passes one point in a circuit every second.
14. **Voltage (E):** force that moves electrons through a conductor is called electromotive force (EMF). EMF is measured in volts.
    1 volt = force required to move 1 coulomb/second
    through a resistance of 1 Ω
15. **Potential:** whenever there are 2 poles of different charges, a potential for producing current exists.
16. **Resistance:** resistance to current flow in a circuit. Measured in ohms.
    1 Ω = resistance when 1 volt maintains a current of 1 ampere
17. **Resistor:** electronic component that impedes current flow.
18. **Capacitor:** device used to store a quantity of electrical charge.
19. **Dielectric:** insulating material.
20. **Transformer:** changes the input voltage to the voltage needed by the instrument, i.e., 240 volts to 110 volts.
21. **Switch:** turns current on or off by completing or breaking the circuit.

B. Voltammetric Methods

1. **Principle:** an electrochemical method where the current generated from the electrochemical reaction is measured versus the reference electrode.
2. **Electrodes** are a combination of two or three electrodes.
3. **The 3 electrode combination:** working electrode, reference electrode, and auxiliary electrode (not very common).
4. **The 2 electrode combination:** working electrode and a reference electrode are present. The oxygen electrode is a specific type of voltammetry called **amperometry, i.e., oxygen electrode.**
   a. **Amperometry**

1) **Current generated** at a fixed potential by an electroactive analyte in solution.
2) A platinum cathode covered by a thin layer of electrolyte and an Ag/AgCL anode.
3) The electrode is isolated from the sample by an oxygen permeable membrane.
4) Oxygen diffuses through the membrane, then is reduced at the platinum electrode.
5) The current generated at the platinum electrode is directly proportional to the concentration of oxygen.
   b. **Glucose electrode:** also an **amperometric** electrode.
5. **Potentiometric electrodes:** measure of the potential difference between an indicator electrode and a reference electrode.
   a. Composed of semipermeable glass that allows H^+ ions through.
   b. The electrode extends into a bulb.
   c. The migration of hydrogen into the electrode bulb creates a **potential** between the inside and the outside of the electrode and that potential is measured.

C. Electrophoresis
1. Primary method used to analyze proteins.
2. **Definition:** the movement of charged molecules in an electric field. An electric field, a charged particle, and a medium where movement occurs are needed.
3. **Zone electrophoresis:** electrophoresis in a solid medium.
4. **Media:** any solid material that can absorb or hold an electrolyte, i.e., paper, agarose, starch, acrylamide, and cellulose acetate.
5. Movement of charged particles through a medium **depends** on the nature of the charged particle, the character of the buffer, and the intensity of the electric field.
   a. Nature of the charged particle: **proteins are amphoteric** and may be charged positively or negatively depending on the pH of the buffer solution. The pH at which negative and positive charges are equal on a protein is the **protein's isoelectric point.**
   b. An excess of positive ions neutralizes the negative charge, leaving a net positive charge on the proteins.
   c. An excess of negative ions leaves a net negative charge on the group. Because positively charged protein molecules absorb media, electrophoresis of proteins is done with negatively charged groups.
   d. **On cellulose acetate,** the net charge on the protein is responsible for its movement through the medium.
   e. **Buffers with a pH over 8.0, usually 8.6,** are generally used for protein electrophoresis.
6. **Character of the buffer** (ionic atmosphere and zeta potential)
   a. Ions of opposite charge hover in the vicinity of charged macromolecules and form a double layer of charges called an ionic atmosphere.
   b. **Zeta potential:** the electrical potential produced around a molecule that influences the movement of ions in an electric field.

7. The **intensity** of the electric field alters the charges on the macromolecules and influences the movement of macromolecules.
8. **Support media**
   a. **Bulk flow (convection):** when a liquid or less than solid medium is used for electrophoresis, dense zones that are heavier than the solvent will "fall through" and cause blurring of the electrophoresis zones.
   b. A **supporting medium** allows the material to be electrophoresed to flow freely, but will prevent convection.
   c. Most **media** have a pore size that allows materials of specific sizes to flow through easily.
   d. **Capillary tubes** may also be used as a support medium. This type of electrophoresis is called **capillary zone electrophoresis.**
   e. **Electro-osmosis** occurs when ions in the support medium become charged and produce a net flow of solvent in a particular direction. This is also called endo-osmosis. This is a very general effect.
   f. **Types of supporting materials**
      1) Sucrose-density gradient
      2) Polyacrylamide
      3) Agarose
      4) Cellulose acetate
   g. **Molecular sieving**
      1) The average pore size of a medium is usually fixed, but there are some that can be controlled.
      2) The pore size can be controlled to produce molecular sieving (straining out by pore size) by varying the concentration of the support medium used.
9. **Selection of support media and buffers**
   a. Selecting a media is based on whether one is comparing many samples and will control many adverse effects such as convection, endo-osmosis, and resolution.
   b. **Paper and cellulose acetate** are usually used for low-molecular weight substances.
   c. **Gels** can be used for higher molecular weight substances such as proteins, lipoproteins, and hemoglobin A_{1C}.
10. **Electroblotting**
    a. **Western blot**
       1) Determines if a serum contains one or more antibodies to a complex antigenic material, i.e., human immunodeficiency virus (HIV).
       2) The virus or other complex antigenic material is separated through electrophoresis.
       3) The separated components (antigens) are transferred from the gel to a nitrocellulose media by blotting them from the gel to the new media, and the patient's serum is added.
       4) If the serum contain antibodies to the antigens, immune complexes form.

5) Unbound proteins are washed away, and immune complexes precipitate at characteristic locations.

   b. Western blots are very sensitive.

11. **Conditions**
    a. **Position:** electrophoresis can be done horizontally or vertically.
    b. **Sample application:** samples are applied to surface and soak in, or are applied in, slots or holes.
    c. **Current and voltage:** electrophoresis can use a constant voltage, constant current, or constant power. It is best to conduct the separation as quickly as possible to avoid interfering processes.
    d. **Separation time**
       1) **Isotachophoresis:** electrophoresis is stopped when the trailing ion emerges.
       2) **Isoelectric focusing:** stopped when the gradient is formed and the current becomes stable.
       3) **Zone electrophoresis:** when the tracking dye reaches a certain point.

12. **Locating the analyte**
    a. **Measurement of a physical property,** staining with colorimetric dyes or fluorescent dyes. Ninhydrin stain is used for proteins, periodic acid-Schiff stain is used for carbohydrates, fat-soluble dyes are used for fats, etc.

13. **Clinical applications**
    a. **Specific protein electrophoresis (done on serum):** used to separate serum proteins and determines if there is monoclonal gammopathies, polyclonal gammopathies, or any other abnormal conditions.
    b. **Isoenzyme analysis:** to better determine the source of a disease.
    c. **Western blot:** to identify specific proteins (HIV).
    d. **Southern blot:** to identify nucleic acids (RNA and DNA).

14. **Commonly encountered problems in electrophoresis**
    a. **No migration:** can be caused by not connecting instrument to electrical outlet, wrong pH buffer, or electrodes connected backward.
    b. Bowed electrophoretic pattern of edges of support: overheating or drying out of support.
    c. **Tailing of bands:** chemical reaction or salt in sample.
    d. **Holes in staining pattern:** analyte present in too high a concentration.
    e. **Very thin, sharp bands:** molecular weight of sample very high for support presize.
    f. **Very slow migration:** high molecular weight, low charge, ionic strength too high, voltage too low.
    g. **Sample precipitates in support:** pH too high or low, and too much heating.

X. CHROMATOGRAPHY

A. Techniques Used to Separate Chemical Compounds in a Solution

B. Gas Chromatography

1. A technique used to **separate a mixture of gases** or **volatile liquids.**

   a. A mixture of gases or volatile liquids is heated and injected into an inert gas.

   b. The gases are forced through the instrument and over a phase that will separate the mixture as it exits the instrument.

2. **Gas-solid chromatography** uses a solid phase to separate the gases—the gas is passed over a solid structure and adsorbed by the solid.

3. **Gas-liquid chromatography** uses a liquid phase to separate the gases—the gas is passed over a liquid and the liquid attracts the gas (most common method).

4. **Choosing a carrier gas:** consider efficiency of system, stability of column and compounds, type of detector, purity of gas, possible risks or hazards

5. **Solid phases** are in two types of columns: packed and capillary.

   a. In packed columns, the column itself is inert, and the material inside the column is the solid phase.

   b. Capillary columns need only a fraction of the sample as a full-size column.

6. Once the gases are separated, they will be carried to a detector to be identified. **Types of detectors** include thermal conductivity, flame ionization, nitrogen-phosphorus, and electron capture.

C. Liquid Chromatography

1. **Advantages** over gas chromatography

   a. Separates any compound soluble in liquid phase

   b. Operates at a lower temperature

   c. Depends on interaction of compounds with both mobile and stationary phases

   d. **Disadvantage:** less efficient than gas chromatography

D. Column Chromatography

1. Uses large, nonrigid support materials

2. Gives long separation with broad peaks and poor limits of detection

3. Mobile phase flows by gravity

4. Applications: sample purification and removal of interferences

E. High-Performance Liquid Chromatography (HPLC)

1. Uses small, uniform, rigid supports

2. Produces narrow peaks

3. Resulting in improved limits of detection and shorter separation times

4. High pressure moves the mobile phase (pump)

F. Thin-Layer Chromatography

1. Example is paper chromatography (paper is the stationary phase). Good screening test.

key concepts

Compare and contrast gas and liquid chromatography and thin layer chromatography and clinical applications.

G. Definitions

1. **Strong mobile phase:** solvent elutes quickly from the column; occurs when mobile phase is chemically similar to the stationary phase.
2. **Weak mobile phase:** solvent that slowly elutes compounds from the column; occurs when mobile phase is not chemically similar to the stationary phase.
3. **Gradient elution:** begin by using a weak mobile phase, then switch to a strong mobile phase.
4. **Isocratic elution:** constant mobile phase.
5. **Liquid-solid (adsorption) chromatography:** liquid mobile phase that interacts with a solid stationary phase, i.e., paper chromatography.
6. **Liquid-liquid (partition) chromatography:** two types:
   a. **Normal-phase liquid chromatography:** stationary phase is polar.
   b. **Reversed-phase liquid chromatography:** nonpolar stationary phase.
7. **Ion-exchange chromatography:** separation based on charge, i.e., cation and anion exchangers.
8. **Ion-pair chromatography:** a hybrid type; combines reversed-phase with ion-exchange chromatography
9. **Affinity chromatography:** based on the binding of an enzyme with substrate or antibody with antigen.
10. **Size-exclusion chromatography:** solid phase allows only particles of a particular size to pass through.
11. **Liquid chromatography detectors:** refractive index detector, absorbance detector, variable wavelength detector, diode array detector, fluorescence detector, conductivity detector, and electrochemical detector.

XI. MASS SPECTROMETRY

A. Mass Spectrometer—an instrument that uses the principle of charged particles moving through a magnetic or electric field can be separated from other charged particles according to their mass-to-charge ratios.

B. Instrument Components

1. **Vacuum system:** enhances collision efficiency and ion formation.
2. **Sampling device:** introduces the sample to the instrument.
3. **Ionization source:** samples enter the ion source and are bombarded by the ionization beam.
   a. Varying magnitude and polarity of electronic potentials, the ions can be stored, accelerated, and directed to exit slit.
   b. Samples are ionized by electrons that possess enough energy to displace electrons.
4. **Mass filter:** uses either electronic or magnetic separation; occurs in a quadrupole.
   a. A quadrupole is 4 parallel rods that provide specific radio frequency—voltage is applied that creates a unique oscillating field where a positive ion injected into the region will oscillate between poles

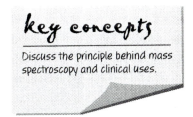

key concepts

Discuss the principle behind mass spectroscopy and clinical uses.

5. **Magnetic separation:** as ions enter the magnetic mass filter, they experience a force that causes them to move in a curved path. Ions of different mass-to-charge ratios will vary the curvature according to the accelerating voltage applied.

6. **Ion collection:** area that collects the ions to be discarded.

7. **Mass fragmentation:** occurs when ionization beam collides with the sample.
   a. The sample will release an electron to form a positively charged ion.
   b. The charged ion still has the molecular weight of the compound.
   c. A stable ion will last longer, thereby generating an intense peak.
   d. A short-lived ion will generate a small peak.
   e. Fragmentation provides much structural information and a unique spectrum for identification.

8. **Mass spectrometry** is the best technique for identifying drugs or drug metabolites. Each unique spectrum is analyzed by a database and can be matched to identify the sample.

XII. IMMUNOCHEMICAL TECHNIQUES

A. These are used to detect extremely small amounts of analytes by using antibodies and various tags.

B. Methods

1. **Competitive-binding:** based on noncovalent, reversible binding of an antigen to an antibody.
   a. Mix labeled and unlabeled antigen together in an antibody-coated tube.
   b. The sample and labeled antigen **compete** for antibody binding sites on the tube.
   c. There will be an excess of labeled antigen in the tube compared to the number of available binding sites.
   d. The concentration of the antibody binding sites is limited with respect to total antigens leading to less antibody bound when sample concentration of antibody is high.
   e. This is an **inverse relationship:** the higher the sample concentration, the lower the labeled concentration.
   f. Type of competitive assays
      1) **Heterogenous** require that antibody-bound labeled antigen be physically removed from the free-labeled antigen.
      2) **Homogenous** do not require physical removal of bound and unbound free-labeled antigen.
   g. **Techniques** used to separate bound and unbound antigens
      1) Adsorbents: nonspecific, specific, and chromatography
      2) Precipitation by ammonium sulfate
      3) Double antibody
   h. **Labels** used for competitive binding assays include **chromagenic** substrates, **fluorogenic** substrates, **luminogenic** substrates, **radioactive** isotopes, **microparticles**, and **enzyme substrates.**

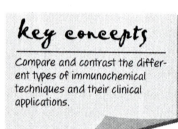

key concepts

Compare and contrast the different types of immunochemical techniques and their clinical applications.

i. **Detection limits:** immunochemical techniques detect very small amounts of substances. Monoclonal antibodies increase the specificity of the procedure.

j. Examples

1) **Immunoradiometric assay (IRMA)** uses a radiolabeled antibody. The antigen in the sample competes with the antigen attached to a solid surface for the binding sites of the labeled antibody **(noncompetitive).**

2) **Enzyme-linked immunosorbent assays (ELISA)** are heterogenous nonisotopic assays that use an antibody immobilized onto a solid support. Useful because they are highly specific, easily coupled to antigens, stable, absent in fluid or tissue, and tend to retain their activity for a specified time (noncompetitive).

3) **Enzyme-multiplied immunoassay (EMIT):** a homogenous immunoassay where binding of antibody to the enzyme-antigen conjugate limits the enzyme substrate's access to the active site (competitive).

4) **Fluorescence polarization immunoassay (FPIA):** uses the rotation of the complex to allow light to be transmitted to a detector on a particular plane **(competitive).**

k. **Polyclonal antiserum:** a pool of antibodies that are specific for the antigen.

l. **Monoclonal antiserum:** absolutely specific and are completely homogenous because all cells producing the antibodies are cloned.

m. **Limitations of monoclonal antiserum**

1) React only with a single antigen and will not **crosslink**.

2) **Avidity** cannot be manipulated because the antibodies react only with 1 antigen.

3) Reaction mechanism for antigen and antibody binding.

Not Static

$Antigen_n + Antibody \leftrightarrow Antigen_n\ Antibody \leftrightarrow Antigen_n\ Antibody_b$

Antibody Excess

All antigenic sites are covered with antibody and lattice formation is inhibited.

$Antigen + Antibody \leftrightarrow Soluble\ complexes$

Equivalence Zone

$Antigen + Antibody \leftrightarrow Insoluble\ complexes$

Optimal proportion. Occurs when 2–3 antibody molecules are present for each antigen molecule, produces maximum lattice formation and therefore maximum precipitate.

Antigen Excess

All antibody sites are saturated by antigen. Triplets (2 Ag + 1 Ab) are maxi-

Antigen + Antibody ↔ Soluble complexes

mum size of particles. No precipitate. Ionic species and ionic strength affect the binding of antigen and antibody.

XIII. MOLECULAR TECHNIQUES

A. Overview

1. All genetic information in prokaryotic and eukaryotic cells is contained in **deoxyribonucleic acid (DNA).**
2. This information is transferred within the cell via the pathway **DNA → RNA → Proteins.**
3. The **genetic information** is transferred from cell to cell and parent to daughter by DNA replication.

B. Components of Nucleic Acids

1. **A nucleic acid is a polynucleotide**, a linear polymer of nucleotides, made up of three components.
   a. **Nitrogenous heterocyclic base (purines and pyrimidines)** attached to the 1′ carbon atom of the sugar by a N-glycosidic bond.
      1) **Purines** include **adenine (A)** and **guanine (G).**
      2) **Pyrimidines** include **cytosine (C), thymine (T), and uracil (U).**
      3) Both DNA and RNA contain A, G, and C. **T is only found in DNA, and U is only found in RNA.**
   b. Cyclic 5-carbon sugar residue.
      1) RNA contains a **ribose sugar.**
      2) DNA contains a **deoxyribose sugar**.
   c. A phosphate is attached to the 5′ carbon atom of the sugar by a phosphoester linkage. This phosphate is responsible for the strong negative charge of both nucleotides and nucleic acids.
2. The nucleotide in nucleic acids are joined to one another by a second phosphoester bond.
   a. Between the 5′ phosphate of one nucleotide and the 3′ OH group of the adjacent nucleotide.
   b. Such a doubly esterified phosphate is called a phosphodiester group.

C. Physical and Chemical Structure of DNA

1. **Base pairing**
   a. Even though the base composition of DNA varies from organism to organism, **A always pairs with T (U in RNA) and C always pairs with G.**
   b. Therefore, the concentration of purines always equals the concentrations of pyrimidines.
2. **Double helix**
   a. In 1953, Watson and Crick introduced the **double helix** structure for DNA: two polynucleotide strands are coiled around one another to form a double-stranded helix.
      1) Sugar-phosphate backbones of each strand follow a helical path at the outer edge of the molecule, and bases are in **a helical array in the central core.**

2) Each base in one strand is hydrogen-bonded to a complementary base in the other strand. **This forms the purine-pyrimidine base pairs (AT and GC).**

b. The helix has 2 external helical grooves.

1) A deep wide one (the major groove) is the site of binding of various protein molecules to DNA.

2) A shallow narrow one (the minor groove).

3. **Complementary strands**

a. Due to pairing rules, the two strands are complementary. If one strand has the sequence GATACC, its complementary pair is CTATGG (read in the same direction).

G – C
A – T
T – A
A – T
C – G
C – G

b. **The two strands of the DNA double helix are anti-parallel in the sense that the chemical orientations are different.**

1) The 3′ OH end of the strand is opposite the 5′ P end of the other strand. This structural feature has important consequences for DNA replication.

2) By convention, a base sequence is usually written with the 5′P terminal end at the left.

4. **Miscellaneous information**

a. Although at physiological temperatures the DNA base pairs are stable, they break and reform rapidly. This process is known as "breathing of the DNA."

b. There are two forms of DNA possible.

1) A right-handed form that follows a clockwise path as it moves away from the observer.

2) A left-handed form, which follows a counterclockwise path as it moves away from the observer.

D. Chromosomes

1. DNA of all eukaryotic cells is organized into chromosomes. Each chromosome contains only a single, long DNA molecule, so the DNA must be greatly folded.

2. DNA molecules in chromosomes are bound to basic proteins called **histones.** The complex comprising the DNA and histone is called **chromatin.**

3. DNA shape

a. DNA in eukaryotes is helical.

b. DNA in prokaryotes is circular.

1) Circular DNA molecules of great practical importance are called plasmids.

2) Plasmids contain genetic information that is separate from chromosomal DNA. They are able to replicate in cells and hence are carried from one generation to the next.

E. Denaturing/Melting Curves

1. Determination of the 3-dimensional structure
   a. The 3-dimensional structure of DNA, RNA, and proteins are determined by weak noncovalent interactions. The principle interactions are hydrogen bonds and hydrophobic interactions.
   b. The free energy of these interactions are not much greater than the energy of thermal motion at room temperature. **At elevated temperatures, the structures of these molecules are disrupted.**
2. **Denaturation**
   a. A macromolecule in a disrupted state is denatured. The ordered state that is presumed present in nature is called **native**.
   b. When double-stranded DNA is heated, the bonding forces between the strands are disrupted, and the two strands separate. Thus denatured DNA is single-stranded.
3. **Renaturation**
   a. **A solution of denatured DNA can be treated such that native DNA reforms by a process called renaturation or annealing.**
   b. In molecular biology, annealing can be used to:
      1) Determine whether certain sequences occur more than once in DNA of a particular organism.
      2) Locate specific base sequences in a DNA molecule.
      3) Detect particular species of RNA.
   c. **Two requirements are necessary for the annealing to occur:**
      1) The salt concentration must be high enough that the electrostatic repulsion between phosphates in the 2 strands is eliminated.
      2) The temperature must be high enough to disrupt the random, intrastrand hydrogen bonds (optimal temperature for annealing is 20–25°C).

F. DNA Replication, Repair, and Mutagenesis

1. DNA replication is an essential step in the production of "daughter cells" and organisms.
2. Replication is a complex and incompletely understood process owing to:
   a. A requirement for energy to unwind the helix.
   b. The tendency of single-stranded DNA to form intrastructure base pairs.
   c. The antiparallel structure of DNA.
   d. The existence of systems to minimize replication errors.
   e. The great length of DNA compared with the cell size.
3. **Errors in replication occasionally occur and are corrected by 2 major repair systems.**
   a. The base sequence of DNA is subject to change via attack by chemical reagents and environmental agents.
   b. A variety of repair mechanisms also exists for restoring the original sequence.
   c. Occasionally, the repair doesn't occur, and the new sequences persist, giving rise to mutant "offspring."

4. **Replication**
   a. The prime role of any replication mechanism is the duplication of the base sequence of the parent DNA molecule.
   b. During DNA replication, DNA molecules are created that are identical to the parent molecule.
   c. Each parental DNA strand serves as a template for one daughter strand.
      1) As each new strand is formed, it is hydrogen bonded to its parental template.
      2) As replication proceeds, the parental double helix unwinds and then rewinds again in two new double helices. Each helix has one parental strand and one newly formed daughter strand.

G. Replication Mechanism
   1. **Unwinding**
      a. **Unwinding** the double helix presents somewhat of a mechanical problem.
         1) The two daughter branches at the "Y" fork must revolve around each other.
         2) Winding in the reverse sense somewhere "downstream" from the fork compensates for the unwinding at the fork, which must be accompanied by forward movement.
      b. In order for the unwinding to occur, hydrogen bonds and hydrophobic interactions must be eliminated, and this requires energy.
   2. **Polymerization reaction of DNA**
      a. **Enzymes called DNA polymerases catalyze polymerization of DNA.**
         1) These enzymes select the nucleotide to be added to the end of the growing chain and form a phosphodiester bond.
         2) DNA polymerases are able to synethsize DNA from 4 precursor molecules (the [4] deoxynucleoside-5'-triphosphates) as long as a DNA molecule to be copied (a template) is provided.
      b. DNA polymers cannot catalyze the reaction between two free nucleotides (even if one has a 3'-OH group and the other has a 5'-triphosphate).
         1) Polymerization occurs only if the nucleotide with the 3'-OH group is hydrogen-bonded to the template strand.
         2) **This nucleotide is called a primer.** The primer can be either a single nucleotide or the terminus of a hydrogen-bonded oligonucleotide.
      c. DNA replication requires not only an enzymatic mechanism for adding nucleotides to the growing chains but also a means of unwinding the parental double helix.
         1) Unwinding the helix is closely related to the initiation of synthesis of precursor fragments.
         2) Energy needed to eliminate hydrogen bonds and hydrophobic interactions can be obtained as the polymerase enzyme and utilizes the free energy of hydrolysis of the triphosphate

for unwinding as it synthesizes a DNA strand in a way other polymerases cannot. This enzyme is called a helicase.

H. Nucleases and Restriction Enzymes

1. A variety of enzymes called nucleases break phosphodiester bonds in nucleic acids (they usually exhibit chemical specificity).
   a. **DNAses—Deoxyribonucleases**
      1) Many act on either single stranded or double stranded DNA only.
      2) Some act on both single and double strands.
   b. **RNAses—Ribonucleases**
   c. **Exonucleases:** cut only at the end of a nucleic acid, removing a single nucleotide at a time.
2. **Restriction enzyme: endonucleases that recognize a specific base sequence in a DNA molecule. It makes 2 cuts, 1 in each strand, generating a 3′-OH and a 5′P termini.**
   a. Several classes of restriction enzymes are known.
      1) **Type II enzymes,** which make cuts within the recognition site, are the greatest utility for recombinant DNA experiments.
      2) A particular restriction enzyme generates a unique family of fragments for a particular DNA molecule.
      3) A different enzyme generates a different family of fragments from the same DNA molecule.

I. Fragment Identification

1. Identifying a fragment that carries a particular gene or base sequence can be done by denaturing the fragments and measuring the ability of the separated strands to renature with a denatured labeled DNA (called a probe) carrying the same sequence or a part thereof.
2. Hybridization
   a. **Nucleic acid hybridization: the process of forming base pairs between 2 different nucleic strands is called nucleic acid hybridization.**
   b. Blotting techniques have been used to establish the presence of DNA or RNA and to determine their approximate size.
   c. Types of blotting
      1) **Southern blot**
         a) DNA fragments obtained by using restriction enzymes are size separated by gel electrophoresis, and then the strands are separated in the gel by denaturation.
         b) Single strands are blotted and permanently bound onto a specially modified paper support such as nitrocellulose or nylon.
         c) This support sheet is incubated in a solution containing DNA or RNA complementary to the DNA or RNA on the paper support.
         d) **The complementary sequence, called a probe,** has been radioactively labeled.
         e) The complementary sequences are allowed to hybridize; the paper support is washed free of unhybridized probe and placed in contact with x-ray film.

      f) The DNA fragments which are complementary to the nucleotide sequence of the probe will show up as dark bands on the autoradiograph or x-ray film.

    2) **Northern blot**

      a) RNA is blotted onto nitrocellulose or nylon paper so that RNA becomes permanently bound.

      b) Like the Southern blot, a radioactive DNA probe is used to localize the complementary RNA on the blot.

    3) **Western blot (see Section IX.C.10, Electroblotting)**

  d. Nonradioactive labels, such as fluorescent or colorimetric labels, may also be used in the different blotting techniques.

J. Restriction Fragment Length Polymorphism (RFLP)

1. **Background**

  a. About 25 percent of all human genes occur in multiple allelic forms that are called polymorphisms.

  b. Restriction enzyme sites are also polymorphic in human populations, so that the pattern of DNA fragments produced by a particular restriction enzyme digest of DNA sometimes differs from person to person.

2. **RFLP**

  a. Restriction fragment length polymorphisms have become extremely useful in constructing a map of the human genome and for screening and diagnosing hereditary diseases.

  b. A major achievement of RFLPs has been the construction of a linkage map of the human genome.

  c. Another rapidly growing use of RFLPs is in the fields of forensic pathology and criminology.

    1) A particular set of probes, called Jeffrey's probes, detect hypervariable sequences in the human genome.

    2) The Southern blot patterns of these short, inherited hypervariable sequences are characteristic for each individual and constitute a unique "genetic fingerprint."

K. Genetic Engineering

1. **Recombinant DNA technology (genetic engineering):** a method for covalent joining of two DNA molecules from any sources and propagation of the joint molecule.

2. **Gene therapy is the replacement of defective genes in the somatic cells of the human body to correct genetic diseases.**

  a. Joining a DNA segment of interest to a vector DNA molecule that is able to replicate carries this out.

  b. **Then, it is inserted into cells in which the DNA fragment of interest is cloned and amplified.**

L. DNA probes

1. Used in four main disciplines: **microbiology, immunology, forensics,** and **genetics.**

2. **Definition:** single-stranded piece of DNA where bases are complementary to those of the target.

3. Produced by synthesis of oglionucleotides or **cloning.**

4. **Probes** are labeled with radioisotopes, colorimetric substrates, chemiluminescent compounds, or ELISA techniques.
5. Traditional method: **Southern blot.**
   a. **Procedure**
      1) **Extract** DNA.
      2) **Digest** DNA into fragments.
      3) **Separate** fragments by electrophoresis.
      4) **Denature** and separate into single-stranded DNA (ssDNA).
      5) ssDNA transferred to solid support.
      6) Support is **treated** with labeled probe.
      7) **Probe is usually ^{32} P.**

M. Polymerase Chain Reaction (PCR)
   1. **Definition:** method used to exponentially increase the amount of DNA found in a sample—also called DNA amplification.
   2. **PCR** is used to **amplify target DNA** to make DNA probes more sensitive.
   3. **Technique**
      a. **Denature** sample DNA by heating.
      b. **Add** primers.
      c. Cool to **anneal** primers.
      d. Add polymerase to **replicate** DNA.
      e. **Denature** by heating.
      f. **Add** primers.
      g. Cool to **anneal.**
      h. **Repeat cycle 20–30 times to produce amount of DNA needed.**

XIV. AUTOMATION

A. Types of Instruments
   1. **Centrifugal analysis** uses centrifugal force to mix specimens and reagents in separate cuvettes. This type of instrument is very good in batch analysis.
   2. **Discrete analysis** involves running multiple tests where the sample and reagents are in a separate container for each test.
   3. **Random access:** specimens can be analyzed independently of other samples on the analyzer. Programmed to run a test ahead of other specimens.

B. Principles of Automation—automated instruments use robotics and fluidics to replicate manual tasks.
   1. **Specimen preparation** includes clot formation, centrifugation, and identification

C. Specimen Aliquotting and Mixing—most automated instruments require an **operator to load** the samples onto the instrument. Some instruments have **level-sensing probes and allow bar-coded serum separator tubes** to be loaded onto the instrument. Other instruments require the operator to **manually enter** the position of the patient sample and order the tests.

D. Reagents
   1. **Dry reagents** can be packaged as

      a. **Lyophilized powder** that must be reconstituted with a buffer or water

      b. A **tablet form** that must be crushed and mixed with the specimen and diluent in the analyzer

      c. Or **spread over thin plastic strips** and assembled into a single use slide

  2. **Liquid reagents** may be purchased in bulk or single use packs. Liquid reagents are pipetted by the instrument and mixed with the specimen.

E. Testing Phase—this is where the **reagents are mixed with the specimen**, then **allowed to react** for a specified time at a specified temperature.

  1. **Mixing** occurs in a container called a **cuvette.** Some instruments have **permanent, nondisposable cuvettes** that are opaque and made of Teflon. Usually cuvettes are clear and made of plastic.

  2. **Reaction temperatures and times** vary for each analyte. The most common reaction temperatures are 37°C and 30°C.

      a. **Kinetic assays** are incubated for a short period of time, and **many readings are taken.** The concentration is based on a **change in absorbance.**

      b. **Endpoint assays** are incubated for a specific time, then the absorbance is determined. **The absorbance is directly proportional to the concentration of the analyte.**

F. Determining Absorbance or Change in Absorbance

  1. Instruments contain a light source and a **monochromator** to provide many wavelengths.

  2. The incident light that makes it through the sample fall on a **photodetector** that transforms the incident light into electrical energy.

G. Data Management

  1. Most instruments have data management modules that allow operators **to analyze QC values and patient values before releasing patient results.**

  2. Instruments/laboratory information systems (LIS) also archive patient results and QC values. These archived results are stored by the laboratory for various lengths of time.

H. Total Laboratory Automation—systems exist for laboratories that receive specimens, centrifuge them, then distribute specimens to particular sections of the lab and/or instruments. This kind of automation is not widely used at this time.

I. Point-of-Care Testing (POCT)

  1. **Definition:** performing diagnostic tests outside the main laboratory and at or near patient caregiving areas.

  2. **Applications:** designed for immediate laboratory test results for immediate patient assessment and determination of appropriate care. POCT can be used in neonatal intensive care, coronary care, intensive care, or even the emergency room.

  3. **Operators:** only waived laboratory tests can be performed using point-of-care instruments. Medical laboratory technicians and med-

ical technologists must operate instruments that perform complex or high-complex laboratory tests.

4. **Point-of-care instrument evaluations:** all POC instruments must be evaluated in accordance with CLIA 88. The values obtained from POC instruments must correlate with values obtained from larger laboratory instruments. Linearity testing, calculation of control ranges, correlations of data, and reference ranges must be done for each instrument.

5. **Training:** all POC instrument operators must be trained, and it must be documented.

6. **Quality control:** all effective quality control systems must be set up for each POC instrument. The program must use appropriate standards and controls, statistical analyses, and a proficiency testing system.

7. The **logs must contain** patient's name, identification number, test results, units, operator initials, lot numbers of reagents, controls and standards, expiration dates, and action logs.

8. **Cost:** POC instruments have a higher cost per test than large laboratory instruments. Overall cost of POC instruments should be taken into consideration before setting up a POC program.

XV. TEST METHODOLOGIES

A. Calcium

1. Decreased ionized calcium levels cause muscle spasms or uncontrolled muscle contractions called **tetany.**

2. Regulation: **3 hormones regulate serum calcium:** parathyroid hormone (PTH), vitamin D, and calcitonin.

  a. **Parathyroid hormone** (PTH)

    1) A decrease in serum calcium stimulates the release of PTH by the parathyroid gland, and a rise in calcium terminates PTH release.

    2) In bone, PTH activates osteoclasts to break down bone to increase serum calcium.

    3) In the kidney, PTH increases tubular reabsorption of calcium and stimulates hydroxylation of vitamin D to the active form.

  b. **Vitamin D (cholecalciferol)**

    1) Obtained by diet or exposure to sunlight.

    2) Initially, vitamin D goes to the liver when it is hydroxylated but still inactive, then to the kidney where it is converted to its active form: 1,25-dihydroxycholecalciferol.

    3) Calcium absorption in the intestines is enhanced by vitamin D, as well as the effect of PTH on increasing tubular reabsorption of calcium in the kidneys.

  c. **Calcitonin**

    1) Released by the parafollicular cells of the thyroid gland when serum calcium level increases

    2) Inhibits vitamin D and parathyroid hormone activity to decrease serum calcium

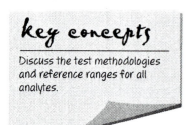

key concepts

Discuss the test methodologies and reference ranges for all analytes.

3. **Clinical significance**
    a. Hypercalcemia: primary **hyperparathyroidism** (parathyroid adenoma) or malignancy.
    b. Hypercalcemia: secondary hyperparathroidism–renal failure. Ionized calcium is most sensitive for diagnosing asymptomatic or subtle **hyperparathyroidism**.
    c. Hypocalcemia: primary **hyperphosphatemia,** altered vitamin D metabolism, or hypoparathyroidism.
    d. Hypocalcemia: sepsis, burns, and cardiac insufficiency.

4. **Test method**
    a. Atomic absorption (reference method)
    b. Ion-selective electrodes
    c. Orthocresolphthalein complexone + Ca → purple complex
    d. Arsenazo

5. **Reference range**
    Total calcium: 8.7–10.2 mg/dL
    Ionized calcium: 4.6–5.3 mg/dL

B. Magnesium

1. Magnesium is an **activator** for many enzymes.
2. **Regulation:** controlled by the kidney through reabsorption and excretion of magnesium.
3. Clinical significance
    a. **Hypomagnesmia:** coronary vasospasm, acute cardiac infarction, and sudden death
    b. **Hypomagnesmia**
        1) Drugs, i.e. diuretics, gentamicin, cisplatin, and cyclosporine
        2) Diabetics (can aggravate neuromuscular and vascular complications of diabetes)
        3) Alcoholics due to dietary magnesium deficiency, ketosis, diarrhea, and hyperaldosteronism
4. **Test method**
    a. Mg + calmagite reagent → calmagite-Mg complex
    b. Atomic absorption spectrophotometry
5. **Reference range:** 1.6–2.4 mg/dL

C. Phosphorus

1. **Regulation**
    a. **Phosphate** in the blood can be absorbed from dietary sources, released from cells, or lost from bone. Regulation occurs by reabsorption or excretion by the kidneys.
    b. Most important regulatory hormone is **parathyroid hormone (PTH)** which increases renal excretion of phosphate.
2. **Clinical significance**
    a. **Hyperphosphatemia**
        1) Renal failure
        2) Severe infections
        3) Intense exercise
        4) Neoplastic diseases

  b. **Hypophosphatemia**
1) Infusion of dextrose solution
2) Nutritional recovery syndrome
3) Antacids
4) Alcohol withdrawal
3. **Test methods**

$$\text{Phosphomolybdenum} \xrightarrow{\text{+electrons}} \text{molybdenum blue}$$

4. **Reference range:** 2.7–4.5 mg/dL

D. Bilirubin

1. **Regulation**
   a. Bilirubin is produced by breaking down hemoglobin from old RBCs.
   b. Bilirubin is conjugated to bilirubin diglucoronide in the liver, stored in the gallbladder, secreted into the duodenum, and excreted in the stool as urobilin.
2. **Clinical significance**
   a. Many diseases affect the production, uptake, storage, metabolism, and excretion of bilirubin. Some diseases and their affect on total bilirubin, conjugated bilirubin, and unconjugated bilirubin can be found in the following table:

Disease	Total Bilirubin	Conjugated Bilirubin	Unconjugated Bilirubin
Physiological jaundice	Increased	Normal	Increased
Crigler-Najjar syndrome	Increased	Normal	Increased
Gilbert's syndrome	Increased	Normal	Increased
Intrahepatic cholestasis	Increased	Increased	Normal
Dubin-Johnson syndrome	Increased	Increased	Normal

3. **Test methodology**
   a. **Jendrassik-Graf total bilirubin test**
      Bilirubin + sodium acetate + caffeine-sodium benzoate (alcohol) + diazotonized sulfanilic acid → purple azobilirubin (high pH)
   b. **Evelyn-Malloy Total Bilirubin Test**
      Bilirubin + sodium acetate + caffeine-sodium benzoate (alcohol) + diazotonized sulfanilic acid → purple-blue azobilirubin (low pH)
   c. For newborns, bilirubin concentration is directly proportional to absorbance at 455 nm.
4. Reference range:
   Infants: 1–6 mg/dL
   Adults: 0.2–1.0 mg/dL

E. Urobilinogen

1. **Regulation**
   a. Anaerobic bacteria in the gut convert the bilirubin to urobilinogens (stercobilinogen, mesobilinogen, and urobilinogen).
   b. A small amount of urobilinogens in the gut are reabsorbed and secreted in the urine.

2. **Clinical significance**
   a. Urobilinogen formation is decreased in all conditions that impair bilirubin excretion.
   b. This is evidenced by a clay-colored or chalky white stool found in complete obstructive jaundice.
3. **Test methodology**
   a. **Urine**

   urobilinogen + p-dimethyl aminobenzaldehyde →
   red colored complex

4. **Reference range:** 0.1–1.0 mg/dL/2 hours

F. Total Protein

1. **Regulation**
   a. Most proteins are synthesized in the liver.
   b. Injury or inflammation causes the liver to increase synthesis of the acute phase reactant proteins.
   c. Severe or chronic liver diseases cause a decrease in plasma protein production.
   d. Immunoglobulins are synthesized in plasma cells.
2. **Clinical significance**
   a. **Prealbumin**
      1) Decreased: hepatic damage, acute phase inflammatory response, tissue necrosis, and poor nutritional status
      2) Increased: patients receiving steroids, alcoholism, and chronic renal failure
   b. **Albumin**
      1) Decreased: muscle-wasting diseases, malnutrition, liver disease, gastrointestinal loss, and renal disease (nephrotic syndrome, glomerulonephritis)
   c. **α_1-antitrypsin**
      1) Decreased: severe, degenerative, emphysematous pulmonary disease; juvenile hepatic cirrhosis
      2) Increased: inflammatory reactions, pregnancy, and contraceptive use
   d. **α_1-fetoprotein (AFP)**
      1) Peaks in the fetus at 13 weeks' gestation and recedes at 34 weeks' gestation.
      2) Elevated AFP conditions (in maternal serum): neural tube defects, including spina bifida, atresia of the gastrointestinal tract, and fetal distress, as well as multiple babies.
      3) Decreased: Down syndrome
      4) AFP is measured between 15 and 20 weeks' gestation and is reported out as multiples of the mean (MoM).
      5) Extremely elevated levels of AFP can also be indicative of hepatocellular carcinoma and gonadal tumors.
   e. **α_1-acid glycoprotein (orosomucoid)**
      1) Increased: inflammation, pregnancy, cancer, pneumonia, rheumatoid arthritis, and conditions associated with cell proliferation

    f. **α_1-antichymotrypsin (α_1-ACT)**
      1) Elevations: inflammation
      2) Deficiency: asthma and liver disease

    g. **Inter-α-trypsin Inhibitor (ITI)**
      1) Elevated: inflammatory disorders

    h. **Haptoglobin**
      1) Increased: inflammatory conditions, burns, nephrotic syndrome
      2) Decreased: intravascular hemolysis

    i. **Ceruloplasmin**
      1) Increased: females, pregnancy, inflammatory processes, malignancies, oral estrogen, and contraceptives
      2) Decreased: Wilson's disease, malnutrition, malabsorption, severe liver disease, and nephrotic syndrome

    j. **α_2-macroglobulin**
      1) Increased: nephrosis, contraceptive use, pregnancy, diabetes, and liver disease

    k. **Transferrin**
      1) Function: transport iron and prevent iron loss through the kidney
      2) Decreased: liver disease, malnutrition, or nephrotic syndrome
      3) Increased: iron deficeiency anemia, hemachromatosis (bronze skin, cirrhosis, diabetes mellitus, and low plasma transferrin levels)

    l. **Hemopexin**
      1) Function: remove circulating heme
      2) Increased: pregnancy, diabetes mellitus, Duchenne muscular dystrophy, and malignancies (melanomas)
      3) Decreased: hemolytic disorders

    m. **β-microglobulin**
      1) Elevated: impaired clearance by the kidney, rheumatoid arthritis, and systemic lupus erythematosus (SLE)

    n. **Complement**
      1) Increased: inflammatory states
      2) Decreased: malnutrition, systemic lupus erythematosus, DIC, and inherited deficiencies

    o. **Fibrinogen**
      1) Increased: inflammatory process, pregnancy, and contraceptive use
      2) Decreased: hereditary disorders (afibrinogenemia) and DIC

    p. **C-reactive protein (CRP)**
      1) Increased: tissue necrosis, rheumatic fever, bacterial infections, myocardial infarction, rheumatoid arthritis, carcinomatosis, gout, and viral infections

    q. **Immunoglobulins**
      1) 5 major groups: IgA, IgD, IgE, IgG, and IgM
      2) Synthesized in plasma cells
      3) IgG increased: liver disease, infection, and collagen disease

       4) IgG decreased: monoclonal gammopathies of another group

       5) IgA increased: liver disease, infections, and autoimmune diseases

       6) IgA decreased: depressed protein synthesis, ataxia-telangiectasia, and hereditary immune disorders

       7) IgM increased: toxoplasmosis, cytomegalovirus, rubella, herpes, syphilis, various bacterial and fungal diseases, and Waldenström's macroglobulinemia

       8) IgM decreased: protein-losing conditions and immunodeficiency diseases

       9) IgD increased: infections, liver disease, and connective tissue disorders

     10) IgE increased: allergies, asthma, and hay fever

  r. **Myoglobin**

       1) Elevated; muscle damaging disorders, i.e., rhabdomyolysis

  s. **Hypoproteinemia**

       1) **Causes:** increased urinary excretion, gastrointestinal tract inflammation, liver disorders, inherited immunodeficiency disorders, and loss of blood in open wounds, internal bleeding, or extensive burns

  t. **Hyperproteinemia**

       1) **Causes:** dehydration, increased protein production, and chronic diseases

3. **Test methodology**

  a. **Refractometry**

       1) Velocity of light is changed as it passes through the boundary between 2 transparent layers and the light is bent.

  b. **Biuret**

       1) **Principle:** cupric ions complex with the peptide bonds in an alkaline medium producing a purple-colored complex. The amount of purple complex produced is directly proportional to the number of peptide bonds present and reflects the amount of protein.

  c. **Dye binding**

       1) The protein binds to the dye and causes a shift in the maximum absorbance of the dye. The increase in absorbance is used to determine protein concentration.

  d. **Quantitating specific proteins**

       1) **Globulins** = total protein − albumin

       2) **Albumin**

          a) Dye binding principle: albumin binds to the dye and shifts the absorption maximum of the free dye. The amount of shift is proportional to the amount of albumin present. Bromcresol green dye and bromcresol purple are most common.

       3) **Electrophoresis**

          a) **Separates proteins** on the basis of electrical charge. Proteins move according to their net charge, which is determined by the pH of the surrounding buffer.

b) The speed of the migration is based on the degree of ionization of the protein in a particular buffer.

c) **Serum protein electrophoresis:** serum is applied close to the cathode end of a gel saturated with a buffer of pH = 8.6. All serum proteins migrate toward the anode with albumin traveling the farthest, followed by α_1-globulins, α_2-globulins, β-globulins, and γ-globulins. The proteins are fixed, stained, then quantitated using a densitometer.

d) **High resolution protein electrophoresis** uses a higher voltage, a cooling system, and a more concentrated buffer to separate proteins into as many as 12 zones. The most common support used is agarose gel.

4) Immunochemical protein quantitation (*see* Chapter 5)

a) **Radial immunodiffusion (RID)**

b) **Immunofixation**

c) **Electroimmunodiffusion**

5) **Turbidimetry and nephelometry (see Section VI, Nephelometry)**

a) Use light scattering to measure the amount of light scattering by the antibody-antigen complexes.

6) **Isoelectric focusing (IEF)**

a) Zone electrophoresis that separates proteins at their isoelectric point.

b) **Isoelectric point** is where the pH of the gel equals the isoelectric point of the protein (where the protein is neutral).

c) **Clinical applications:** phenotyping α_1-antitrypsin deficiencies, determining genetic variations of enzymes and hemoglobins, detection of paraproteins in serum, and oligoclonal bands in CSF.

G. Cholesterol Test Methodology

1. **Regulation**

   a. Cholesterol concentrations in the body are regulated by a feedback mechanism—increased dietary cholesterol tends to slow cholesterol synthesis.

2. **Clinical significance**

   a. The body uses cholesterol extensively—cell membranes, lipoproteins, and bile acids to mention a few uses.

   b. **Elevated cholesterol concentrations have been linked to atherosclerosis, coronary artery disease, and increased risk for myocardial infarction.**

   c. Decreased cholesterol levels are present in various forms of liver disease—most notably alcoholic cirrhosis.

3. **Test Methodology**

   a. **Reference method: Lieberman-Burchard**

Sulfuric acid + acetic acids + acetic anhydride + cholesterol → Complex with a blue-green color

   b. **Enzymatic**

Cholesterol ester + H_2O $\xrightarrow{\text{cholesterol esterase}}$ cholesterol + fatty acid

$$\text{Cholesterol} + O_2 \xrightarrow{\text{cholesterol oxidase}} \text{cholesterol} + H_2O_2$$

$$H_2O_2 + \text{ethanol} \xrightarrow{\text{catalase}} \text{acetyaldehyde} + 2H_2O$$

$$\text{Acetyldehyde} + \text{NADP} \xrightarrow{\text{aldehyde dehydrogenase}} \text{acetaldehyde} + \text{NADPH}$$

    4. **Reference range:** male: 146–270 mg/dL; female: 140–242 mg/dL

H. Triglyceride

1. **Regulation**
   a. Transported by chylomicrons
   b. Broken down by lipoprotein lipases
2. **Clinical significance**
   a. Increased in Fredrickson's Type I, IIb, IV, and V hyperlipoproteinemias, pancreatitis, alcoholism, obesity, hypothyroidism, nephrotic syndrome, and storage diseases (Gaucher's, Niemann-Pick)
3. **Test methodology**

$$\text{Triglyceride} + 3\ H_2O \xrightarrow{\text{lipase}} \text{Glycerol} + 3 \text{ fatty acids}$$

$$\text{Glycerol} + \text{ATP} \xrightarrow{\text{glycerol kinase}} \text{glycerol-3-phosphate} + \text{ADP}$$

$$\text{Glycerol-3-phosphate} + O_2 \xrightarrow{\text{glycerophosphate oxidase}}$$
$$\text{dihydroxyacetone-phosphate} + H_2O_2$$

$$H_2O_2 + \text{Dye} \xrightarrow{\text{peroxidase}} \text{colored product} + H_2O$$

    4. **Reference range**: male: 50–321 mg/dL; female: 52–262 mg/dL

I. HDL Measurement

1. **Regulation:** HDL is produced by the liver and intestine and is secreted into the plasma.
2. **Clinical significance**
   a. HDL decreases the atherosclerotic process. Increased HDL decreases the risk of coronary artery disease, and decreased HDL increases the risk of coronary artery disease.
3. **Test methodology**
   a. Precipitation with dextran sulfate (50,000 MW recommended) or heparin-manganese chloride, then test for total cholesterol present. Cholesterol present is HDL.
4. **Reference range**: male: 28–75 mg/dL; female: 33–92 mg/dL

J. LDL

1. **Regulation**: the exact mechanism of regulation is not known, but LDL is synthesized in the liver.
2. **Clinical significance: LDL is directly associated with artherosclerosis and coronary heart disease.**
3. **Test methodology**
   a. **Friedwald formula** (indirect; not valid for triglycerides over 400 mg/dL):

$$\text{LDL cholesterol} = \text{total cholesterol} -$$
$$[\text{HDL cholesterol} + \text{triglycerides}/5]$$

   b. Direct LDL cholesterol by Sigma.

   c. **Reference range**: male: 70–186 mg/dL; female: 71–206 mg/dL

K. Apo A-1, Apo B, and Lp(a)

1. **Regulation**
   a. Since the apolipoproteins are integral parts of lipoprotein molecules, they are regulated by the amount of lipoproteins in the blood.
   b. Lp(a) is inherited and is regulated by synthesis in the liver.

2. **Clinical significance**
   a. **Apo A-1** is the major protein found in HDL. It is thought to activate lecithin-cholesterol acyltransferase (LCAT) and remove free cholesterol from extrahepatic tissues.
   b. **Apo B** is the major protein found in all lipoproteins except HDL. It is associated with increased risk of coronary artery disease.
   c. **Lp(a)** is an independent risk factor associated with impaired plasminogen activation and thus decreased fibinolysis. A high level suggests increased risk for stroke and myocardial infarction.

3. **Test methodology**
   a. Apo-A, Apo-B, and Lp(a) are measured by immunochemical methods

4. **Reference range**
   a. Apo-A: 120–160 mg/dL
   b. Apo-B: < 120 mg/dL
   c. Lp(a): < 30 mg/dL

L. Glucose

1. **Regulation:** glucose is regulated by insulin and glucagons (see Section XXV, B).

2. **Clinical significance:** an increased blood glucose level the hallmark of diabetes mellitus, but can also indicate Cushing's disease and other hormonal problems.

3. **Test methodology**
   a. **Glucose oxidase**

   $$\beta\text{-glucose} + O_2 \xrightarrow{\text{glucose oxidase}} \text{D-glucono-}\delta\text{-lactone} + H_2O_2$$

   $$H_2O_2 + \text{reduced dye} \xrightarrow{\text{peroxidase}} \text{oxidized dyes (colored)}$$

   b. **Glucose hexokinase**

   $$\text{Glucose} + \text{ATP} \xrightarrow[\text{Mg}^{++}]{\text{hexokinase}} \text{Glucose-6-PO}_4 + \text{ADP}$$

   $$\text{Glucose-6-PO}_4 + \text{NADP}^+ \xrightarrow{\text{glucose-6-phosphate dehydrogenase}}$$
   $$\text{6-phosphogluconate} + \text{NADPH} + H^+$$

4. **Reference range: fasting** 70–115 mg/dL

M. BUN

1. **Regulation:** blood urea nitrogen (BUN) is the major nitrogen-containing compound resulting from protein catabolism. Almost all the urea is excreted through and regulated by the kidneys (90%).

2. **Clinical significance:** increased BUN: glomerular, tubular, interstitial, or vascular damage such as kidney stones and kidney disease.

3. **Test methodology**
   a. **Berthelot's reaction**

   $$\text{urea} + 2\,H_2O + H^+ \xrightarrow{\text{urease}} (NH_4)_2CO_3 + H^+ \rightarrow 2NH_4 + HCO_3^-$$

   $$NH_4 + OH^- \rightarrow NH_3 + H_2O$$

   NH_3 + NaOCl + 2phenol (alkaline medium with sodium nitroprusside)
   $\rightarrow$ indolphenol

   b. **Fearon reaction**

   diacetyl monoxime + H_2O $\rightarrow$ diacetyl + hydroxylamine
   diacetyl + urea (acid medium) $\rightarrow$ diazine derivative

4. **Reference range: 7–18 mg/dL**

N. Uric Acid

1. **Regulation:** uric acid is the major waste product from adenosine and guanosine, and it is regulated by the kidney.
2. **Clinical significance:** uric acid increased: renal failure, myeloproliferative disorders, hypothyroidism, poisons, and organic aciduria.
3. **Test methodology**
   a. **Carraway method**

   uric acid + phosphotungstic acid + O_2 $\rightarrow$
   allantoin + CO_2 + tungsten blue

   b. **Uricase method**

   uric acid $\xrightarrow{\text{uricase}}$ allantoin + H_2O_2 + CO_2

4. **Reference range: 3.5–7.2 mg/dL**

O. Creatinine

1. **Regulation:** creatinine levels are regulated by kidney excretion.
2. **Clinical significance:** increased creatinine levels are associated with renal disease and renal failure.
3. **Test methodology**
   a. **Jaffe reaction**

   creatinine + picric acid (alkaline solution) $\rightarrow$
   creatinine picrate (red tautomer)

   b. **Enzymatic reaction**

   creatinine + H_2O $\xrightarrow{\text{creatinine amidohydrolase}}$ creatine

   creatine + H_2O $\xrightarrow{\text{creatine amidohydrolase}}$ sarcosine + urea

   sarcosine + O_2 $\xrightarrow{\text{sarcosine oxidase}}$ glycine + formaldehyde + H_2O_2

   H_2O_2 + dye $\xrightarrow{\text{peroxidase}}$ colored dye + H_2O

4. **Reference range: 0.7–1.2 mg/dL**

P. Na, K, Cl, CO$_2$

1. **Regulation:** electrolytes are regulated by the kidneys and the lungs.
2. **Clinical significance** (see Section XXI Electrolytes and Water Balance, B Electrolytes)
3. **Test methodology**
   a. All measured by ion selective electrodes (**ISE**).
4. **Reference range:**
   K^+: 3.5–5.1 mmol/L
   Na^{++}: 135–145 mmol/L

XVI. ENZYMES

A. General Properties

1. **Definition: biological catalysts** that appear in the serum in increased amounts after cellular injury or tissue damage.
2. **Isoenzyme:** different forms of the same enzyme that exist in the body.
3. **Cofactor:** a nonprotein compound that may be necessary for enzyme activity.
4. **Activators:** nonorganic enzyme activators such as Mg or CL.
5. **Coenzyme:** organic cofactor.
6. **Prosthetic group:** organic cofactor tightly bound to the enzyme.

B. Enzyme Kinetics

1. **Activation energy:** energy required to raise all molecules to the transition state in a chemical reaction so that products may be formed.
2. **Enzymes** increase the speed of chemical reactions by **providing an alternate pathway** that requires a lower activation energy to reach the product stage.

C. Factors That Influence Enzyme Reactions

1. **Substrate concentration**
   a. The **substrate:** binds to free enzyme at low substrate concentration. As long as the enzyme exceeds the amount of substrate, the reaction rate increases as more substrate is added. The reaction is directly proportional to substrate concentration **(first-order kinetics)**.
   b. When the **substrate** concentration is high enough to bind with all available enzyme, the reaction velocity is at its maximum and when the product is formed, the enzyme reacts with more substrate **(zero order kinetics)**.
2. **Enzyme concentration:** as long as the substrate concentration exceeds the enzyme concentration, the velocity of the reaction is proportional to the enzyme concentration.
3. **pH:** this variable must be controlled very carefully because extreme pHs can denature an enzyme, change its ionic state and possibly its active site, and change its activity completely.
4. **Temperature:** increasing the temperature increases the rate of a chemical reaction by increasing molecular energy. Enzymes have optimal reaction temperatures which is usually 37°C.
5. **Inhibitors**
   a. A substance that **interferes** with an enzyme-catalyzed reaction.
   b. **Competitive inhibitor:** compete with substrate for the active site. This inhibition is reversible.
   c. **Noncompetitive inhibitor:** binds with the enzyme at a site other than the active site and prevents the enzyme catalyzed reaction from taking place. This inhibition may be reversible or irreversible. It may be irreversible if it destroys part of the enzyme or renders the active site inaccessible.
   d. **Uncompetitive inhibitor:** binds to the enzyme-substrate complex so that increasing the substrate concentration leads to more enzyme-substrate complexes and more inhibition.

D. Measuring Enzyme Activity

1. Enzyme reactions are performed in **zero-order kinetics**, with enough substrate in excess to ensure only 20 percent is converted to product.
2. It is extremely important in enzyme reactions that the pH, temperature, and additives (i.e., cofactors, coenzymes, activators) **remain constant.**
3. There are **two methods** used to measure enzyme reactions: end-point and kinetic.
   a. **Endpoint:** these reactions combine reactants and at a fixed time (i.e., 5 minutes) the products are measured. Concentration of the enzyme is based on the final absorbance reading.
   b. **Kinetic:** these reactions combine reactants, then measure the change in absorbance at specific time intervals (i.e., 30 seconds) over a specific time interval. Concentration of the enzyme is based on the change in absorbance over time.

E. Calculation of Enzyme Activity

1. Enzymes are reported in activity units because they are reported relative to their activity instead of their true concentration.
2. **International unit:** the amount of enzyme that will catalyze the reaction of one micromole of substrate per minute under specified conditions of temperature, pH, substrates, and activators.

F. Specific Enzymes

1. **Creatine kinase (CK) and CK isoenzymes**
   a. **Regulation**
      1) CK is regulated by excretion by the kidneys. CK concentration is influenced by sex, muscle mass, physical activity, and race.
      2) CK isoenzymes are regulated by the cells that break down and liberate these isoenzymes into the blood.
         a) CK consists of two subunits: M for muscle and B for brain.
         b) Each CK isoenzyme is a dimer with three possible types: CK-MM, CK-BB, and CK-MB.
   b. **Clinical significance**
      1) Elevations of CK and CK isoenzymes are summarized in the following table:

Disease	Total CK	CK-MM	CK-BB	CK-MB
Muscular dystrophy	Increased	Increased	Normal	Small increase
Viral myositis	Increased	Increased	Normal	Small increase
Polymyositis	Increased	Increased	Normal	Small increase
Myasthenia gravis	Normal	Normal	Normal	Normal
Multiple sclerosis	Normal	Normal	Normal	Normal
Poliomyelitis	Normal	Normal	Normal	Normal
Malignant hyperthermia	Increased	Increased	Normal	Small increase
Crush injuries	Increased	Increased	Normal	Small increase
Strenuous exercise	Increased	Increased	Normal	Small increase
Paroxysmal myoglobinuria	Increased	Increased	Normal	Small increase
Myocardial infarction	Increased	Normal	Normal	Increased
Cardiac surgery	Increased	Normal	Normal	Increased
Subarachnoid hemorrhage	Increased	Normal	Increased	Normal
Reye's syndrome	Increased	Normal	Increased	Normal

    c. **Test methodologies**
      1) **CK isoenzymes**
        a) **Measured by** electrophoresis, ion-exchange chromatography, ELISA, and RIA.
      2) **Oliver-Rosalki CK test methodology**

$$\text{Creatine phosphate} + \text{ADP} \xrightarrow{\text{CK}} \text{creatine} + \text{ATP}$$

$$\text{ATP} + \text{glucose} \xrightarrow{\text{hexokinase}} \text{ADP} + \text{glucose-6-phosphate}$$

$$\text{Glucose-6-phosphate} + \text{NADP}^+ \xrightarrow{\text{glucose-6-phosphate dehydrogenase}} \text{6-phosphogluconate} + \text{NADPH}$$

        a) **Sources of error** include hemolyzed serum.
    d. **Reference range:** male: 15–160 IU/L; female: 15–130 IU/L.

2. **Aspartate aminotransferase (AST)**
    a. **Highest concentrations:** cardiac tissue, liver, and skeletal muscle.
    b. AST is used to evaluate acute myocardial infarction (AMI), **hepatocellular disorders,** and skeletal muscle disorders.
    c. In **AMI,** AST rises within 6 to 8 hours, peaks at 24 hours, then returns to normal within 5 days.
    d. **AST is usually elevated in pulmonary embolisms,** extremely elevated in **liver disease** (100 times normal in viral hepatitis and 4 times normal in cirrhosis), **skeletal muscle disorders,** and **inflammatory** conditions.
    e. **Assay**

$$\text{aspartate} + \alpha\text{-ketoglutarate} \xrightarrow{\text{AST}} \text{oxaloacetate} + \text{glutamate}$$

$$\text{Oxaloacetate} + \text{NADH} + \text{H}^+ \xrightarrow{\text{malate dehydrogenase}} \text{malate} + \text{NAD}^+$$

    f. Sources of error-hemolyzed serum.
    g. Reference range: 5–30 IU/L.

3. **Alanine aminotransferase** (ALT)
    a. High concentrations in the **liver**.
    b. **Diagnostic significance:** liver disorders, hepatocellular disorders (hepatitis, cirrhosis) are higher than intra- or extrahepatic obstruction.
    c. **Assay**

$$\text{Alanine} + \alpha\text{-ketoglutarate} \xrightarrow{\text{ALT}} \text{pyruvate} + \text{glutamate}$$

$$\text{Pyruvate} + \text{NADH} + \text{H}^+ \xrightarrow{\text{LD}} \text{lactate} + \text{NAD}^+$$

    d. **Sources of error**—none.
    e. **Reference range**: 6–37 IU/L.

4. **Alkaline phosphatase (ALP)**
    a. **Highest concentrations** found in intestines, liver, bone, spleen, placenta, and kidney.
    b. **Clinical significance**
      1) Increased: hepatobiliary and bone disorders; in hepatobiliary disorders, the increased levels are due to obstructive disorders.

    2) **In biliary tract obstruction**, ALP levels are 3 to 10 times normal

    3) **Highest elevations** of ALP: Paget's disease.

    4) ALP levels **decreased:** hypophosphatasia.

    5) ALP levels are also increased in children and the elderly.

  c. **Assay**

$$p\text{-nitrophenylphosphate} \xrightarrow{\text{ALP}} \text{p-nitrophenol + phosphate ion}$$
$$\text{(colorless)} \qquad\qquad\qquad \text{(yellow)}$$

    1) **Sources of error:** hemolysis

    2) **Reference range:** 30–90 IU/L

5. **Acid phosphatase (ACP)**

  a. Found in high concentrations in the **prostate**

  b. **Clinical significance**

    1) Diagnosing prostate cancer.

    2) More common in men over 50 years of age; classified in **4 stages**: **stage A and stage B** tumors are **confined** to the prostate; **stage C has spread beyond the prostate**, but is still in the pelvic area, and **stage D is metastatic**.

$$\text{Prostatic ACP} = \text{Total ACP} - \text{ACP after tartrate inhibition}$$

  c. **Assay**

$$p\text{-nitrophenylphosphate} \xrightarrow{\text{ACP}} \text{p-nitrophenol + phosphate ion (pH = 5)}$$

    1) **Sources of error:** separate serum from clot ASAP because RBCS and platelets contain ACP.

    2) **Reference range:** total ACP: males: 2.5–11.7 IU/L; females: 0.3–9.2 IU/L. Prostatic ACP: males: 0.2–5.0 IU/L; females: 0.0–0.8 IU/L.

6. **Gamma-glutamyltransferase**

  a. **Increased** levels in all **hepatobiliary** diseases.

  b. Higher levels observed in biliary tract obstruction.

  c. **Sensitive indicator of alcoholism:** enzyme elevations are from 2 to 3 times normal.

  d. Levels can be increased in pancreatitis, diabetes mellitus, and AMI.

  e. **Assay**

$$\gamma\text{-Glutamyl-}p\text{-nitroanilide + glycylglycine}$$
$$\xrightarrow{\text{GGT}} \gamma\text{-Glutamyl-glycylglycine + }p\text{-nitroaniline}$$

  f. **Reference range**: male: 6–45 IU/L; female: 5–30 IU/L.

7. **Amylase**

  a. Serum amylase produced by pancreas and salivary glands.

  b. **Clinical significance**

    1) **Diagnosis: acute pancreatitis**.

    2) **Increased:** mumps, perforated peptic ulcer, intestinal obstruction, cholecystitis, ruptured ectopic pregnancy, mesenteric infection, and acute appendicitis.

    3) Amylase has **isoenzymes** originating from the pancreas (P type) and the salivary glands (S type).

    c. **Assay**
- 1) **Amyloclastic:** measures the decrease in the starch substrate.
- 2) **Saccharogenic:** measures the increase of the product produced (maltose).
- 3) **Chromogenic:** measures the increase of the product that is coupled with a chromogenic dye.
- 4) **Enzymatic:** combines several enzyme assays to monitor activity.

    d. **Reference range:** serum: 95–290 IU/L; urine: 35–400 IU/h.

8. **Lipase**
- a. **Hydrolyses dietary triglycerides**
- b. **Clinical significance:** confirms diagnosis of acute pancreatitis
- c. **Assay**

$$\text{triglyceride} + 2H_2O \xrightarrow{\text{LPS}} \text{2-monoglyceride} + \text{2 fatty acids}$$

- d. **Reference range:** 0–1.0 U/L

9. **Cholinesterase**
- a. Group of two enzymes: **acetylcholinesterase (AChE)** and **pseudocholinesterase (SChE)**
- b. **Clinical significance**
  - 1) **Pseudocholinesterase:** indicator of complications in hepatocellular disease and of prognosis in cancer
  - 2) Decreased SChE: fertilizer and insecticide poisonings
- c. **Assay**

$$\text{butyrylthiocholine} \xrightarrow{\text{SChE}} \text{thiocholine} + \text{butyric acid}$$

$$\text{thiocholine} + \text{5,5'-dithiobis-(2-nitrobenzoic acid)} \longrightarrow$$
$$\text{5-thio-nitrobenzoic acid}$$

  - 1) **Sources of error:** hemolysis
  - 2) **Reference range:** acetylcholine: 4.7–11.8 IU/mL

10. **Glucose-6-Phosphate Dehydrogenase (G-6-PD)**
- a. **Very little G-6-PD** in healthy individual's serum
- b. **Clinical significance**
  - 1) **Deficiency:** RBC hemolysis
  - 2) **Increased:** megaloblastic anemias and AMI
- c. **Assay**

$$\text{Glucos-6-phosphate} + NADP^+ \xrightarrow{\text{G-6-PD}}$$
$$\text{6-phosphogluconate} + NADPH + H^+$$

- d. **Reference range:** serum 0–0.18 IU/L

11. **Lactate dehydrogenase (LD)**

$$\text{Lactate} + NAD^+ \xrightarrow{\text{LD}} \text{pyruvate} + NADH + H^+$$

- a. **Clinical significance**
  - 1) **Elevated:** cardiac, hepatic, or skeletal muscle disease
  - 2) **Highest elevation:** pernicious anemia
- b. **Sources of error:** hemolyzed serum
- c. **Reference range:** 100–225 IU/L

XVII. THERAPEUTIC DRUG MONITORING

  A. **Definition**—evaluation (including analysis and interpretation) of circulating concentrations of drugs.

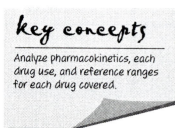

key concepts

Analyze pharmacokinetics, each drug use, and reference ranges for each drug covered.

B. **Purpose**—to establish maximum benefits with minimal side effects for drugs whose correlation between dosage and effect or toxicity is weak.

C. **Routes of Administration**—IV (intravenous), IM (intramuscular), and oral.

D. **Absorption**
   1. **Liquids absorbed more quickly** than oral route.
   2. Most are **absorbed consistently from GI tract** in healthy people.
   3. **First-pass metabolism:** all drugs absorbed from the GI tract must go through the liver before entering the general circulation.

E. **Free vs. Bound Drug**
   1. Only **free drugs** can **interact with target sites and produce a response**.
   2. **Therapeutic range:** range of drug concentration that produces benefits.
   3. **Free drug measurements** need to be considered for highly protein bound drugs or when clinical response is inconsistent with total drug concentrations.

F. **Drug Distribution**
   1. **Free drugs can diffuse into interstitial and intercellular spaces.** This occurs with hydrophobic or lipid soluble drugs
   2. **Polar drugs** (not ionized) diffuse easily out of circulation but do not gather in the lipid compartments.

G. **Drug Elimination**
   1. Hepatic metabolism, renal filtration, or both methods eliminate drugs.
   2. **Hepatic metabolism:** main mechanism converts drugs to water soluble substances, and the body eliminates them through the kidneys.
   3. **Renal clearance:** drug clearance is directly proportional to the creatinine clearance rate.

H. **Pharmacokinetics**
   1. **Definition:** mathematical model of changes in blood concentrations of drugs.
   2. **As a drug enters circulation, it is already being metabolized and secreted.** To increase serum concentration, concentrations of a drug must exceed elimination and metabolism.
   3. **Drugs are usually administered on a scheduled basis,** and this produces a high and low variation in drug concentration. The aim is to keep the level from dropping below a concentration that does not produce therapeutic benefits and to keep the concentration from rising above the toxic level. 5–7 doses are required to achieve a steady state.

I. **Sample Collection**
   1. **Sample collection timing is critical in therapeutic drug monitoring.**
   2. **Trough levels** are drawn right before next dose.
   3. **Peak levels** are drawn:

a. 2 hours after oral administration

b. 1 hour after intramuscular administration

c. 0.5 hours after completion of IV administration

J. Cardiovascular Drugs

1. **Digoxin**

a. Cardiac glycoside use to treat **congestive heart failure.**

b. Therapeutic range: 0.2–2.0 ng/dL.

c. **Mechanism:** inhibits membrane Na^+-K^+-ATPase that causes a decrease in intracellular K^+ and an increase in intracellular calcium. Increased calcium improves cardiac contraction.

d. **Toxicity symptoms:** nausea, vomiting, visual disturbances, premature ventricular contractions (PVCs), and atrioventricular node blockage.

e. Requires monitoring to ensure blood concentrations are therapeutic because absorption of the drug is variable.

f. **Serum concentrations at 8 hours after an oral dose** correlate with tissue concentrations.

2. **Lidocaine**

a. **Purpose:** correct ventricular arrhythmias and prevent ventricular fibrillation.

b. Usually given by **continuous IV administration** after a loading bolus because it is quickly removed from circulation by the liver.

c. **Therapeutic range:** 1.5–4 µg/mL.

d. **Toxicity:** 4–8 µg/mL = CNS depression; 8 µg/mL = seizures and severe hypotension.

3. **Quinidine**

a. **Purpose:** correct cardiac arrhythmias.

b. **Peak serum concentrations** occur 2 hours after oral ingestion.

c. **Toxic symptoms:** nausea, vomiting, abdominal discomfort, and PVCs.

d. Usually only the trough level is monitored to ensure achievement of therapeutic levels.

e. **Therapeutic range:** 2–5 µg/mL.

4. **Procainamide**

a. **Purpose**: treat cardiac arrhythmias, tachycardia.

b. **Peak levels** at 1 hour after ingestion.

c. **Increased levels** cause cardiac depression and arrhythmia.

d. **Must assess procainamide and N-acetyl procainamide** (metabolite) when assessing serum concentration because both drug and metabolite produce same activity of heart.

e. **Therapeutic range**: 4–8 µg/mL.

5. **Disopyramide**

a. **Purpose:** treat cardiac arrhythmias.

b. **Therapeutic range:** 3–5 µg/mL.

c. **Toxic symptoms:** at > 4.5 µg/mL, anticholinergenic effects (dry mouth and constipation) but at higher levels (> 10 µg/mL) bradycardia, atrioventricular node blockage.

K. Antibiotics

1. **Aminoglycosides**
   a. Includes gentamicin, tobramycin, kanamycin, and amikacin.
   b. **Purpose:** kill gram negative rods in conjunction with other drugs or alone.
   c. Nephrotoxicity and ototoxicity most common.
   d. Usually administered IV and IM.

2. **Vancomycin**
   a. **Purpose:** eliminate gram positive cocci.
   b. **Administered by IV** (oral vancomycin is given, but not monitored).
   c. **Therapeutic range:** 5–10 µg/mL.
   d. Toxic effects are "red-man syndrome" (erythemic flushing of extremities), nephrotoxicity, and ototoxicity.

L. Antiepileptic Drugs

1. **Phenobarbital**
   a. **Purpose:** slow-acting drug that controls seizures.
   b. Peak serum concentration occurs at **10 hours after an oral dose.**
   c. **Toxicity** effects are drowsiness, fatigue, depression, and reduced mental capacity.
   d. Mostly removed by **hepatic metabolism.**
   e. **Therapeutic range:** 10–40 µg/mL

2. **Phenytoin**
   a. **Purpose:** treat seizure disorders to keep the brain from swelling and injuring tissue during brain traumas.
   b. Toxic effects can occur within therapeutic range.
   c. Toxicity includes seizures, hirsutism, gingival hyperplasia, and vitamin D and folate deficiency.
   d. **Therapeutic range:** 1–2 µg/mL.
   e. **Fosphenytoin: injectable form of drug.**

3. **Valproic acid**
   a. **Purpose:** to treat petit mal and absence seizures.
   b. Eliminated by **hepatic metabolism.**
   c. **Therapeutic range:** 50–120 µg/mL
   d. **Toxic effects:** nausea, lethargy, weight gain, pancreatitis, hyperammonemia, and hallucinations associated with concentrations > 200 µg/mL.

4. **Carbamazepine**
   a. **Purpose:** treat seizure disorders.
   b. Eliminated by **hepatic metabolism.**
   c. **Therapeutic range:** 4–12 µg/mL.
   d. **Toxic effects:** rashes, leukopenia, nausea, vertigo, febrile reactions, aplastic anemia, mild liver dysfunction.

5. **Ethosuximide**
   a. **Purpose:** treats petite mal seizures.
   b. **Therapeutic range:** 40–100 µg/mL

M. Psyochoactive Drugs

1. **Lithium**

    a. **Purpose:** treat bipolar disorders.

    b. **Therapeutic range:** 0.8–1.2 mmol/L.

    c. **Toxic effects** at 1.2–2.0 mmol/L include apathy, lethargy, speech difficulties, and muscle weakness; at > 2.0 mmol/L there is muscle rigidity, seizures, and coma.

2. **Tricyclic antidepressants**

    a. **Purpose:** treat depression, insomnia, extreme apathy, and loss of libido.

    b. Includes **amitriptyline, imipramine, doxepin,** as well as the **metabolites desimpramine** and **nortriptyline.**

    c. **Peak concentrations** occur 2–12 hours after ingestion.

    d. **Therapeutic effects** occur after 2–4 weeks of therapy.

    e. **Toxic effects:** drowsiness, constipation, blurred vision, memory loss, seizure, cardiac arrythmia, and unconsciousness.

N. Bronchodilators

1. **Theophylline**

    a. **Purpose:** treat asthma and other chronic obstructive pulmonary disorders (COPD).

    b. **Therapeutic range:** 10–20 µg/mL, toxic > 20 g/mL.

    c. **Toxic effects:** nausea, vomiting, diarrhea, cardiac arrythmias, and seizures.

O. Immunosuppressive Drugs

1. **Cyclosporine**

    a. **Purpose:** suppress graft-versus-host disease in allogenic transplants.

    b. **Therapeutic range:** differs with organ transplanted; liver requires 300 ng/mL.

    c. **Toxic** at > 350 ng/mL and produces renal tubular and glomerular dysfunction.

2. **Tacrolimus**

    a. 100 times more potent than cyclosporine.

    b. Purpose: suppress graft vs. host disease in allogenic transplants

    c. Therapeutic range is variable.

XVIII. TOXICOLOGY

A. Definition—study of poisons.

B. Exposure to toxins may be due to suicide attempt, accidental exposure, or occupational exposure.

C. Routes of Exposure include ingestion, inhalation, and transdermal absorption.

D. Dose Response Relationship

1. **Central toxicology theme:** any substance can cause harm if enough is administered.

2. Toxicologists have developed a relative toxicity index to rate the potential harm a substance can cause.

3. **Toxic response:** the amount of damage done to an organism when the substance is administered at less than the lethal dose.

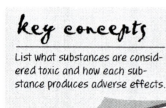

key concepts

List what substances are considered toxic and how each substance produces adverse effects.

E. Acute and Chronic Toxicity

1. **Acute toxicity:** a single, short-term exposure to a substance that causes a toxic response.
2. **Chronic toxicity:** repeated exposure for extended time periods at a dosage that will not cause an acute response.

F. Analysis of Toxic Agents

1. **Screening test performed first:** usually a qualitative procedure.
2. **Confirmatory test** is usually very specific and quantitative.

G. Toxicology of Specific Substances

1. **Alcohol**
   a. Effects are general and specific.
      1) **General:** disorientation, confusion, and euphoria that can lead to unconsciousness, paralysis, and death.
      2) **Specific**
         a) **Ethanol:** alcoholic hepatitis, cirrhosis
         b) **Methanol:** severe acidosis, blindness, and death
         c) **Isopropanol:** severe acute phase ethanol-like symptoms that last for a long period of time
         d) **Ethylene glycol:** severe metabolic acidosis and renal tubular damage
   b. Laboratory tests
      1) **Ethanol:** enzymatic, gas chromatography, and osmolality

         Enzymatic: ethanol + $NAD^+ \rightarrow$ acetaldehyde + NADH.

         a) Gas chromatography is the reference method.
         b) Osmolality: ethanol concentration is the difference between the calculated serum osmolality and the actual osmolality. This is called the **osmolal gap.** It is not specific for ethanol.

2. **Carbon monoxide**
   a. Toxic because it **binds very tightly to hemoglobin** and does not allow oxygen to attach to the hemoglobin. Forms carboxyhemoglobin.
   b. **Produces hypoxia in brain and heart.**
   c. **Analysis:** reference method is gas chromatography

3. **Caustic agents**
   a. **Aspiration causes** pulmonary edema, shock, and death.
   b. **Ingestion** leads to esophageal and GI lesions, producing hematemesis, abdominal pain, shock, and metabolic acidosis or alkalosis.

4. **Cyanide**
   a. **Supertoxic** substance because exposure can occur by inhalation, ingestion, or transdermal absorption.
   b. Used in industry and insecticides and rodenticides.
   c. **Mechanism:** binds to heme iron and mitochondrial cytochromes.
   d. **Symptoms** include headaches, dizziness, respiratory depression leading to seizures, coma, and death.

5. **Metals**
   a. **Arsenic**
      1) **Binds to thiol groups** in proteins.
      2) **Symptoms** are fever, anorexia, GI distress, peripheral and central nervous system damage, renal effects, hematopoietic effects, and vascular disease leading to death.
   b. **Cadmium**
      1) **Binds** to proteins and accumulates in the kidney.
      2) **Symptoms** are renal tubular dysfunction, tubular proteinemia, glucosemia, and amino aciduria.
   c. **Lead**
      1) **Binds** to proteins, thus changing the structures and functions, including inhibition of many enzymes.
      2) **Symptoms** are cerebral edema, hypoxia, stupor, convulsions, and coma.
      3) **Lab results** include decreased vitamin D, anemia, increased aminolevulinic acid and protophorphyrins, and basophilic stippling.
   d. **Mercury**
      1) **Exposure routes:** inhalation, ingestion.
      2) **Binds** to proteins and inhibits many enzymes.
      3) **Symptoms** include tachycardia, tremors, thyroiditis, glomerular proteinuria, and loss of tubular function.
   e. **Pesticides**
      1) **Contamination** of food is the major route of exposure, but **inhalation, transdermal** absorption, and ingestion due to hand-to-mouth contact are common.
      2) **Symptoms for organophosphates and carbamates** include salivation, lacrimation, involuntary urination and defecation, bradycardia, muscular twitching, cramps, apathy, slurred speech, behavioral changes, and death due to respiratory failure.

6. **Therapeutic drugs**
   a. **Salicylates**
      1) **Purpose:** analgesic, antipyretic, and anti-inflammatory.
      2) **Mechanism:** decreasing thromboxane and prostaglandin formation through inhibition of cyclooxygenase.
      3) **Toxic** effects at high dosages: metabolic acidosis, respiratory center stimulant, ketone body formation; can lead to death.
   b. **Acetaminophen**
      1) **Purpose:** analgesic
      2) **Toxic effect** at high dosages: liver necrosis
      3) **Alcoholic patients are very susceptible to acetaminophen toxicity**

7. **Toxicology of drugs of abuse**
   a. **Amphetamines**
      1) **Effects:** sense of increased mental and physical well-being, restlessness, irritability, and psychosis
      2) **Overdose symptoms:** hypertension, cardiac arrhythmias, convulsions, and death

    b. **Anabolic steroids**
       1) **Effects:** increases muscle mass and athletic performance.
       2) **Abuse effects:** toxic hepatitis, accelerated atherosclerosis, abnormal platelet aggregation, enlargement of the heart, cardiac arrhythmias, testicular atrophy, sterility, impotence, breast reduction, and development of masculine traits.
    c. **Cannabinoids**
       1) **Effects:** sense of well-being and euphoria, impairment of short-term memory and intellectual functions
       2) **Stored in fat cells**
       3) **Half-life of THC** (active ingredient) is 1 day after a single use and 3–5 days after chronic use.
       4) **THC-COOH** (urinary metabolite) is detectable in urine 3–5 days after a single use and up to 4 weeks after chronic use.
    d. **Cocaine**
       1) **Effects:** excitement and euphoria.
       2) **Acute toxic effects:** hypertension, arrhythmias, seizures, and myocardial infarction.
       3) **Urinary metabolites** can be detected in urine 3 days after a single use and 20 days after the last dose in heavy users
    e. **Opiates** (opium, morphine, codeine, heroin, dilaudid, and percodan, demerol, methadone, Darvon, Talwin, and Sublimaze)
       1) **Effects:** analgesic, sedation, and anesthesia.
       2) **Toxic symptoms:** respiratory acidosis, myoglobinuria, increase in CKMB and troponin, and death due to cardiopulmonary failure.
    f. **Phencyclidine (PCP)**
       1) **Effects:** stimulant, depressant, anesthetic, and hallucinogenic.
       2) **Toxic symptoms:** agitation, hostility, paranoia, stupor, and coma.
    g. **Tranquilizers** (barbituates, benzodiazepines, chlordiazepoxide, lorazepam)
       1) **Effect:** CNS depressants
       2) **Toxic symptoms:** lethargy, slurred speech, coma, respiratory depression, hypotension, and death.

XIX. TUMOR MARKERS—not very useful in diagnosis, but are useful in tumor staging, monitoring therapeutic responses, predicting patient outcomes, and detecting cancer recurrence. (*See* Chapter 5 Immunology and Serology, IV. D.)

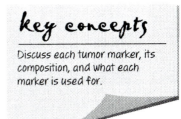

key concepts

Discuss each tumor marker, its composition, and what each marker is used for.

XX. ACID-BASE BALANCE—
A. Acid-Base Theory
    1. **Buffers:** pH varies little when a strong acid or strong base is added.
      a. The **bicarbonate buffer system** uses HCO_3^- and H_2CO_3 to minimize pH changes in the blood.
      b. The **phosphate buffer system** uses the HPO_4^{-2} and $H_2PO_4^-$ in the cell to minimize pH changes in the cell and the blood.

c. The **protein buffer system** uses plasma proteins to minimize pH changes in the blood.

d. The **hemoglobin buffer system** uses the hemoglobin in red blood cells and in plasma to minimize pH changes in the blood.

B. Basic Breathing Mechanisms

1. **Respiration:** process to supply cells with oxygen for metabolic processes and remove the carbon dioxide produced during metabolism.

2. **External respiration:** exchange of oxygen and carbon dioxide that occurs in the lungs.

3. **Internal respiration:** exchange of oxygen and carbon dioxide that occurs at the tissues.

4. **Inspiration:** active process of inhaling.

5. **Expiration:** passive process of exhaling. This process depends on the muscles, rib cartilage, and the elastic tissue of the lungs to contract readily after inspiration.

6. **Partial pressure:** in a mixture of gases, partial pressure is the amount of pressure contributed by each gas to the total pressure exerted by the mixture.

7. **Ventilation:** the physical process of taking air into the lungs and expelling air from the lungs.

8. **Gas exchange:** exchange of gases occurs in the alveoli when the hemoglobin releases the oxygen to the tissues and the hemoglobin also attaches to the carbon dioxide coming from the tissues. The reverse process happens in the lungs: the hemoglobin releases the carbon dioxide into the lungs and takes on the oxygen already in the lungs.

9. **Breathing is controlled by the respiratory control center.** Central chemoreceptors located in the medullary receptors in the brain stem and peripheral chemoreceptors located in the **carotid artery** and **aorta** stimulate involuntary increases in the breathing rate and depth through the medullary respiratory center in the brain stem. **Decreases or increases in** blood pH stimulate the chemoreceptors.

10. **Exchange of gases**
    a. The gradients in partial pressure of oxygen and carbon dioxide control movement of gases between the alveoli and the cells. Oxygen is brought into the lungs from the environment then transported to the cell to aid in cellular metabolism. Carbon dioxide is brought from the tissue to the lungs to be exhaled as a metabolic waste product.

    b. **Oxygen is transported by hemoglobin** present in red blood cells. The **three factors that control oxygen transport** are the pO_2, free diffusion of the oxygen across the alveolar membrane, and the affinity of the hemoglobin for the oxygen. Under normal circumstances, 95 percent of hemoglobin binds oxygen. When the pO_2 is $> 100–120$ mm Hg, 100 percent of hemoglobin binds to oxygen. That is, the hemoglobin is saturated with oxygen or the oxygen saturation is 100 percent. The oxygen saturation can be calculated using the following formula:

$$sO_2\% = [HbO_2] \text{ g/dL} / [Hb] \text{ g/dL} \times 100\%$$

c. When a person's oxygen saturation falls below 95 percent, either the patient is not getting enough oxygen or the patient does not have enough functional hemoglobin available to transport the oxygen. The amount of functional hemoglobin available in the blood can be altered due to decreased red blood cells or nonfunctional hemoglobin. **Nonfunctional hemoglobin** is carboxyhemoglobin, methemoglobin, sulfhemoglobin, or cyanmethemoglobin.

d. **Hypoxia** is decreased pO_2 and decreased sO_2 due to lack of oxygen while **cyanosis** is decreased sO_2 due to high concentrations of nonfunctional hemoglobin.

e. **Clinical significance of pO_2 levels in blood**

1) Increased values (>95%) are observed with supplemental oxygen.

2) Hypoxemia **results in decreased arterial oxygen.** Causes: decreased pulmonary diffusion, decreased alveolar spaces due to resection or compression, and poor ventilation/perfusion (due to obstructed airways—asthma, bronchitis, emphysema, foreign body, secretions).

3) Carbon dioxide is not transported as an undissolved gas, but instead is transported as bicarbonate, carbaminohemoglobin, and dissolved carbon dioxide. Even though these forms transport the carbon dioxide, they also serve as buffers to maintain pH. Carbon dioxide, pH, and pCO_2 are related according to the Henderson-Hasselbalch equation:

$$\textbf{pH} = \textbf{6.103} + \textbf{log } \textbf{[HCO}_3\textbf{]/0.306} \times \textbf{pCO}_2$$

If you know the concentration of bicarbonate and the pCO_2, then you can determine the pH.

f. **Clinical significance of carbon dioxide levels in blood**

1) **Hypercapnia** is increased pCO_2. Causes: decreased alveolar perfusion due to lung diseases, airway obstructions, or breathing CO_2-enriched air. The respiratory center can be depressed by drugs or impaired by poor muscle function, and this can also lead to CO_2 retention.

2) **Hypocapnia** is decreased pCO_2. Causes: increased alveolar perfusion due to abnormally fast rates of mechanically assisted breathing.

11. **Acid-Base Balance**

a. A physiologic balance where the rates of input and output of hydrogen ions are equal for a time interval. Acid-base balance involves balancing carbon dioxide and noncarbonic acids and bases in the blood.

b. The pH of plasma is a function of two independent variables: **the partial pressure of carbon dioxide—regulated by the lungs or** respiratory mechanism—**and the concentration of** bicarbonate (HCO₃)—regulated by the kidneys or renal mechanism.

1) **Respiratory mechanism** involves the speed and the depth of breathing.

2) **Renal mechanism** involves the amount of hydrogen ions excreted into the urine by the kidneys.

   a) **Respiratory mechanism: breathing affects blood pH.** If a person breathes **very slowly**, much carbon dioxide builds up in their lungs, causing more carbon dioxide to be dissolved in the blood. Breathing slowly builds up carbon dioxide in the lungs, turning to carbonic acid in the blood causing a low pH. Conversely, if a person breathes very fast, much carbon dioxide is released from the lungs and this causes the build up of bicarbonate (HCO_3^-) in the blood and the pH goes up.

   b) **Renal mechanism: kidney excretion affects blood pH.** Inorganic and organic acids can build up in the blood due to metabolic processes, and the **kidney affects the blood pH** by secreting or neutralizing the acids with bicarbonate ions. The kidney can also reduce the number of hydrogen ions excreted in response to the blood turning more basic. **By regulating the number of hydrogen ions that are excreted or retained**, the kidney also regulates other electrolytes because hydrogen ions can only be released if another positively charge ion is gained. The **sodium-hydrogen pump** in the kidney exchanges sodium ions for hydrogen ions.

c. **Dissolved carbon dioxide (cdCO₂):** bound carbonic acid and carbon dioxide dissolved in blood.

d. **pCO₂:** the partial pressure of carbon dioxide in blood that is measured in mm Hg.

e. **Total carbon dioxide:** the sum of bicarbonate and dissolved carbon dioxide concentrations.

f. **Base excess:** the **concentration of titratable base** when blood is titrated with a strong acid or base to a pH of 7.40 at a partial pressure of 40 mm Hg at 37°C. **Positive values** show small concentrations of noncarbonic acids. **Negative values** show large concentrations of noncarbonic acids.

12. **Acid-base disorders**

a. **Metabolic acid-base disorders** primarily involve **bicarbonate concentration**.

b. **Respiratory acid-base disorders** primarily involve dissolved **carbon dioxide concentration**.

c. **Acid-base disorders** are classified as **metabolic acidosis, metabolic alkalosis, respiratory acidosis,** and **respiratory alkalosis**.

d. **Metabolic acidosis (nonrespiratory): primary bicarbonate deficit.** Caused by:

1) **Organic acid production exceeds excretion rate.** Acids involved are acetoacetic acid, β-hydroxybutyric acid, and lactic acid: diabetic ketoacidosis.

2) **Reduced acid excretion due** to renal failure or tubular acidosis.

3) **Loss of bicarbonate due to diarrhea.** Bicarbonate is replaced by chloride, phosphate, sulfate, or other organic ions in an attempt to maintain electrical neutrality.

4) Classified as **normal anion gap acidosis** or **increased anion gap acidosis** (normal anion gap acidosis due to hypoaldosteronism, early renal failure; increased anion gap acidosis due to renal failure, ketoacidosis, salicylate intoxication (salicylate levels > 30 mg/dL).

5) **Compensatory mechanism:** respiratory compensation mechanism: a decreased pH triggers hyperventilation that eliminates carbonic acid and causes pCO_2 to decrease resulting as increase in pH.

6) **Laboratory findings:** bicarbonate, total carbon dioxide concentration, and pCO_2 are decreased. *Note:* In **diabetic ketoacidosis,** plasma **sodium,** and **potassium** are **decreased** because they are secreted along with the organic acids.

e. **Metabolic (nonrespiratory) alkalosis: primary bicarbonate excess caused by:**

1) **Ingestion** of excess alkali (antacids).

2) **Loss of hydrochloric acid** from stomach after vomiting, intestinal obstruction, or gastric suction.

3) **Decreased potassium level** in Cushing's syndrome, hyperaldosteronism, licorice intake, or low potassium intake.

4) **Renal bicarbonate retention.**

5) **Prolonged diuretic use.**

6) **Laxative use** and infusion of potassium-poor IV fluids

7) In **metabolic alkalosis,** the **bicarbonate concentration increases,** thus causing the pH to increase. If the pH increases above 7.55, tetany develops.

8) **Respiratory compensation mechanism:** the pH increase slows the person's breathing **(hypoventilation),** thus increasing the amount of CO_2 retained in the lungs. This increases the dissolved CO_2 in the blood, causing more carbonic acid to form. The carbonic acid lowers the pH.

9) **Laboratory findings**
   a) HCO_3 elevated
   b) $cdCO_2$ decreased
   c) pCO_2 decreased

f. **Respiratory acidosis: primary CO_2 excess (hypercapnia)**

1) **Inability of a person to exhale CO_2** through the lungs causing an increase of pCO_2. The increased pCO_2 forms carbonic acid in the blood which drops the pH—chronic obstructive pulmonary disease, emphysema, congestive heart failure, apnea.

2) **Renal compensatory mechanism:** the kidneys increase sodium-hydrogen exchange, ammonia formation, and bicarbonate retention. The increased bicarbonate concentration will raise the blood pH.

3) **Laboratory findings**

a) Dissolved CO_2: **elevated**

b) pCO_2: **elevated**

c) pH: **decreased**

g. **Respiratory alkalosis: primary CO_2 deficit (hypocapnia)**

1) **Decreased pCO_2: caused by** an increased rate or depth of respiration or both. Excessive exhalation of carbon dioxide reduces the pCO_2 and increases the pH in the blood. Anxiety, nervousness, excessive crying, salicylate intoxication.

2) The **renal compensatory mechanism** corrects respiratory alkalosis by excreting bicarbonate.

3) **Laboratory findings**

a) $cdCO_2$ **decreased**

b) pCO_2 **decreased**

c) **pH does not exceed 7.6**

4) Individuals at high altitudes chronically hyperventilate due to hypoxia and have lower pCO_2 values than people at sea level.

XXI. ELECTROLYTES AND WATER BALANCE

A. Colligative Properties

1. **Definition:** a property of a solution that is influenced by size and shape of the molecules, but not the individual composition. There are 4 types of colligative properties: boiling point, freezing point, osmotic pressure, and vapor pressure.

2. **Osmolality definitions**

a. **Osmosis:** water flow across a semipermeable membrane.

b. **Molality:** the number of moles of solute per kg of water.

c. **Osmolality:** the number of moles of particles per kg of water

d. **Osmometry:** measuring all particles or osmolality of a solution.

e. **Calculated osmolality = 2(Na) + glucose/20 + BUN/3.**

1) In healthy individuals, the **calculated osmolality** = the **measured osmolality.**

2) There can be an **osmolal gap** if the person has ingested toxins or alcohol. The osmolal gap can be used to estimate the concentration of alcohol in a person's blood.

3. **Measuring osmolality**

a. Measuring **urine osmolality** can measure the ability of the kidney to concentrate ions and indirectly the function of the kidney. **Major ions** measured by osmolality include **electrolytes, glucose,** and **urea.**

b. **Serum osmolality** is usually measured as a comparison for urine osmolality.

c. **Colloid osmotic pressure** measures only the effect on osmolality by large, essential proteins. Its major use is in detecting conditions leading to pulmonary edema.

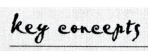

key concepts

Discuss the major electrolytes in the body, how they are measured, how they figure in osmolality, and the reference ranges for each.

    d. **Freezing point depression principle:** solutions cool, then expand when they freeze. By determining the freezing point of a solution, one can determine the amount of particles in that solution based on the freezing curve.

    e. **Vapor pressure** can also be used to measure osmolality: surface molecules in a liquid are in motion. Escaping molecules form a vapor above the liquid that is in equilibrium with liquid molecules. When solutes are added, less solvent can escape into the vapor phase.

B. Electrolytes

1. **Electrolytes:** charged ions that are found in intracellular fluid, extracellular fluid, and interstitial fluid.
2. **Intracellular fluid:** inside cells and contains predominantly potassium ions.
3. **Extracellular fluid:** outside the cells and contains predominantly sodium ions.
4. **Cations:** positively charged ions. Major cations in the body are Na, K, Ca, and Mg.
5. **Anions:** negatively charged ions. Major anions in the body are Cl, HCO_3, HPO_4, SO_4, organic acids, and protein.
6. **Sodium (Na^+)**
   a. **Major cation** of extracellular fluid.
   b. **Normal range:** 136–145 meq/L.
   c. **Changes in sodium** result in changes in plasma volume.
   d. **Largest** constituent of osmolality.
   e. **Helps** maintain acid-base balance through the Na-H pump.
   f. **Works** to excite nerves and muscles.
   g. **Regulation:** sodium is regulated by reabsorption in the proximal convoluted tubules by aldosterone.
   h. **Clinical significance**
      1) **Hyponatremia:** abnormally low sodium levels (< 136 mEq/L)
         a) **Depletional hyponatremia** can be due to diuretics, hypoaldosteronism, diarrhea, or vomiting, and also severe burns or trauma.
         b) **Dilutional hyponatremia** can be due to overhydration, syndrome of inappropriate antidiuretic hormone (SIADH), congestive heart failure, cirrhosis, and nephrotic syndrome.
         c) **Symptoms:** when sodium is >125 mEq/L, there are usually no symptoms. Symptoms occur when Na^+ is <125 mEq/L include nausea and malaise, then 110–120 mEq/L includes headache, lethargy, and obtundation. The severity of the neurologic symptoms are directly proportional to how fast the sodium and osmolality decrease. The severest symptoms occur at <110 mEq/L and include seizures and coma.
      2) **Hypernatremia** occurs when the sodium level is >145 mEq/L.

        a) Usually occurs when water is lost (as through vomiting or diarrhea, or excessive sweating) or sodium gain (as through acute ingestion or infusion of hypertonic solutions containing sodium)

        b) **Conn's syndrome** (primary hyperaldosteronism) results in increased sodium reabsorption and potassium excretion.

7. **Potassium**
   a. **Major** intracellular ion
   b. **Two major physiologic functions**
      1) Neuromuscular excitation
      2) Regulation of cellular processes
   c. **Regulation:** extracellular balance is maintained by the kidneys
   d. **Hypokalemia:** plasma potassium level is < 3.0 mEq/L.
      1) Decreased dietary intake.
      2) Excess insulin causes increased cellular uptake of potassium.
      3) Hyperaldosteronism, diuretics, and licorice ingestion cause renal losses of potassium.
      4) Vomiting, diarrhea, and laxative abuse cause excessive gastrointestinal losses.
      5) **Alkalosis: symptoms** include muscle weakness, paralysis, cramps, paresthesia, tetany, and polyuria. In severe hypokalemia, death can result from respiratory failure.
   e. **Hyperkalemia:** plasma potassium level is > 5.0 mEq/L.
      1) Increased intake of potassium.
      2) Increased cell lysis.
      3) Acidosis and insulin deficiency cause altered cellular uptake.
      4) Renal failure and hypoaldosteronism cause impaired renal excretion.
      5) Leukocytosis, thrombocytosis, and hemolysis cause pseudohyperkalemia.
      6) **Symptoms:** muscle weakness, abnormal cardiac conduction, or even cardiac arrest.
      7) Dehydration

8. **Chloride:** major extracellular anion of the body
   a. **Reference range:** 99–109 mEq/L (serum)
   b. **Major functions:** maintenance of fluid balance and osmotic pressure.
   c. Chloride levels change proportionally with sodium
   d. **Hypochloremia:** chloride < 99 mEq/L.
      1) Prolonged vomiting and nasogastric suctioning increase gastrointestinal losses.
      2) Diuretics and metabolic alkalosis increase renal losses.
      3) Burns also cause increased loss of chloride.
   e. **Hyperchloremia:** chloride < 109 mEq/L
      1) Prolonged diarrhea, loss of bicarbonate, and salicylate intoxication cause renal tubular acidosis and metabolic acidosis.
      2) Dehydration.

      3) Increased sweat chloride results (>35 mmol/L) in diagnostic of cystic fibrosis.

9. **Bicarbonate**
   a. Second largest anion fraction of the extracellular fluid.
   b. It is the major component of the bicarbonate buffer system in the blood.
   c. Decreases result in metabolic acidosis, while increases result in metabolic alkalosis.

10. **Anion gap:** a mathematical formula used to demonstrate the electroneutrality of the fluids.
    a. **Formula**

$$Na^+ - (Cl^- + HCO_3) = \text{anion gap}$$
$$(Na^+ + K^+) - (Cl^- + HCO_3^-) = 10\text{–}20 \text{ mmol/L}$$

   b. **Normal anion gap** is 8–16 meq/L.
   c. **Increased anion gaps** can be caused by
      1) Uremia
      2) Lactic acidosis
      3) Ketoacidosis
      4) Ingestion of methanol, ethylene glycol, salicylate
      5) Large doses of antibiotics
      6) Increased net protein charge
   d. **Decreased anion gaps** can be caused by
      1) Paraproteins
      2) Hypoalbuminemia, hypophosphatemia
      3) Dilution
      4) Increase in potassium, calcium, or magnesium

XXII. RENAL FUNCTION

A. Renal Anatomy

1. Kidneys: bean-shaped organs located on either side of the aorta.
2. Consist of 2 regions: **cortex** and **medulla.**
3. The pelvis is the cavity closest to the ureter where urine is excreted.
4. **Ureters** are thick tubes that connect the kidneys to the bladder.
5. Urine is stored in the **bladder**, then excreted through the **urethra.**
6. Microscopically, the **functional unit of the kidney is the nephron**—this is where blood is filtered and electrolytes balanced. It consists of 5 parts: glomerulus, proximal convoluted tubule, Loop of Henle, distal convoluted tubule, and collecting duct.
   a. **Glomerulus:** capillaries surrounded by Bowman's capsule. The blood to be cleaned goes into the glomerulus through one arteriole and leaves via another arteriole.
   b. **Proximal convoluted tubule** is in the cortex.
   c. **Loop of Henle** begins in the cortex, extends to the medulla, then ends in the cortex.
   d. **Distal convoluted tubule** is in the cortex.
   e. The **collecting duct** carries urine to the renal pelvis.

B. Renal Physiology

1. **Glomerular filtration:** filters blood.

key concepts

Discuss how the kidney filters the blood, where each substance is absorbed in the kidney, and the pathological states of the kidney and their corresponding laboratory values.

a. Large molecules (proteins, cells) stay in the arterioles, while smaller molecules (ions) continue into the nephron
b. These molecules go into the proximal convoluted tubules.
c. The **glomerular filtration rate** is amount of blood filtered per minute by the glomerulus.

2. **The proximal convoluted tubule** decides what molecules need to be reabsorbed and what molecules will be excreted.
   a. **Reabsorbs** 75 percent of water, Na, Cl, and uric acid, all glucose (up to renal threshold), amino acids, vitamins, proteins, Mg, Ca, and bicarbonate. The reabsorption process is active.
   b. **Secretes** hydrogen ions and drugs (i.e., penicillin).

3. **Loop of Henle**
   a. **Ascending loop: Na and Cl reabsorbed** here to decrease urine concentration.
   b. **Descending loop: water absorbed here** to increase urine concentration.
   c. **Urine leaves the loop** and goes into the distal convoluted tubules.

4. **Distal convoluted tubule**
   a. Filtrate that enters this tubule is almost ready to secrete.
   b. Tries to maintain electrolyte and acid-base balance.
   c. **Aldosterone** controls the reabsorption of sodium and secretion of potassium and hydrogen in this tubule.

5. **Collecting duct**
   a. Final site for making urine more dilute or concentrated.
   b. Upper portions controlled by **aldosterone:** Na, Cl, and BUN reabsorbed here.
   c. Also **controlled by ADH:** stimulates water absorption

C. Waste Excretion

1. **Urea:** by-product of protein metabolism
   a. Kidney: only way to excrete urea
   b. Rate of excretion depends on GFR, plasma renal flow, and urine flow rate.

2. **Creatinine**
   a. 20 percent of muscle creatine is converted to creatinine daily.
   b. **The concentration of creatinine is directly proportional to muscle mass and remains constant from day to day.**
   c. Not reabsorbed by the kidneys.

3. **Uric acid**
   a. Major waste product of purine metabolism
   b. Reabsorbed and secreted by the nephron
   c. Formed as sodium urate in urines with pH > 5.75
   d. Can cause stones in urines with pH < 5.75

D. Water Balance

1. Water loss through the kidney is regulated by ADH and increased osmolality stimulates ADH secretion.
2. During dehydration, renal tubules reabsorb water at a maximum rate, and urine becomes more concentrated.

3. During overhydration, water is not reabsorbed, and the urine is more dilute.

E. Electrolyte Balance

1. **Na**
   a. **Primary extracellular cation.**
   b. Excreted through **kidneys.**
   c. Mechanism for control is the renin-angiotensin-aldosterone system.
2. **K**
   a. **Primary intracellular cation.**
   b. Concentration controlled by **renal excretion** which is controlled by aldosterone.
3. **Cl**
   a. **Primary extracellular anion.**
   b. Maintains extracellular fluid balance.
   c. Chloride is **regulated** by the renin-angiotensin-aldosterone system.
4. **Phosphate, calcium, magnesium**
   a. **Phosphate**
      1) Present in equal amounts in intra- and extracellular compartments
      2) Balance determined by PTH
   b. **Ca**
      1) **Primary inorganic cellular messenger.**
      2) Ionized form reabsorption controlled by PTH.
      3) Main regulation occurs with PTH and calcitonin; control of bone resorption and absorption from the gut.
   c. **Mg**
      1) **Acts as enzyme cofactor.**
      2) PTH controls reabsorption in proximal tubule.

F. Acid-Base Balance

1. **Acid wastes excreted by the kidney include** carbonic acid, lactic acid, and ketoacids.
2. Maintains pH by reabsorbing bicarbonate or secreting acids.
3. **Regeneration of bicarbonate ions:** kidney generates bicarbonate ions to replace those lost by metabolism.
4. **Excretion of acids:** kidneys excrete excess hydrogen ions while making urine.
5. **Reaction with ammonia:** ammonia is combined with hydrogen ions in the kidney and excreted as the ammonium ion.
6. **Reactions with HPO_4^{-2}:** this compound combines with hydrogen ions and is excreted; can excrete until urine pH ≈ 4.4.

G. Endocrine Functions

1. **Renin**
   a. The juxtaglomerular cells of the renal medulla secrete renin in response to a decrease in extracellular fluid.
   b. **Function:** vasoconstrictor that increases the blood pressure.
2. **Prostaglandins**
   a. PGA_2, PGE_2, PGI_2, and PG_{12} are secreted.

b. **Function:** increase renal blood flow, sodium and water excretion, and renin concentration.

3. **Erythropoietin**
   a. Produced in **cortex.**
   b. **Regulated by oxygen levels** in the blood.
   c. **Function:** increase the number of red blood cells.

4. Aldosterone acts on the kidneys.

5. Vitamin D, insulin, glucagon, and aldosterone **metabolism occur in the kidney.**

H. Diagnostic Tests

1. **Creatinine clearance (*see* Chapter 1 Urinalysis and Body Fluids, III.B.2)**

2. **Urine protein tests**
   a. **Urine protein increased: renal absorption defects,** glomerular filtering problems, or increase in serum proteins.
   b. **Diseases with markedly increased urine proteins:** acute glomerular nephropathy, tubular proteinemia, multiple myeloma, Waldenström's macroglobulinemia, nephrotic syndrome, diabetes, or systemic lupus erythematosus (SLE).
   c. **Bence Jones proteins** are found in urines of patients with multiple myeloma.
   d. **β_2-microglobulinemia:** indicator of glomerular disease in intermediate diabetic nephropathy or renal transplant status.
   e. **Myoglobin:** early indicator of acute renal failure. Renal failure can be caused by significant cardiac or skeletal muscle injury or release of massive amounts of myoglobin into the blood.
   f. **Microalbumin**
      1) Monitors renal function in diabetics.
      2) Progressive treatment and strict glucose control in patients with elevated microalbumins can reduce the chances for the diabetic to develop end stage renal failure.
      3) **Special dipstick methods** have been developed to detect 10 μg/mL.

I. Diseases of the Kidney

1. **Acute glomerulonephritis**
   a. **Lab results**
      1) Hematuria
      2) Proteinuria (albumin) < 1 g/day
      3) Renal tubular epithelial
      4) Decreased glomerular filtration rate
      5) Anemia
      6) Increased BUN and creatinine
      7) Numerous hyaline, granular casts, and/or RBC casts
      8) Oliguria
   b. **Symptoms**
      1) Oliguria
      2) Water retention (swelling of ankles)
      3) Congestive heart failure

c. **Mechanism**

   1) Immune complexes (e.g., Group A beta Streptococci) settle on the glomerular basement membrane and trigger specific and nonspecific immune responses that damage the basement membrane.

   2) Other causes include drug exposures, SLE, and subacute bacterial endocarditis.

2. **Chronic glomerulonephritis** occurs from prolonged inflammation of the glomerulus, causing destruction of the nephrons. Uremia may be the first clinical sign.

   a. Lab results

      1) Increased RBCs, renal epithelial cells

      2) Increased proteinuria (> 2.5 q/day)

      3) Oliguria → anuria

3. **Nephrotic syndrome**

   a. **Mechanism:** increased permeability of the glomerulus

   b. **Lab results**

      1) **Massive proteinuria (> 3 g/day)**

      2) Hypoalbuminemia

      3) Hyperlipidemia

      4) Lipiduria

      5) Oval fat bodies, free fat

      6) Renal epithelial

   c. **Symptoms:** swelling of ankles, osmotically induced hypovolemia

   d. **Causes:** glomerular disease, SLE, renal vein thrombosis, syphilis, constrictive pericarditis, allergic/toxic reactions, carcinomas, amyloidosis, severe preeclampsia, or transplant rejection

4. **Tubular disease**

   a. **Renal tubular acidosis**

      1) **Distal renal tubular acidosis:** no pH gradient between blood and filtrate

      2) **Proximal renal tubular acidosis:** increased water reabsorption

         a) **Lab findings:** decreased serum phosphate and uric acid, positive glucose and amino acids in urine, WBC, RBCs, proteinuria (< 2g/day), oliguria, and renal function

         b) **Causes:** drug or x-ray toxicity, methicillin hypersensitivity reaction, transplant rejection, infections

5. **Urinary tract infection (UTI)/obstruction**

   a. **Infection**

      1) **Pyelonephritis:** kidney infection

         a) Lab findings: increased WBCs, bacteria, RBCs, renal epithelial

      2) **Cystitis:** bladder infection

         a) Lab findings: increased WBCs, bacteria, RBCs, transitional epithelium

      3) **Lab results:** positive nitrite (for some organisms), positive leukocyte esterase, positive occult blood, and WBC casts (diagnostic for pyelonephritis)

4) **Symptoms:** pain or burning on urination, back pain

b. **Obstruction**

1) **Mechanisms**

a) Increased intratubular pressure so nephrons die and chronic renal failure persists

b) Facilitate frequent UTIs

2) Located in the kidney (in nephrons, collecting ducts, or pelvis), in ureter, or in urethra

3) **Causes:** neoplasms, lymph node tumors, urethral strictures, stones, or congenital abnormalities

4) **Obstructions:** diagnosed by radiologic imaging

5) **Symptoms:** hematuria, extreme pain

6. **Kidney stones**

a. **Renal calculi** are formed by crystallization of organic and inorganic substances. Most common is calcium oxalate.

b. **Symptoms:** hematuria, extreme pain.

7. **Acute renal failure**

a. Definition: sudden decline in renal function due to an insult to the kidneys (GFR = < 10 mL/min)

b. **Prerenal failure**

1) Occurs in blood supply before reaching the kidneys

2) **Causes:** hypovolemia, tubular necrosis, vascular obstructions or inflammations, glomerulonephritis, congestive heart failure

c. **Postrenal failure**

1) Occurs after urine leaves kidney

2) **Causes:** lower urinary tract obstruction, i.e., kidney stone tumor or bladder rupture

d. **Acute kidney failure**

1) Toxic insult to kidney.

2) **Causes:** hemolytic transfusion reactions, heavy metal/solvent poisoning, antifreeze ingestion, analgesic and aminoglycoside toxicities, septic hemorrhagic shock, burns, and cardiac failure.

3) **Symptoms:** oliguria, anuria (< 400 mL/day). If more water retained than sodium, hyponatremia results with the ultimate symptoms being extreme drowsiness, seizures, coma, and death. Hyperkalemia may cause cardiac arrhythmias.

4) **Lab results:** RBC casts, hematuria, proteinuria, metabolic acidosis, uremic syndrome with increased BUN and increased creatinine.

e. **Chronic renal failure**

1) **Progressive disease** that causes a decline in renal function over time and progresses in 4 stages.

a) **1st stage:** BUN and creatinine stay normal while kidney function declines.

b) **2nd stage:** small decrease in renal function. 50 percent loss of function is when BUN and creatinine increase.

c) **3rd stage:** patient becomes acidotic and anemic.

d) **4th stage:** uremic syndrome begins (increased BUN, increased creatinine), oliguria (< 400 mL/day), anuria edema, hypertension, and congestive heart failure (CHF)

f. **Diabetes mellitus**
   1) 45 percent of type I patients develop **diminished kidney function** 15–20 years after diagnosis.
   2) Causes primarily **glomerular** problems.
   3) Associated with glucosuria, polyuria, and nocturia.
   4) **Microalbuminemia** occurs between 10–15 years after diagnosis.

g. **Renal hypertension**
   1) **Causes** decreased blood flow to all or part of an area of the kidney or accumulation of sodium.
   2) Ischemia to the kidney triggers the renin-angiotensin-aldosterone system which causes vasoconstriction.
   3) **Lab results:** aldosterone, sodium and renin levels are high. Urine potassium is elevated; serum potassium is decreased.

XXIII. PROTEINS

A. Proteins

1. **Characteristics**
   a. Molecular weight: 6,000 to several million units
   b. Structure: **proteins are covalently linked polymers of amino acids** (also called polypeptides).
      1) **Primary structure** shows the carbons and the groups linked together.
      2) **Secondary structure:** alpha helixes, and beta sheets, and random coils linked together.
      3) **Tertiary structure:** folding effect due to interactions of the various charged side chains of amino acids.
      4) **Quarternary structure:** two or more peptide chains join to form functional proteins.
   c. **Peptide bond:** carboxyl bond of 1 amino acid links to the amino group of another amino acid.
   d. N-terminal end: end of protein with a free amino group.
   e. C-terminal end: end of protein with a free carboxyl group.

2. **Nitrogen content:** 16 percent nitrogen differentiates proteins from carbohydrates and lipids.

3. **Isoelectric point:** pH where a protein molecule is neutral.

4. **Solubility:** proteins are charged colloids that swell and engulf water.

5. **Synthesis**
   a. Most plasma proteins are synthesized in the liver.
   b. Immunoglobulins are produced by plasma cells.

6. **Classification**
   a. **Simple proteins:** polypeptides that are composed of only amino acids.
      1) **Globular proteins:** symmetrical with compactly folded protein chains (i.e., albumin).

key concepts

List the inborn errors of metabolism states, their characteristics, and how to test for them. Also, understand protein structure, the different types of protein found on a protein electrophoresis, how each protein functions, and the role of each protein in disease.

2) **Fibrous proteins:** elongated, asymmetrical, with a higher viscosity (i.e., collagen and keratin).

b. **Conjugated proteins:** proteins composed of a protein (apoprotein) and a nonprotein (prosthetic group).

1) **Metalloproteins:** a protein with a metal prosthetic group, i.e., ceruloplasmin.

2) **Lipoproteins:** a protein with a lipid prosthetic group.

3) **Glycoproteins:** a protein 10–40 percent carbohydrates attached, i.e., haptoglobin.

4) **Mucoproteins:** a protein with > 40 percent carbohydrates attached, i.e., mucin.

5) **Nucleoproteins:** a protein with nucleic acids attached, i.e., chromatin.

7. **General protein function**

a. **Energy production:** proteins can be broken down into amino acids that can be used in the citric acid cycle to produce energy.

b. **Water distribution:** maintain the colloidal osmotic pressure between different body compartments.

c. **Buffer:** the electronic charges of the individual amino acids of a protein become buffers by absorbing or releasing H^+ ions as needed.

d. **Transporter:** allow movement of hormones and other compounds around in the body.

e. **Glycoproteins:** antigens and assist the body in recognizing "self" from "nonself" cells.

f. **Antibodies:** proteins that protect the body against "foreign" invaders.

g. **Cellular proteins:** act as receptors that activate cellular components or allow specific compounds into the cells.

h. **Structural proteins:** maintain structures in all body parts.

i. **Enzyme:** catalyst

8. **Plasma proteins**

a. **Prealbumin**

1) Migrates ahead of albumin on a serum protein electrophoresis on agarose gel.

2) Transports thyroxine, triiodothyronine, and retinol.

b. **Albumin**

1) Highest concentration of any plasma protein.

2) Synthesized in the liver.

3) Major contribution to maintenance of colloid osmotic pressure of intravascular fluid.

4) Binds with substances in the blood such as bilirubin, salicylic acid, fatty acids, calcium, magnesium, cortisol, and some drugs.

c. α_1**-antitrypsin**

1) Acute phase reactant that neutralizes trypsinlike enzymes.

2) Migrates immediately following albumin in a serum protein electrophoresis on agarose gel.

d. α_1-**fetoprotein (AFP)**
  1) Synthesized in the fetal yolk sac, then by the liver.
  2) Electrophoretic mobility is between albumin and α_1-globulin.
  3) ELISA is the test of choice for AFP.
e. α_1-**acid glycoprotein (orosomucoid)**
  1) Forms certain membranes and fibers with collagen.
  2) Immunodiffusion is used to quantitate this molecule.
f. α_1-**antichymotrypsin (α_1-ACT)**
  1) Serine proteinase.
  2) Migrates between the α_1 and α_2 regions on serum protein electrophoresis on agarose gel.
g. **Inter-α-trypsin inhibitor (ITI)**
  1) Three units: two heavy chains and a light chain.
  2) Light chain inhibits trypsin, plasmin, and chymotrypsin.
  3) Migrates between α_1 and α_2 regions on serum protein electrophoresis on agarose gel.
h. **Haptoglobin**
  1) Composed of two α and one β chain.
  2) Radial immunodiffusion and immunonephelometric methods are used for quantitation.
  3) Function: binds free hemoglobin in the blood to prevent its loss in the urine.
i. **Ceruloplasmin**
  1) Copper-containing α_2-glycoprotein with enzyme activities.
  2) Synthesized in the liver.
  3) 90 percent or more of serum copper is in ceruloplasmin.
  4) Quantitate using radial immunodiffusion or nephelometry.
j. α_2- **Macroglobulin**
  1) Synthesized by hepatocytes.
  2) Inhibits proteases.
  3) Quantitate with radial immunodiffusion and immunonephelometry.
k. **Transferrin**
  1) Synthesized by the liver.
  2) Migrates at the β-globulin fraction on serum proteins electrophoresis on agarose gel.
  3) Quantitated by radial immunodiffusion and immunonephelometry.
l. **Hemopexin**
  1) Synthesized in the liver.
  2) Migrates in the β-globulin region on serum protein electrophoresis on agarose gel.
  3) Function: removes circulating heme.
m. β-**microglobulin**
  1) Part of the major histocompatibility complex.
  2) Measured by immunoassay.
n. **Complement**
  1) Several proteins that participate in the immune response.

2) Quantitated by radial immunodiffusion, nephelometry, and complement activity.

3) Increased in inflammatory states.

o. **Fibrinogen**

1) Synthesized in the liver.

2) Seen as a distinct band between the β and γ globulins on serum protein electrophoresis on agarose agar.

3) Quantitated by coagulation methods, immunoassay, radial immunodiffusion, and nephelometry.

p. **C-reactive protein (CRP)**

1) Appears in the blood of patients with inflammatory diseases.

2) Measured by latex slide precipitation, nephelometry, and enzyme immunoassay (EIA)

q. **Immunoglobulins**

1) 5 major groups: IgA, IgD, IgE, IgG, and IgM.

2) Synthesized in plasma cells.

r. **Myoglobin**

1) Oxygen-binding protein in skeletal and myocardial muscle.

9. Proteins in other body fluids

a. **Urinary proteins**

1) Performed on 24-hour urine specimens.

2) Test methods

a) Sulfosalicylic acid

b) Coomassie blue

3) **Clinical significance of proteinuria**

a) Results from tubular or glomerular dysfunction.

b) Glomerular membrane can be damaged in diabetes, amyloidosis, dysglobulinemia, and collagen diseases.

c) Glomerular dysfunction can be detected in its early stages by microalbumin. Microalbumin is not detectable by urine dipsticks, but exceeds normal ranges.

d) Tubular dysfunction can be of two types—overflow and dysfunction.

e) Overflow proteinuria: high serum proteins result in a high concentration of protein in the tubules that cannot be totally absorbed. This type of proteinuria is seen in multiple myeloma.

b. **CSF proteins**

1) CSF is formed in the choroid plexus of the ventricles of the brain.

2) **Reference range = 15–45 mg/dL.**

3) **Test methods** include sulfosalicylic acid, trichloroacetic acid, Coomassie Blue.

4) **Clinical significance**

a) Increased: bacterial, viral, and fungal meningitis, traumatic tap, multiple sclerosis, obstruction, neoplasm, disk herniation, and cerebral infarction

b) **Decreased:** hypothyroidism

c) Proteins present in adult: prealbumin, albumin, α_1-globulin composed mostly of α_1-antitrypsin, α_2 band, β_1 band

composed mostly of transferrin, and a CSF-specific
transferrin

XXIV. CARBOHYDRATES

A. Normal Carbohydrate Metabolism

1. During a fast, the blood sugar level is kept constant by mobilizing the glycogen stores in the liver which are metabolized by glucose-6-phosphate dehydrogenase (not found in muscle glycogen stores).
2. During long fasts, gluconeogenesis is required to maintain blood sugar levels because glycogen stores are used up in about 48 hours.

B. Hormones Affecting Blood Glucose Levels

1. **Insulin:** produced by the β cells of the pancreatic islets of Langerhans; promotes the entry of glucose into liver, muscle, and adipose tissue to be stored as glycogen, and fat; also inhibits the release of glucose from the liver; promotes ANABOLIC (or storage) functions. *Note:* Overweight individuals with normal carbohydrate metabolism require more insulin than do normal weight individuals.
2. **Somatostatin:** A polypeptide concentrated in the hypothalamus and the D cells of the pancreatic islets of Langerhans. It inhibits secretion of insulin and glucagon.
3. **Growth hormone and ACTH:** polypeptides secreted by the pituitary that counteract insulin and raise blood glucose.
4. **Cortisol:** It is secreted by the adrenal cortex and stimulates gluconeogenesis.
5. **Epinephrine:** secreted by the adrenal medulla and stimulates glycogenolysis. Physical or emotional stress cause increased secretion of epinephrine and an immediate increase in blood glucose levels.
6. **Glucagon:** Secreted by the α cells of the pancreatic islets of Langerhans. Increases blood glucose by stimulating glycogenolysis and lipolysis (principal counterregulatory hormone).
7. **Thyroxine:** Secreted by the thyroid gland. Stimulates glycogenolysis and increases glucose absorption from the intestines.
8. **Human placental lactogen:** Secreted by the placenta and has anti-insulin activity.
9. **Somatomedins: Somatomedin A and Somatomedin C** mediate the action of the growth hormone on the skeleton and other tissues. They have insulinlike activity.

C. Absorption of Ingested Glucose

1. After the intake and absorption of glucose, 60 percent goes to the liver while 40 percent goes into the circulation.
2. As the blood glucose rises, the liver and brain cells increase their uptake of glucose. Then insulin is released, more glucose is put into storage (glycogen and fat), while glucagon secretion is inhibited. These activities bring blood glucose levels back to fasting levels.
3. An individual with a fasting blood glucose level > 100 mg/dL is said to be hyperglycemic. An individual with a fasting blood glucose level < 50 mg/dL is said to be hypoglycemic.

D. Renal Threshold for Glucose

1. Glucose is filtered by the glomeruli and totally reabsorbed by the tubules. If an individual's blood glucose is elevated, glucose appears in the urine.
2. An individual's **renal threshold** for glucose varies widely (160–180 mg/dL), but it is that concentration of glucose in the blood that causes glucose to "spill" into the urine. A person's kidney can only reabsorb so much glucose.

E. Abnormal Carbohydrate Metabolism

1. **Diabetes mellitus**
   a. In the diabetic, glucose production is increased, and metabolism is decreased. In the fasting state, diabetics have greatly increased glucose levels.
   b. Both the release of insulin and the cellular response to insulin are decreased.
   c. Decreased insulin control leads to decreased utilization of glucose for energy.
   d. In the diabetic, the body utilizes triglycerides, fats, and proteins for energy.
   e. After a meal, the diabetic's body does not control the hepatic output as well as a normal individual.
   f. Coupled with decreased insulin and increased insulin resistance in the cells, **the blood glucose level of a diabetic increases** more than a normal person and falls only slightly after about 3 hours.

2. **Classification of diabetes mellitus**
   a. **Type 1 diabetes**
      1) **Insulin dependent:** no insulin production at all
      2) **Ketosis-prone:** can produce excess ketone resulting in diabetic ketoacidosis.
      3) **Etiology:** an autoimmune disorder where the β cells of the islets of Langerhans are destroyed by the body.
   b. **Type 2 diabetes**
      1) **Noninsulin dependent:** some insulin production and also cellular resistance to insulin.
      2) **Non-ketosis prone:** Without exogenous insulin or oral hypoglycemic medication, these individuals will have an elevated glucose, but will not go into diabetic ketoacidosis.
      3) Associated with obesity and sedentary lifestyle.
   c. **Gestational diabetes**
      1) Onset of diabetes during pregnancy. After delivery, patient may no longer be diabetic or may have diabetes mellitus. Even if the woman reverts to normal after delivery, there is an increased chance that she may develop Type 2 diabetes later in life.

3. **Glycogen storage diseases**
   a. Inherited diseases involving the deficiency of particular enzymes
      1) von Gierke's: G-6-PD deficiency

2) Pompe's: α-1,4-glucosidase

3) Cori's: amylo-1,6-glucosidase

F. Laboratory Diagnosis of Hyperglycemia

1. **Fasting glucose**
   a. This is the preferred method for diagnosing diabetes.
   b. Fasting glucose levels of more than 126 mg/dL on at least 2 different days is diagnostic for diabetes mellitus.

2. **Random glucose test**
   a. A random glucose level of 200 mg/dL indicates diabetes.
   b. This test result must be confirmed on another day with a fasting glucose or oral glucose tolerance test.

3. **Glucose tolerance test**
   a. Serial measurement of serum and urine glucose before and after ingesting a specific amount of glucose.
   b. Patient preparation: diet of at least 150 g of carbohydrates for 3 days before the test.
   c. Fasting glucose and urine collected after a 10–12-hour fast.
   d. Patient ingests 75 grams of glucose.
   e. Urine and serum glucose specimens are collected at 30 minutes, 1 hour, 2 hours, and 3 hours after ingestion of glucose.
   f. Interpretation of GTT results
      1) Normal response: 2-hour glucose level below 140 mg/dL and all values between 0 and 2 hours less than 200 mg/dL.
      2) **Impaired glucose tolerance (IGT):** fasting glucose less than 126 mg/dL and the 2-hour glucose level between 140 and 199 mg/dL.
      3) Diabetes: diagnosed when two diagnostic tests done on different days meet the criteria for DM.
      4) Gestational diabetes: diagnosed when a woman has two of the following: a fasting plasma glucose >95 mg/dL, a 1-hour glucose >180 mg/dL, a 2-hour glucose >155 mg/dL, or a 3-hour glucose >140 mg/dL.

4. **Hemoglobin A_{1C}**
   a. Principle: glucose attaches to hemoglobin A_{1C}.
   b. Measured by affinity chromatography and colorimetrically.
   c. Reflects blood glucose levels for the last 2–3 months.

5. **Fructosamine**
   a. Forms a ketoamine linkage between the glucose and protein.
   b. Reflects blood glucose levels for 2–3 weeks before sampling.

XXV. LIPOPROTEINS

A. Lipoprotein Structure

1. **Fatty acids:** short, medium, and long chains of molecules that are major constituents of trigylcerides and phospholipids

2. **Triglycerides**
   a. One glycerol molecule with 3 fatty acids molecules attached.
   b. If they contain saturated fatty acids, they are solid at room temperature. If they contain unsaturated fatty acids, they are liquid at room temperature.

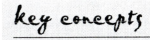

key concepts

Analyze the different types of lipids in the body, the composition of the body lipids, and all the abnormal states of lipid metabolism.

c. 95 percent of all fats stored in adipose tissues are triglycerides.

d. Triglycerides are transported through the body by chylomicrons and VLDL (very low density lipoproteins).

e. Metabolism involves releasing the fatty acids to the cells for energy, then recycling the glycerol into triglyceride.

f. Lipase, lipoprotein lipase, epinephrine, and cortisol break down triglycerides.

3. **Cholesterol**

a. Unsaturated steroid alcohol found exclusively in animals.

b. **Functions:** manufacture and repair cell membranes, synthesis of bile acids and vitamin D, precursor of progestins, glucocorticoids, mineralocorticoids, steroids, androgens, and estrogens.

c. 70 percent of stationary cholesterol is in skin, adipose tissue, and muscle cells.

d. 30 percent is transported via lipoproteins.

4. **Phospholipids**

a. Contain both hydrophilic and hydrophobic fatty acid chains.

b. Are major constituents of cell membrane and outer shells of lipoprotein molecules.

c. **Sphingomyelin** is not made from glycerol but from sphingosine.

5. **Glycolipids**

a. **Ceramides:** lipids that contain sugar and sphingosine molecule.

b. **Gangliosides:** complex glycolipids that are found in the brain.

6. **Prostaglandins:** long, chained polysaturated fatty acids called eicosanoids.

7. **Apoliproteins**

a. Proteins associated with lipoproteins.

b. These allow lipoproteins to be soluble and carried in the blood.

B. Classification of Lipoproteins

1. **Lipoproteins** are molecules that combine water insoluble dietary lipids and water soluble proteins so that lipids can be transported throughout the body. Micelles are spherical and have an inner core of neutral fat.

2. **Chylomicrons** are the lightest lipoprotein that carries **triglycerides** after a meal. **Chylomicrons** are composed of 90 percent triglycerides, 5 percent cholesterol, 3 percent phospholipids, and 2 percent protein. In **normal lipid metabolism,** they are absorbed by the intestine and broken down by adipose tissue and muscle. **Chylomicrons** have **apoproteins** B-48, C, and A-I on their surface.

3. **Very low density lipoproteins** (VLDL): these carry **triglycerides** and fats and are synthesized in the liver. **VLDL** molecules are composed of **60 percent triglycerides,** 20 percent cholesterol, 14 percent phospholipid, 2 percent protein and have apoproteins B-100, C, and E on their surface. In **normal lipid metabolism,** these molecules are secreted into the blood by the liver, then broken down by adipose tissue and muscle.

4. **Low density lipoproteins** (LDLs): also know as **"bad choles-terol."** **LDLs** are the body's major cholesterol carrier. They are composed of **40 percent cholesterol,** 22 percent phospholipids, 20 percent triglycerides, 18 percent protein, and have apoprotein B-100 on its surface. In **normal lipid metabolism,** this lipoprotein brings cholesterol to peripheral cells for membrane synthesis and forma-tion of adrenal and reproductive hormones.

5. **High density lipoproteins** (HDL) are also know as **"good choles-terol."** **HDL** is synthesized in the intestine and liver cells. **HDL** molecules are recycled chylomicron and VLDL molecules. **HDL** is composed of **44 percent protein**, 26 percent phospholipids, 25 per-cent cholesterol, and 5 percent triglycerides. HDL has apoproteins A-I and A-II on their surface. In **normal lipid metabolism**, HDL removes "excess" cholesterol from cells and transports it to other catabolic sites.

6. **Other lipoproteins**

   a. **Lp(a) or sinking pre-β-lipoprotein** migrates at the pre-beta position. It may be an **independent risk factor** for premature coronary heart disease, myocardial infarction, and cerebrovas-cular disease.

C. Abnormal Lipoprotein Metabolism

1. Normal lipid metabolism can be altered genetically or can be acquired.

2. **Hyperlipoproteinemias (Friedrickson-Levy classification):**

   a. **Elevated chylomicrons (familial chylomicronemia)** (Type I hyperlipoproteinemia)

      1) **Serum appearance:** creamy layer over clear serum.
      2) **Cholesterol test values:** LDL and HDL normal.
      3) **Triglyceride test values:** extremely high.
      4) Apo B48 increased, Apo A IV decreased, and Apo C II decreased.

   b. **Increased LDL (primary hypercholesterolemia)** (Type IIa hyperlipoproteinemia)

      1) **Serum appearance:** clear.
      2) **Cholesterol:** LDL very elevated; HDL normal.
      3) **Triglyceride:** normal.
      4) Apo B 100 increased.

   c. **Type IIb hyperlipoproteinemia**

      1) **Serum appearance:** clear or cloudy.
      2) **Cholesterol:** elevated LDL and VLDL.
      3) **Triglyceride:** elevated.
      4) Apo B 100 increased.

   d. **Increased IDL (familial dysbetalipoproteinemia)** (Type III hyperlipoproteinemia)

      1) **Serum appearance:** creamy layer sometimes present over a cloudy layer.
      2) **Total cholesterol:** elevated.
      3) **Triglyceride:** elevated.
      4) Apo E II decreased, Apo E III decreased, and Apo E IV decreased.

e. **Increased VLDL (familial hypertriglyceridemia)** (Type IV hyperlipoproteinemia)
   1) **Serum appearance:** cloudy or hazy.
   2) **Cholesterol:** normal.
   3) **Triglyceride:** elevated.
   4) Apo C II is either increased or decreased, and Apo B 100 is increased.
f. **Increased VLDL with increased chylomicrons** (Type V hyperlipoproteinemia)
   1) **Serum appearance:** cloudy and creamy (looks like milk).
   2) **Cholesterol:** very high.
   3) **Triglyceride:** very high.
   4) Apo C II increased or decreased, Apo B 48 increased, and Apo B 100 increased.

3. **Secondary lipoproteinemia**
   a. Many conditions cause lipoproteins to be abnormally metabolized
      1) **Diabetes:** normal to elevated cholesterol, very high triglycerides, mimics lipoprotein phenotypes IIb, IV, and V
      2) **Hypothyroidism:** very high cholesterol, slightly elevated triglycerides, mimics lipoprotein phenotypes I, IIb
      3) **Obesity:** slightly elevated cholesterol, slightly elevated triglycerides, mimics lipoprotein phenotype IV
      4) **Pregnancy:** slightly elevated cholesterol, slightly elevated triglycerides, mimics lipoprotein phenotype IV or V
      5) **Nephrotic syndrome:** very elevated cholesterol, slightly elevated triglycerides, mimics lipoprotein phenotypes IIa, IIb, IV, V

4. **Abetalipoproteinemia**
   a. **Symptoms:** fat malabsorption, retinis pigmentosa, neuromuscular dysfunction
   b. **Laboratory findings:** cholesterol and triglyceride levels very low, chylomicrons, VLDL, LDL, and Apo B-100 absent from serum

5. **Hypobetalipoproteinemia**
   a. **Symptoms:** no significant symptoms
   b. **Laboratory findings:** cholesterol, triglycerides, and apo B-100 reduced

6. Hypoalphalipoproteinemia **or analphalipoproteinemia:** also known as **Tangier's** disease)
   a. **Symptoms:** cataracts, neuropathy, hepatosplenomegaly, and enlarged orange tonsils
   b. **Laboratory findings:** no HDL, cholesterol level is half of normal, and triglycerides normal

7. **Clinical implications of hyperlipidemia**
   a. **Coronary artery disease:** the **Framingham** study that followed a cohort of men for 20 years concluded that increased LDL leads to increased coronary heart disease. In 1988, the **National Cholesterol Education Program** set cutoff values for cholesterol levels:

1) **Total cholesterol:** desirable: < 200 mg/dL; borderline: 200–239 mg/dL; high: >240 mg/dL

2) **LDL cholesterol:** desirable: < 130 mg/dL; borderline: 130–159 mg/dL; high risk: > 160 mg/dL

3) **HDL cholesterol:** Desirable: > 60 mg/dh; high risk: <35 mg/dL

4) **Triglycerides:** Desirable: < 250 mg/dL; borderline: 200–400; high: > 400 mg/dL

XXVI. CARDIAC FUNCTION

A. Enzymes of Clinical Significance

1. **Creatine kinase (CK)**

   a. Associated with ATP regeneration in contractile or transport systems. Biggest function is in muscle cells where it stores high energy creatine phosphate.

   b. **Sources:** widely distributed in all tissues. Highest concentrations in skeletal muscle, heart muscle, and brain tissue.

   c. CK is elevated in skeletal and cardiac muscle disease.

   d. **Considered a sensitive indicator for AMI (acute myocardial infarction).**

   e. CK elevated: cerebral vascular accidents, seizures, nerve degeneration, central nervous system shock, hypothyroidism, malignant hyperpyrexia, and Reye's syndrome.

   f. CK is separated into its 3 isoenzymes to specifically pinpoint the source of the elevated enzyme levels.

      1) CK has 3 isoenzymes: **CK-BB** (brain), **CK-MM** (skeletal muscle), and **CK-MB** (cardiac muscle). Healthy people have the CK-MM as the major isoenzyme.

      2) **CK-MB** usually is less than 6 percent of the total CK. Any CK-MB value greater than 6 percent of total CK is diagnostic for AMI. Following AMI, CK-MB levels rise within 4–8 hours, peak at 12–24 hours, then return to normal within 48–72 hours.

      3) CK-BB is elevated in central nervous system damage, tumors, and childbirth.

2. **Lactate dehydrogenase (LD)**

   a. **Very high concentrations** found in the heart, liver, skeletal muscle, kidney, and RBCs.

   b. **Elevated:** cardiac, hepatic, skeletal muscle, and renal diseases.

   c. **Highest levels of LD:** pernicious anemia.

   d. In AMI, LD levels rise within 12 to 24 hours, peak at 48 to 72 hours, then remain elevated for 10 days.

   e. Highest LD: viral hepatitis, cirrhosis, AMI, pulmonary infarct, skeletal muscle disorders, leukemias.

3. **Troponin**

   a. Three proteins that bind to thin filaments of striated muscle and regulate muscle contraction.

   b. TnT (troponin T) used as an AMI indicator because its concentration starts to rise within 4 hours of an AMI.

key concepts

Discuss the indicators of cardiac function, the elevations of these indicators during heart attacks, and the methods used to detect the cardiac indicators.

c. TnT remains elevated for 10 to 14 days after an AMI.

d. Quantitated by ELISA test.

XXVII. LIVER FUNCTION

A. Liver Structure

1. Lobule: cord of hepatocytes from a central vein

2. Sinusoid: vascular space between lobules

3. Kupffer cells: phagocytic macrophages that line the sinusoids

B. Physiology

1. Excretory and secretory functions

a. **Liver secretes bile** to assist in the digestion. Bile salts are composed of cholic acid and chenodeoxycholic acid conjugated with glycine or taurine.

b. **Bilirubin:** principal pigment in bile that is derived from hemoglobin breakdown.

c. **Bilirubin is transported** to the liver by albumin.

d. **Bilirubin is conjugated** in the hepatocyte endoplasmic reticulum with glucuronic acid to form bilirubin diglucuronide (conjugated bilirubin). Conjugated bilirubin is water soluble.

e. **Jaundice (icterus)** occurs when the bilirubin concentration in the blood rises and the bilirubin is deposited in the skin and sclera.

f. **Prehepatic jaundice occurs** when a large amount of bilirubin is brought to the liver for metabolism. Unconjugated hyperbilirubinemia is characteristic of this condition. Prehepatic jaundice: 1) hemolysis (hemolytic anemias), 2) increased RBC turnover, 3) neonatal physiologic jaundice.

g. **Hepatic jaundice** occurs when the liver cells cannot take up or conjugate the bilirubin or secrete too much bilirubin.

   1) **Gilbert syndrome:** cells cannot take up the bilirubin, and patients have mild icterus and a bilirubin of less than 3 mg/dL which is unconjugated.

   2) **Crigler-Najjar:** a complete absence (Type I) or decreased (Type II) of uridyldiphosphate glycuronyl transferase. No or little conjugated bilirubin is formed.

   3) **Dublin-Johnson's and Rotor's syndromes** are characterized by conjugated hyperbilirubinemia due to defective liver cell excretion of bilirubin.

h. **Posthepatic jaundice** occurs when an obstruction blocks the flow of bile into the intestines. Serum conjugated bilirubin increases, conjugated bilirubin is found in the urine, and the stool is clay-colored.

2. **Synthesis:** liver produces proteins, coagulation factors, ammonia, carbohydrates, fat, ketones, vitamin A, somatomedin, angiotensin, and enzymes.

3. **Detoxification and drug metabolism:** this is the primary site in the body that converts toxins and drugs to harmless substances.

C. Disorders of the Liver

1. **Jaundice**

a. **Yellow discoloration of skin and sclera** due to excess bilirubin (> 2–3 mg/dL).

    b. **Kernicterus:** elevated bilirubin levels that affect the central nervous system in infants, resulting in mental retardation.

    c. **Hypercarotenemia:** skin discoloration caused by elevated vitamin A levels due to ingestion of a large amount of vitamin A.

2. **Cirrhosis**

    a. Result of **chronic scarring** of hepatocytes turning them into nodules. Usually classified as micronodular or macronodular.

    b. **Alcoholism causes micronodular cirrhosis.**

    c. **Other causes** of cirrhosis are hemochromatosis, postnecrotic cirrhosis, and primary biliary cirrhosis.

    d. **A cirrhotic liver causes portal hypertension,** resulting in splenomegaly, esophageal varices, reduced synthesis of proteins and clotting factors, and accumulation of ascites in the abdomen. Esophageal varices can rupture resulting in life-threatening hemmorhage.

3. **Tumors**

    a. Hepatocellular cancer, hepatocarcinoma, or hepatoma: primary cancer of the liver.

    b. **Hepatoma:** from a previous hepatitis infection.

    c. **Metastatic tumors:** from cancers of the lung, pancreas, gastrointestinal tract, or ovary.

4. **Reye's syndrome**

    a. **Cause is unknown** but the **symptoms include** encephalopathy, neurologic abnormalities including seizures or coma, and abnormal liver function tests due to hepatic destruction.

    b. Usually occurs after a viral infection (varicella or influenzae) and aspirin therapy (mainly in children).

5. **Drug- and alcohol-related disorders**

    a. Toxins: hepatic necrosis leading to coma and death.

    b. **Most important toxin is ethanol.** Ingesting small amounts causes mild, asymptomatic injury, heavy drinking leads to serious damage, and prolonged heavy drinking leads to cirrhosis.

    c. Drugs such as phenothiazines, antibiotics, antineoplastic drugs, and anti-inflammatory drugs **cause liver damage**.

    d. **Acetaminophen can produce fatal liver necrosis when ingested in large quantities**.

6. **Hepatitis A**

7. **Hepatitis B (HBV, serum hepatitis)**

8. **Hepatitis C (HCV)**

9. **Delta Hepatitis (HDV)**

10. **Hepatitis E (*See* Chapter 5 Immunology and Serology, Section XXIII, Viral Hepatitis)**

11. **Chronic hepatitis**

    a. **Defined** by elevated liver enzymes for more than 6 months.

    b. The **severity** of the initial illness does not determine if a patient will develop chronic hepatitis

    c. **Chronic hepatitis** may produce a severe acute illness or an asymptomatic illness

XXVIII. ENDOCRINOLOGY
A. Hormones
1. **Definition:** chemical compound secreted into the blood by organ that causes a specific response in a target.
2. There are three classes of hormones—**steroids, peptide,** and **amines**
   a. **Steroids**
      1) Synthesized by the gonads, placenta, and adrenal glands.
      2) Produced from **cholesterol.**
      3) Not stored, but produced as needed.
      4) **Need a carrier protein** to circulate in the blood.
      5) Hormones include cortisol, aldosterone, testosterone, estrogen, and progesterone.
      6) **Mechanism of action:** steroid hormones interact with an intracellular receptor that initiates protein synthesis to produce proteins to carry out the hormone action.
   b. **Peptides/glycoproteins**
      1) **Hormones** include follicle stimulating hormone (FSH), leutinizing hormone (LH), thyroid stimulating hormone (TSH), β-HCG, insulin, glucagon, parathyroid hormone, growth hormone, and prolactin.
      2) **Synthesized, then stored** in the gland until needed.
      3) **Do not need carrier proteins** to enter blood.
      4) **Mechanism of action:** peptide hormones and epinephrine and norepinephrine interact with a cell membrane receptor. This activates a second messenger system and then cellular action.
   c. **Amines:** hormones include epinephrine, norepinephrine, thyroxine, and triiodothyronine.
3. **Control**
   a. **Endocrine hormones are controlled by** regulation of hormone synthesis through a feedback loop where **negative feedback** stops hormone release.
   b. **Indirect negative feedback** stops the tropic hormone from stimulating release of the target hormone.
   c. **Assays:** RIA, IRMA, ELISA, EMIT, FPIA, fluorescent immunoassay, HPLC, colorimetry

B. Overview and Clinical Significance
1. **Hypothalamus**
   a. Hormones produced
      1) **Anterior hypothalamus** produces thyrotropin-releasing hormone, gonadotropin-releasing hormone, somatostatin, corticotropin-releasing hormone, prolactin-inhibiting factor, and growth hormone-releasing hormone
      2) **Supraoptic and paraventricular nuclei** produce antidiuretic hormone, vasopressin, and oxytocin.
   b. **Diseases:** tumors, inflammatory or degenerative processes, and congenital problems
2. **Anterior pituitary**

---

key concepts

Discuss the hormones that regulate the body, how they function, and the disease states and corresponding hormone levels.

a. **Hormones secreted** are ACTH, GH, prolactin, TSH, LH, and FSH.
b. Excessive pituitary secretions are due to a tumor of 1 type of cell.
c. **Growth hormone**
   1) Hypothalamus controls the release of growth hormone with growth-hormone releasing hormone and somatostatin.
   2) **Reference range:** male < 2 ng/mL; female < 10 ng/mL.
   3) **Increased levels**
      a) In severe malnutrition, chronic liver or kidney disease, uncontrolled diabetes mellitus, growth failure, or a pituitary adenoma.
      b) In childhood: **giant.**
      c) In adulthood: **acromegaly** (widening of the bones in the extremities, impaired glucose tolerance, hypertension, and galactorrhea).
   4) **Decreased levels**
      a) Adults: decreased muscle mass, increased body fat, and decreased bone density.
      b) Children: **pituitary dwarfism.** They retain all the normal proportions, but shorter.
      c) If the growth hormone deficiency is part of an overall pituitary deficiency, then the dwarfism will be accompanied by **no sexual development, hypothyroidism,** and **hypoadrenocorticism.**
d. **Prolactin**
   1) **Function:** initiation and maintenance of lactation.
   2) **Reference range:** male: 0–20 ng/mL; females: 5–40 ng/mL.
   3) **Increased prolactin levels**
      a) After delivery, may reach 200–300 ng/mL.
      b) Can also occur in renal failure, hypothyroidism, and adrenal insufficiency.
      c) Pituitary adenomas that produce prolactin.
   4) **Decreased prolactin** levels are seen in panhypopituitarism.
3. **Posterior pituitary (neurohypophysis)**
   a. The **hormones released by the posterior pituitary are synthesized** in the hypothalamus, then secreted by the posterior pituitary.
   b. **Antidiuretic hormone (ADH, vasopressin)**
      1) Function: makes the distal convoluted tubule and collecting tubule of the kidney permeable to water.
      2) Increases plasma osmolality and decreases blood volume and blood pressure.
      3) **Increased levels**
         a) Relative hypersecretion of ADH occurs when a decreased blood volume stimulus overrides osmolality stimulus for triggering ADH secretion.
         b) When blood volume is normal and serum osmolality is low, ADH is released in the **syndrome of inappropriate ADH (SIADH).** Usually caused by ectopic tumor production of ADH. Is common in oat-cell carcinoma of the lung, CNS trauma or infections, administration of certain

drugs (opiates, barbituates, clofibrate, chlorpropamide), sarcoidosis, and tuberculosis.

4) **Decreased levels:** diabetes insipidus resulting in a severe polyuria and polydipsia.

c. **Oxytocin** stimulates contractions during delivery and causes ejection of milk.

4. **Parathyroid glands**

a. **Function: Parathyroid hormone** (PTH) increases the serum calcium level by increasing calcium resorption from bone, stimulating calcium retention in the renal tubules, and increasing vitamin D production in the kidney.

b. **Hyperparathyroidism**

1) Increased PTH released from parathyroid tumors or hyperplasia, due to a vitamin D deficiency, renal failure, or secondary hyperparathyroidism.

2) **Primary hyperparathyroidism:** increased PTH released from a pituitary adenoma.

a) Major complications occur in kidneys and bones—kidney stones, renal colic, and increased calcium resorption from bone.

b) **Other complications:** peptic ulcer disease and central nervous system symptoms.

3) **Secondary hyperparathyroidism:** increased PTH secretion due to decreased serum calcium and hyperplasia of the parathyroid glands.

a) Causes: vitamin D deficiency and chronic renal failure.

b) **Complications:** severe osteoporosis.

4) **Tertiary hyperparathyroidism:** patients with a vitamin D deficiency and hyperplasic parathyroid glands develop a parathyroid adenoma or the parathyroid glands function on their own.

c. **Hypoparathyroidism**

1) Causes: injury to the glands during thyroid or neck surgery, removal of the glands with the thyroid glands, or idiopathic atrophy.

2) **Severe hypocalcemia** develops and complications include altered neuromuscular activity **(tetany).** If the serum calcium falls below 6 mg/dL, laryngeal stridor and grand mal seizures may result.

3) **Pseudohypoparathyroidism (hereditary):** end organs are resistant to PTH. Patients with this disorder have round facies and deformities of the hand bones.

5. **Adrenal glands**

a. **Adrenal cortex**

1) Outermost layer: zona glomerulosa: secretes mineralocorticoids, with aldosterone the major hormone.

a) **Controlled by the renin-angiotension axis:** renin produced by the kidney when sodium levels are low, or in response to low renal pressure. Renin acts on angiotension to produce antiotension I. Angiotension-converting enzyme converts angiotensin I to angiotensin II. **Angiotensin II** stimulates the secretion of aldosterone and is a **potent vasoconstrictor.**

b) **Function** of aldosterone is to increase renal tubular retention of sodium and increase excretion of potassium.

c) **Hyperaldosteronism**

   (i) **Primary:** uncommon and due to an aldosterone-secreting tumor.

   (ii) **Secondary:** due to excess production of renin and can be caused by narrowing of the renal arteries, malignant hypertension, or a renin-secreting renal tumor.

d) **Hypoaldosteronism:** destruction of the adrenal glands.

e) **Reference range:** male: 6–22 pg/dL, female: 5–30 pg/dL.

2) Second layer (zona fasciculata): secretes **glucocorticoids** with cortisol as the major hormone.

a) Actions of cortisol: anti-insulin effects on carbohydrates, fat, and protein metabolism, suppression of inflammatory and allergic reactions, and water and electrolyte balance.

b) **Regulation of cortisol:** a feedback loop to the pituitary to decrease production of ACTH and corticotropin-releasing hormone.

c) ACTH and cortisol exhibit **diurnal variation.**

d) **Hypercortisolism** (also called **Cushing's syndrome**) adrenal adenoma or carcinoma production of excessive cortisol, excessive production of ACTH, ectopic tumor production of ACTH, or exogenous administration of cortisol.

e) **Symptoms of Cushing's syndrome:**

   (i) Weight gain in the face, neck, shoulders, and abdomen (including a "buffalo hump" at the base of the neck)

   (ii) Hyperglycemia

   (iii) Muscle wasting, purple striae, poor wound healing

   (iv) Hypertension

   (v) Decreased immune response

f) **Hypocortisolism:** primary adrenal disease or secondary to pituitary hypofunction.

g) **Primary adrenal disease:** atrophy of the gland.

h) **Symptoms:** weight loss, weakness, and GI problems.

i) **Adrenal insufficiency:** low sodium, low bicarbonate, low glucose, high potassium, and high BUN.

j) **Reference range:** A.M. 5–23 µg/dL, P.M. 3–16 µg/dL

3) Third layer (zona reticularis) **secretes sex steroids.**

a) Excessive production of androgens causes virilizaton.

b. **Adrenal medulla**

1) Produces catecholamines—dopamine, norepinephrine, and epinephrine.

2) **Function of epinephrine and norepinephrine:** mobilize energy stores, increase heart rate, blood sugar, and blood pressure.

3) Epinephrine and norepinephrine are **metabolized into metanephrines and vanillylmandelic acid.**

4) Increased levels of epinephrine and norepinephrine: **pheochromocytomas** (tumors of the adrenal medulla that produce large amounts of epinephrine and norepinephrine).

5) **Neuroblastomas** are malignant adrenal medulla tumors that occur in children. These also produce epinephrine and norepinephrine.

6. **Islets of Langerhans**
   a. **Insulin**
      1) Released when blood glucose levels increase, ingestion of amino acids, vagal stimulation.
      2) **Inhibited by** epinephrine and norepinephrine release and certain drugs (thiazide, dilantin, diazoxide).
      3) **Function:** promotes the storage of carbohydrates, fats, and amino acids; increases glycogenesis, decreases glycogenolysis.
      4) **Elevated:** hypoglycemia, insulomas (insulin-producing tumors of the β cells of the pancreas).
      5) **Hypoinsulinemia:** lack of insulin or ineffective insulin (diabetes mellitus).

7. **Glucagon**
   a. **Increase:** high-protein meals, acute hypoglycemia, and exercise.
   b. **Decrease:** a high carbohydrate meal.
   c. **Function:** hepatic glycogenolysis, gluconeogenesis, and lipolysis.
   d. **Hyperglucagonemia:** glucagon-secreting tumors of the pancreas. These tumors are malignant and have usually metastasized by the time they are diagnosed.

8. **Reproductive system**
   a. **Ovaries**
      1) Secrete estrogen, progesterone, and small amounts of androgen.
      2) Primary estrogen hormone is **estradiol.**
      3) **Estrogen** is responsible for promoting growth in the uterus, fallopian tubes, vagina, breasts, external genitalia, and depositing fat in the female distribution.
      4) **Progesterone** prepares the uterus for pregnancy and the breast for lactation.
      5) **Hormone changes in the female reproductive cycle**
         a) Follicle-stimulating hormone (FSH) promotes growth of follicles and an increase in estrogen in the first part of the cycle.
         b) Rising estrogen levels decrease the FSH, but cause LH to be released.
         c) The luteinizing hormone (LH) triggers ovulation → estrogen and LH levels to decrease rapidly.

    d) The follicle becomes the corpus luteum, which produces estrogen and progesterone that peak 8–9 days after ovulation.

    e) Lack of fertilization causes the corpus luteum to degenerate, and decreases the estrogen and progesterone levels.

    f) Menstruation results, then the cycle begins all over again.

6) **Estrogen:** abnormalities of estrogen production may occur and can cause accelerated or delayed puberty and/or infertility.

7) **Hyperestrinism:** Childhood—early onset of puberty; adulthood—irregular and/or excessive menses; menopause—resumption of uterine bleeding.

8) **Precocious puberty:** puberty occurs in the United States between the ages of 10 and 14. Changes occur in this order: breast development, pubic hair development, and beginning of menses. If these changes occur before 8 or 9, this is precocious puberty. Most cases are idiopathic.

9) **Infertility and irregular menses:** at the beginning and end of their reproductive years, women can have a cycle where no ovum is released. When a female has repeated cycles where no ovum is released, she is considered infertile

10) **Postmenopausal bleeding:** serious symptom of a cervical or endometrial carcinoma.

11) **Hyperestrinism** in males results in testicular atrophy and enlargement of the breasts. Usually caused by decreased testosterone production.

12) **Ovarian insufficiency** can be primary or secondary to gonadotropin secretion.

13) **Delayed puberty:** failure of puberty to occur by age 16.

    a) **Primary amenorrhea:** breasts and pubic hair have developed, but menses have not started.

    b) **Turner's syndrome:** a genetic defect occurs when the ovaries do not develop properly. Exogenous estrogen can be administered to develop secondary sex characteristics, but the patients are sterile.

14) **Amenorrhea** is due to ovarian failure during menopause (between 48 and 55 years of age).

15) **Hyperprogesteronemia** occurs when a corpus luteum does not degenerate after no fertilization occurs. Uncommon.

16) **Hypoprogesteronemia** is when the corpus luteum does not produce progesterone. Common and causes irregularities in menses, but the cycle is regular.

b. **Placenta**

1) Makes and secretes estrogen, progesterone, β-human chorionic gonadotropin, and human placental lactogen.

2) Human chorionic gonadotropin (HCG) secretion maintains progesterone synthesis by the corpus luteum in early pregnancy. The placenta then takes over HCG secretion to maintain the pregnancy.

3) **HCG levels are also useful in detecting** ectopic pregnancy, predicting spontaneous abortion, detecting multiple fetuses, and diagnosing and monitoring HCG-producing tumors.

4) **Human placental lactogen** acts to produce estrogen and progesterone from the corpus luteum. Also stimulates mammary gland development.

5) **Steroids:** placenta produces progesterone and estrogen during the pregnancy.

c. **Testes**

1) FSH stimulates spermatogenesis, LH stimulates production of testosterone from the Leydig's cells.

2) **Produce testosterone**

3) **Function:** promote growth and development of the male reproductive system, prostate, and external genitalia. At puberty, testosterone produces development of pubic, axillary, and facial hair, growth of internal and external genitalia, deepening voice, and development of sex drive and potency.

4) **Hyperandrogenemia:** in adults, there are no observable symptoms; in children, it causes early puberty (in males usually indicates a benign or malignant tumor).

5) **Hypoandrogenemia:** in children, delayed puberty results; in adults, loss of secondary sex characteristics result.

6) **Klinefelter's syndrome:** the patient possesses an extra X chromosome (XXY). Characteristics include tall with long extremities, small firm testes, gynecomastia, and decreased sperm count. Many have a low IQ.

7) **Primary testicular failure** in adults is due to infections, mumps, or irradiation.

8) **Alcoholism** is associated with testicular atrophy, loss of secondary sex characteristics, and gynecomastia.

9. **Gastrointestinal hormones**

a. **Gastrin:** secreted by the stomach in response to food entering the stomach.

1) **Hypergastrinemia:** decreased acid production by gastric parietal cells or by an islet-cell carcinoma of the pancreas.

2) **Zollinger-Ellison syndrome:** an elevated gastrin level accompanied by gastric hyperacidity.

b. **Serotonin:** secreted by the enterochromaffin cells in the gastrointestinal tract.

1) **Function:** binds to platelets and is released during coagulation. Liver metabolizes it to 5-hydroxyindole acetic acid (5-HIAA).

2) **Tumors** from the enterochromaffin cells occur in the appendix and ileum.

3) **Carcinoid syndrome:** large amounts of serotonin, histamine, kallikrein, and prostaglandins are secreted into the blood. Consists of attacks of diarrhea, flushing, tachycardia, and hypotension.

10. **Pancreas and gastric function**
    a. **Pancreas physiology**
       1) **Endocrine function:** secretes insulin, glucagon, gastrin, and somatostatin.
       2) **Exocrine function:** secretes digestive enzymes into the duodenum. Digestive enzymes include trypsin, chymotrypsin, elastase, collagenase, leucineaminopeptidase, lipase, amylase, and nucleases.
    b. **Secretion** is regulated by nerves and endocrine hormones.
       1) Nerves stimulate secretion of enzymes when food is smelled or ingested; controlling hormones include secretin and cholecystokinin.
    c. **Pancreatic diseases**
       1) **Cystic fibrosis**
          a) **Definition:** a dysfunction of mucus and exocrine glands of the body
          b) **Mechanism:** blocks pancreatic secretions from entering the duodenum
       2) **Pancreatic cancer**
          a) Usually an adenocarcinoma
          b) **Symptoms**: pain, jaundice, weight loss, anorexia, and nausea
       3) **Islet cell tumor**
          a) In β cells, result is **hyperinsulinemia**.
          b) In α cells, result is **gastrinoma** or **Zollinger-Ellison syndrome**, resulting in watery diarrhea, recurring peptic ulcers, gastric hypersecretion, and hyperacidity.
       4) **Pancreatitis:** inflammation of the pancreas.
          a) **Causes:** alcohol abuse, biliary tract disease, hyperparathyroidism, hyperlipidemia, mumps, biliary obstruction, gallstones, pancreatic tumors, tissue injury, artherosclerotic disease, shock, pregnancy, hypercalcemia, hypersensitivity, and postrenal transplantation
          b) **Symptoms:** severe abdominal pain—especially in upper quadrants radiating toward the back or down left or right side
          c) Chronic pancreatitis: **excessive alcohol consumption**
          d) **Lab results:** increased amylase, increased lipase, increased triglycerides, hypercalcemia, and hypoproteinemia
    d. **Lab tests**
       1) **Fecal fat**
          a) **Qualitative**
             (i) Slide 1: mix a small amount of stool with a fat-soluble stain (Sudan III, Sudan IV, Oil Red O, or Nile Blue), then coverslip and look for orange-red colored oil droplets. This indicates there is undigested fat (neutral fats, triglyceride) in the stool.

   (ii) Slide 2: add acetic acid and heat, fat drop. Indicate neutral fats (triglycerides), fatty acid salts (soap) and fatty acids.

   b) **Quantitative:** performed on a 72-hour stool and reported as grams excreted per 24 hours.

2) **Amylase**

   a) **Values rise within a few hours** of the onset of symptoms, peak in 24 hours, then return to normal in 3–5 days.

   b) Elevated in mumps, cholecystitis, hepatitis, cirrhosis, and ruptured ectopic pregnancy.

3) **Gastrin secretion**

   a) **Secretion caused** by neurogenic brain impulses, stomach expansion caused by food or fluids, contact of protein products with gastric mucosa, and gastrin.

   b) **Inhibition caused** by gastric acidity, gastric inhibitory peptide (secreted in response to fats, glucose, and amino acids), and vasoactive intestinal polypeptide.

   c) **Gastric analysis:** to detect acidity, hypersecretion of gastrin that is present in Zollinger-Ellis syndrome and to determine how much acid is secreted.

4) **Intestinal function tests**

   a) **Lactose tolerance test**

      (i) Lactase cleaves lactose into glucose and galactose.

      (ii) Acquired lactase deficiency is present in 10–20 percent whites and 75 percent African Americans.

      (iii) Procedure: patient ingests 50 g lactose, then blood specimens are obtained at 0, 30, 60, and 120 minutes. Blood glucoses are done, and increase in blood glucose level of 30 mg/dL or more is positive for a lactase.

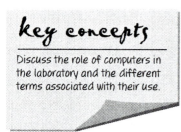

key concepts

Discuss the role of computers in the laboratory and the different terms associated with their use.

XXIX. COMPUTERS IN THE LABORATORY

A. Definitions

1. **Laboratory information system:** PC-based or based on a server or mainframe. To manage laboratory data, form an interface between instruments to translate data into patient results, evaluate quality control data, and store preventive maintenance records.

2. **Personal computer** (PC): a stand-alone computer that contains a central processing unit, monitor, disk drives, etc., and can be used for word processing, spreadsheets, databases, presentations, etc.

3. **Server:** a computer with an extremely large memory that directs signals and stores data from other computers. Servers can also have programs stored on them.

4. **Mainframe:** a very large capacity computer that is based on an operating system such as UNIX.

5. **LAN:** Local area network: many PCs that are connected to at least one server through cabling—RJ45 or fiber optic. The PCs are able to send e-mail and share files with others.

6. **Intranet:** a linkage that occurs between a set number of users and is not accessible to anyone outside that organization or office.
7. **HIS** (hospital information system): a large computer with a software package installed that is responsible for storing patient data, business data, employee data, etc., transmitting patient results from ancillary departments to the unit or even a totally electronic patient record.
8. **Parallel transmission:** transfer of data over parallel lines.
9. **Synchronous communication:** parallel transmission that requires the receiver and sender to be synchronized.
10. **Serial transmission:** transmission of 1 bit of data after another on 1 line.
11. **Asynchronous communication:** serial transmission that does not require the receiver and sender to be synchronized.

B. Laboratory Information Systems

1. **Data: raw facts** that have no meaning until grouped together or organized.
2. **Information:** data that are organized and grouped to increase a user's knowledge.
3. **Laboratory information system (LIS):** computers that are linked together to manage, sort, store, process, and send laboratory data and information.
   a. **Components of an LIS**
      1) Keyboards, barcode readers, computer links, and data converters
      2) **Central Processing Unit (CPU):** may be a minicomputer, server, or personal computer
      3) **Printers** and **screens**
   b. **Information provided by an LIS**
      1) Patient demographics
      2) Test information
      3) Work lists
      4) Reports
      5) Master test lists
      6) Business functions: cost per billable test calculations, test volume, employee hours, etc.
      7) Workload data
      8) Quality control
      9) Interfaces with other computers
4. **System design**
   a. **Process begins** with a laboratory needs assessment where data are collected on the information needs of the laboratory.
   b. **Needs are analyzed** to determine feasibility of a system.
   c. **System specifications flow from the needs,** i.e., what is needed to get the job done.
   d. **Computer specialists** translate the specifications into hardware and software requirements.
   e. The **software** will determine how the LIS will be used. It will have specific screens for entering data, sending reports, report-

ing results, etc. The software will have features such as security, access control, file maintenance, etc.

5. **Selecting an LIS**

   a. Laboratory managers contact vendors and **request information** about a particular LIS. This information may include interface capabilities to hospital information systems, remote user access, system requirements, costs, custom features, etc.

   b. Next, **vendor demonstrations, site assessments, reference checks,** and **visits to laboratories using the system** help narrow the choices.

   c. Selection is based on the systems that can best **meet the laboratory's needs at the lowest cost.**

6. **Installation**

   a. Important and very time-consuming

   b. **American Association of Blood Banks (AABB) operating procedures for installing, evaluating and running a computer system**

      1) **Bring up the computer** as part of the work flow. Make sure a time table, standard operating procedures, and work flow analysis are done.

      2) The **process steps** involving the computer in the daily work flow need to be identified.

      3) **Manual procedures:** if the computer system goes down, a contingency plan for manual procedures and forms needs to be in place.

      4) **System backup:** procedures need to be in place that back up the data daily so if the records are lost, there is another copy.

      5) **Disaster recovery:** every laboratory needs a plan to restore the system after system disruption by a storm, fire, or other hardware damaging situation.

      6) **System shutdown:** this procedure should be in place for routine maintenance and data downloading.

      7) **System startup:** procedures detailing the boot procedures and how to load programs on the LIS.

      8) **Hardware and software maintenance:** contracts for routine and emergency repairs need to be in place.

      9) **System security:** ongoing procedures to ensure the security of patient data and user profiles.

      10) **Software validation:** software must be validated to ensure with high confidence that the software performs as the vendor specifies and meets the laboratory's needs.

      11) **Quality assurance:** computer performance and quality must be monitored constantly.

      12) **Planning needs:** these include hardware and software upgrades, repairs, and fixing bugs.

      13) **Training and competency:** must be planned at the onset and must include implementation, operation, and upgrades for all users.

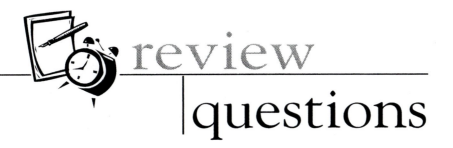

review questions

DIRECTIONS Each of the questions or incomplete statements below is followed by suggested answers or completions. Select the **one answer** that is best in each case.

1. A sample analyzed at 10 A.M. had a value for total bilirubin of 15 mg/dL. The sample was left on the counter and late that afternoon the specimen was analyzed again. This time the total bilirubin was 9 mg/dL. Which of the following is the probable cause of the discrepancy between the two readings?
   a. The wrong sample was analyzed the first time.
   b. The sample was stored at too warm a temperature.
   c. Bilirubin was lost due to photo-oxidation.
   d. The sample was hemolyzed, and the hemoglobin deteriorated.

2. A 23-year-old woman enters the hospital with dark urine and yellow eyes. She complained of lethargy and general malaise for 2 previous weeks. Her total serum bilirubin is 9.5 mg/dL, conjugated bilirubin is 6.0 mg/dL, ALP is 220 mU/mL, LD is 8040 IU/L, and ALT is 3000 IU/L. Her most probable diagnosis is:
   a. hepatitis.
   b. obstructive jaundice.
   c. cystic fibrosis.
   d. hemolytic anemia.

3. The presence of HBsAg, anti-HBc, and HBeAg is characteristic of
   a. convalescent HBV hepatitis.
   b. acute HBV hepatitis.
   c. carrier state of HBV hepatitis.
   d. recovery phase of HBV hepatitis.

4. If the direct bilirubin is 1.1 mg/dL and the total bilirubin is 4.3 mg/dL, what is the unconjugated bilirubin?
   a. zero
   b. 5.4 mg/dL
   c. 3.2 mg/dL
   d. 1.1 mg/dL

5. A 7-year-old boy comes to the emergency room (ER) semiconscious. His mother is hysterical. She tells the ER physician that her son had flulike symptoms and vomiting yesterday. This morning he continued to vomit, then became lethargic before he passed out. The lab results are ALT—700 IU/L, AST—500 IU/L, ammonia—1000 μg/L, total bilirubin—1.0 mg/dL, uric acid—12.0 mg/dL, and glucose—50 mg/dL. What is the most probable diagnosis?
   a. Gilbert's syndrome
   b. cholestasis
   c. Reye's syndrome
   d. Wilson's disease

6. The compounds produced by the liver that regulate cholesterol secretion into the bowel and also facilitate intestinal absorption of lipids into the circulation are known as:
   a. amino acids.
   b. bile acids.
   c. fatty acids.
   d. ketoacids.

7. This disease leads to a fatty liver and encephalopathy.
   a. Reye's syndrome
   b. Crigler-Najjar disease
   c. Wilson's disease
   d. Gilbert's sydrome

8. A 6-year-old came to the ER complaining of lethargy, nausea, and vomiting for 3–4 days. The mother said the child was urinating frequently, thirsty all the time, and eating a lot. The patient's WBC was 12,500, Hgb—11.2 g/dL, acetone—large, glucose—800 mg/dL, pH—7.183, pO_2—120 mmHg, pCO_2—20.1 mmHg, HCO_3—12 mmol/L, and base excess—14.7. What is the patient's diagnosis?
   a. NIDDM
   b. hypoglycemia
   c. hypothyroidism
   d. diabetic ketoacidosis

9. This hormone plays a critical role in stimulating gluconeogenesis and ketogenesis in IDDM patients.
   a. ACTH
   b. glycogen
   c. glucagon
   d. growth hormone

10. A 50-year-old male (obese) comes to the ER complaining of general lethargy of 3 weeks' duration. It is 3 P.M. and the man ate lunch at 12:30 P.M. The lab results for the man are WBC—8,500, Hgb—16.5 g/dL, Na—140 mmol/L, K—4.2 mmol/L, Cl—100 mmol/L, CO_2—13 mmol/L, and glucose—225 mg/dL. What is the doctor's probable diagnosis?
    a. hypoglycemia
    b. gestational diabetes
    c. NIDDM
    d. IDDM

11. In kinetic enzyme assays:
    a. Samples are added and read continuously.
    b. Samples are added and read 1 time after an incubation period.
    c. Samples are added and read at specific time intervals.
    d. Samples are added and one reading is made after addition of the sample.

12. The following results were obtained for a 56-year-old female patient admitted to the hospital through the ER:

    CK—550 IU/L
    LD—normal, but beginning to rise
    ALT—66 IU/L
    AST—20 IU/L

    What is the most likely cause for the observed laboratory data?
    a. liver disease
    b. myocardial infarction
    c. Paget's disease
    d. Muscle disease, muscular dystrophy

13. A 48-year-old man is brought to the ER unconscious and seizing. His EKG is normal, as is his heart rate. His lab results are CK—150 IU/L, AST—25 IU/L, LD—205 IU/L, ALT—20 IU/L, GGT—50 IU/L, ALP—75 IU/L, and phenytoin—35 mg/dL. What is wrong with this man?
    a. Nothing we can detect.
    b. cirrhosis
    c. viral hepatitis
    d. Paget's disease

14. A 35-year-old woman goes to her doctor complaining of bone pain. Her ALP is 500 IU/L. After inactivation at 56 C for 10 minutes, her ALP was 10 IU/L. What is her diagnosis?
    a. liver disease
    b. Paget's disease
    c. intestinal disease
    d. carcinoma

15. An electrophoretic serum protein pattern indicates a bridging effect between the β and γ fractions. What is the most likely disease to cause this pattern?
    a. nephrotic syndrome
    b. cirrhosis
    c. hepatitis
    d. acute inflammation

16. A patient visits the ER complaining of being sick for 2 weeks. The patient's symptoms include fever, cough, postnasal drainage, and sinus pressure. Further investigation reveals the patient has been sick on and off for the

last 3 months. A serum protein electrophoresis (SPEP) was done and the gamma portion was markedly decreased. What is the probable diagnosis?
a. hyperimmunoglobulinemia
b. defective T-cell function
c. HIV disease
d. immunoglobulin deficiency

17. This disease state is characterized by a hyperviscosity syndrome and Bence Jones protein is present in the patient's urine.
a. multiple sclerosis
b. glomerularnephritis
c. scarlet fever
d. multiple myeloma

18. A 45-year-old woman consulted a physician after blood pressure screening at a health fair revealed mild-to-moderate hypertension. The patient had central obesity, thin limbs, and a round, ruddy face. She was not taking any medication. Her blood pressure was 160/100 mmHg. A fasting blood glucose performed by fingerstick in the doctor's office was 120 mg/dL.

The physician ordered serum cortisols to be drawn at 8 A.M. and 4 P.M. and a 24-hour urine collection for 17-hydroxycorticosteroids and 17-ketosteroids. Laboratory results are below:

8 A.M. cortisol—32 ug/dL
4 P.M. cortisol—30 ug/dL
17-OH–corticosteroids—10 mg/24 hour
17-ketosteroids—15 mg/24 hr

What is the patient's probable diagnosis?
a. Addison's disease
b. Hashimoto's disease
c. Cushing's disease
d. Graves' disease

19. A 30-year-old woman presents with restlessness, inability to sleep well, and bulging eyes. These symptoms have occurred during the last 5 months. She tires easily and is always hungry, but never seems to gain weight. In fact, she has lost 10 pounds in the last 2 months. The results for her lab work are below:

Glucose—95 mg/dL
T_3Uptake—25 ug/dL
T_4—25 µg/dL
TSH—0.5 (µ) IU/mL
Free T_4—8.0 ng/dL
FTI—8.8 µg/dL

What is the most probable diagnosis?
a. Addison's disease
b. Hashimoto's disease
c. Graves' disease
d. Cushing's disease

20. Which hyperlipoproteinemia is characterized by an increase in cholesterol, an increase in the LDL, normal triglycerides, and the absence of chylomicrons?
a. Familial chylomicronemia
b. Primary hypercholesterolemia
c. Familial dyebetalipoproteinemia
d. Familial hypertriglyceridemia

5 Immunology and Serology

contents

➤ COMPREHENSIVE KEY CONCEPTS

1. Analyze how the human body responds to foreign invaders.

2. Discuss how serological tests can detect antibodies for specific diseases.

I. INTRODUCTION TO IMMUNOLOGY

A. Definition—immunity includes the body processes that occur to defend the body against foreign antigens:

1. Inflammation
2. Phagocytosis
3. Antibody synthesis
4. Effector T-lymphs
5. Removal of dying cells

B. Types of Immunity

1. **Innate (Nonspecific)** Natural
   a. Born with it; doesn't need prior exposure to antigen to occur.
   b. First line of defense.
   c. Physical barriers, i.e., epithelial cells, pH of skin surface, trapping of bacteria in mucus.
   d. Age determines immune system function.
   e. **Chemicals** secreted by cells and tissues, i.e., complement type 1 interferon (IFN).
   f. **Phagocytosis:** the process of a macrophage or neutrophil engulfing bacteria.
   g. **Inflammation:** body processes such as
      1) Cellular movement
      2) Tissue repair
      3) Chemical release
      4) Elimination of foreign material

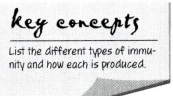

key concepts

List the different types of immunity and how each is produced.

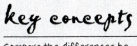

key concepts

Compare the differences between the structure of antigens and antibodies.

2. **Adaptive (specific or acquired)**
   a. Acquired only after a specific challenge is encountered and responds only to a **specific challenge.**
   b. **Two responses**
      1) **Humoral**
         a) Extracellular
         b) Antibody production by β lymphocytes and plasma cells
      2) **Cell-mediated**
         a) Intracellular
         b) Infected cell or tumor cell
         c) T-lymphocyte-cytotoxic T-cell
         d) Cytotoxins
   c. **Active immunity**
      1) Host is exposed to foreign antigen as a result of infection, and the host's immune cells manufacture specific products to eliminate foreign antigen.
      2) Vaccination-immune system responds to an altered (noninfectious) organism.
      3) Active immunity endures for life.
   d. **Passive (natural) immunity**
      1) Immune products injected into the host.
      2) Passive immunity is short term (no memory cells produced).
   e. **Antigens and antibodies**
      1) **Antigens**
         a) **Immunogen:** a substance capable of producing an immune response.
         b) **Antigen:** a substance that interacts with cells or substances of the immune system. Immunogens are also considered as antigens, but all antigens do not produce an immune response.
         c) **Epitope:** the portion of a molecule that the body recognizes as an antigen.
         d) **Thymic-dependent immunogens:** antigens that must be processed, then brought to T-helper cells.
         e) **Thymic-independent immunogens:** antigens that initiate antibody production without stimulating T-cells.
         f) **Immunogenicity characteristics**
            (i) **Foreign:** must be recognized by the body as "not self."
            (ii) **Size:** must weigh more than 10 kilodaltons.
            (iii) **Chemical composition:** proteins and carbohydrates are most immunogenic, whereas lipids and nucleic acids are weakly immunogenic
            (iv) **Complexity:** the more complex a molecule, the more immunogenic it becomes.
            (v) Route of entry into the host also determines immunogenicity.
            (vi) Dose of immunogen determines immunogenicity.
            (vii) Ability to degrade the immunogen.

2) **Haptens:** low-molecular weight molecules that can combine with another molecule to produce an antibody response.
3) **Adjuvants:** compounds that enhance an immune response. They are not immunogenic and cannot produce an antibody response alone. Types of adjuvants include:
   a) **Insoluble complex, salts:** aluminum hydroxide, aluminum potassium tartrate (alum), and calcium phosphate
   b) Slow release of antigen, oil in water: Freund's incomplete, mineral oil, Freund's complete mineral oil with mycobacteria
   c) Increase in IgM production: lipopolysaccharide, endotoxins
   d) Lysosomal release: vitamin A, beryllium salts, toxic forms of silica, and quarternary forms of ammonium salts
4) **Antibody** (immunoglobulin): protein that binds to antigens. There are 5 classes: **IgG, IgM, IgE, IgA, and IgD.**
   a) Immunoglobulins are composed of 2 heavy polypeptide chains and 2 light polypeptide chains which are joined by carbohydrate.
      (i) **Light chains**
         (a) 2 types: **kappa and lambda**.
         (b) Antibodies can have only one type of chain present: **kappa or lambda**.
      (ii) **Heavy chains**
         (a) **Immunoglobulin classes are defined by a unique heavy chain:**
            IgM- mu-μ   IgG- gamma-γ   IgA- alpha-α
            IgD- delta-δ   IgE- epsilon-∈
   b) Chains are joined by disulfide bonds.
   c) Every heavy chain and light chain consists of one variable domain and one or more constant domains.
   d) Variable domain defines the specificity of an antibody.
   e) The hinge region is made up of the first and second constant domains of the heavy chain. This region changes the shape of an antibody from a "T" shape in the free form and a "Y" shape when attached to an antigen.
   f) When mixed with papain, an enzyme that cleaves the antibody molecule at the hinge region, three fragments are produced—2 Fab and 1 Fc. (Fab = fragment antigen binding) and (Fc = fragment crystallizable).
   g) Antibody heterogeneity
      (i) **Isotypes**
         (a) Variations between light and heavy chains.
         (b) Defined by constant regions of all immunoglobulins and kappa and lambda.
         (c) Species specific.
      (ii) **Allotypes**
         (a) Species specific variations in the constant domains of heavy or light chains.

(b) 3 markers for κ chain (Km allotypes).

(c) 2 markers for α2 heavy chain (2m).

(d) Up to 25 markers for γ heavy chain (γm).

(iii) **Idiotypes**

(a) Variation in the variable region.

(b) A single clone expresses a single idiotype.

(c) Anti-idiotype antibodies are found in autoimmune disease.

h) **J chain:** multiple polymers of IgM and IgA are linked by a J chain. One J chain is needed for each IgM or IgA molecule that is linked together.

i) **Antibody classes**

(i) **IgG**

(a) On serum protein electrophoresis, IgG migrates in the gamma region. The gamma region is broad because it represents many IgG classes, subclasses, and variable regions.

(b) **85 percent of immunoglobulins** in the blood and has a long half-life.

(c) Hypervariable regions on the gamma chain are located at nearly the same position as on the light chain.

(d) Produced in secondary antibody response.

(e) Antitoxin antibody.

(f) Only immunoglobulin to cross the placenta.

(g) IgG activates the classical complement pathway.

(h) Subclasses include IgG1, IgG2, IgG3, and IgG4.

(ii) **IgM**

(a) **5 antibody molecules linked together by a J chain and interchain disulfide bonds.**

(b) **10 percent of total serum immunoglobulins.**

(c) First antibody produced against an antigen.

(d) Produced in both primary and secondary immune responses.

(e) Activates the classical pathway of complement best—only 1 molecule required.

(iii) **IgA**

(a) **Forms: serum and secretory**

(1) Serum IgA is a single immunoglobulin molecule, whereas secretory IgA is a dimer held together by a J chain.

(b) Contains alpha heavy chains.

(c) 2 subclasses: IgA1 and IgA2.

(d) Produced in conjunction with IgG and IgM.

(e) Function of serum IgA is antigen clearance and immune regulation.

(f) Function of secretory IgA is not activating complement, inhibits complement activating activity of IgG, activates alternate complement pathway, and **promotes inflammation**.

(iv) **IgD**

(a) **Single antibody structure**.

(b) Degrades easily using proteolytic enzymes and heat.

(c) Short half-life (2–3 days).

(d) Primarily a cell membrane surface component of B-lymphocytes.

(v) **IgE**

(a) **Responsible for allergic reactions and Type I hypersensitivity reactions**.

(b) Fc portion binds to receptors on mast cells and causes release of histamine and leukotrines. These chemicals cause the symptoms of allergic individuals.

j) **Monoclonal antibodies**

(i) **Definition:** identical antibodies that are produced from a single clone of B-lymphocytes.

(ii) Found in individuals with multiple myeloma which is also called a monoclonal gammopathy.

(iii) Also produced in industry by fusing an antigen-sensitized, splenic B-lymphocyte with nonsecreting myeloma cells, thus creating an immortal cell line that secretes a specific antibody.

k) Quantitation of immunoglobulins

(i) **Function:** to provide information about the functional immune status of a person.

(ii) IgG, IgM, and IgA quantitated using radial immunodiffusion (RID), nephelometry, or turbidimetry.

II. THE IMMUNE SYSTEM

A. Myeloid cells—responsible for nonspecific response

1. **Monocytes and macrophages**

    a. In the peripheral blood, this cell is a monocyte; in the tissue, it is a macrophage.

    b. **Functions**

      1) Phagocytosis of invaders

      2) Activation of immune response by presenting agent to T-cell

    c. Macrophages have MHC Class II, complement, and Ig receptors on their surface.

2. Granulocytes

    a. **Neutrophils**

      1) 70 percent of WBCs in circulation

      2) Function-phagocytosis

    b. **Eosinophils**

      1) 2.5% of circulating WBCs

key concepts

Analyze the cellular immune response mechanism.

2) Mediate IgE allergic response
  c. **Basophils**
    1) 0.5–1.0 percent of circulating WBCs
    2) Has receptors for IgE and granules are responsible for allergic reactions
3. **Lymphocytes**
  a. 20–30 percent of circulating WBCs
  b. **B-lymphocytes**
    1) 5–15 percent of circulating lymphs
    2) B-lymph differentiation: B-cells mature in 2 stages—antigen dependent and antigen independent
      a) **Antigen dependent:** when exposed to an antigen, the B-cell develops into a plasma cell and produces antibodies against a specific antigen.
      b) **Antigen independent:** when a stem cell matures into a pre–B-cell.
  c. **T-lymphs**
    1) 80 percent of circulating lymphs
    2) **Functions**
      a) Lyses cells infected with viruses and tumor targets, lymphokine production.
      b) T-cells increase or suppress other lymphs.
    3) **T-Lymph Maturation**
      a) Pre–T-cells begin in bone marrow and fetal liver.
      b) Cells go to thymus (90% of pre–T-cells die here).
      c) Cells with the ability to recognize self survive and go into circulation.
    4) **Large granular lymphs:** slightly larger than T- or B-cells and have cytoplasmic granules. Thought to be natural killer (NK) cells.
6. **Other cells that assist in immune response**
  a. Dendrites
  b. Langerhans' cells
  c. Mast cell

B. **Cytokines**
  1. **Colony stimulating factors**
    a. **Purpose:** cause proliferation and differentiation of bone marrow cells
      1) **G-CSF** (granulocyte CSF): stimulates bone marrow cells to mature into granulocytes
      2) **M-CSF** (macrophage CSF): stimulates the maturation of cells into monocyte and macrophage cells
      3) **GM-CSF** (granulocyte-macrophage CSF): causes maturation to granulocytes and macrophages
  2. **Interferons**
    a. **3 types: interferon alpha (INF-α), interferon beta (INF-β), and interferon gamma (INF-γ)**
    b. INF-α and INF-β antiviral proteins that inhibit viral replication and activate NK cells

    c. INF-γ: antiviral effects, activates macrophages, NK cells, and stimulates B-cells to produce antibodies

3. **Tissue necrosis factors**
    a. 2 types: α and β
      1) **TNFα:** produced by macrophages, lymphs, and NK cells when encountering bacteria, viruses, tumor cells, toxins, and C5a. Also suppresses myeloid and RBC stem cells, but does not affect differentiation.
      2) **TNFβ (lymphotoxin):** produced by CD4 and CD8 cells after exposure to a specific antigen. Cytotoxic for those antigens.

4. **Interleukins**
    a. **Interleukin 1 (IL-1):** produced by macrophages and fibroblasts. Activates T-cells, increases number of B-cells, increases CSF production in bone marrow, activates vascular endothelium, causes fever and acute phase protein synthesis, and induces T-cells to produce lymphokines, cytokines, and mediators.
    b. **Interleukin 2 (IL-2):** produced by CD4 cells. Causes proliferation of activated T- and B-cells. B-cells produce more antibody, and NK cells activated.
    c. **Interleukin 3 (IL-3):** produced by activated T-cells. Increases number of mast cells in skin, spleen, and liver. Growth differentiation of all cell types.
    d. **Interleukin 4 (IL-4):** produced by activated T-cells. Effects are unknown. Development and differentiation of T-cells.
    e. **Interleukin 5 (IL-5):** produced by activated T-cells and causes B-cells to produce antibodies.
    f. **Interleukin 6 (IL-6):** produced by activated T- and B-cells, monocytes, and fibroblasts. Half-life is 1 hour.
    g. **Interleukin 10 and 12 (IL-10 and IL-12):** IL-10 reduces INFγ production, and IL-12 activates macrophages and NK cells and increases INFγ production.

C. Organs and Tissues of the Immune Cells
1. Immune system housed in reticuloendothelial system—spleen, lymph nodes, bone marrow, liver, and lungs.
2. **Primary lymph tissues**
    a. Bone marrow: lymphs develop into B-cells.
    b. Thymus: pre–T-cells develop into T-cells.
    c. Fetal liver: produce fetal blood cells.
3. **Secondary lymphoid organs**
    a. **Lymph nodes:** cells migrate to the cortex and T-cells to the paracortex.
      1) Primary follicle: many small B-lymphs.
      2) Secondary follicle: after stimulation, primary follicle becomes a secondary follicle. The germinal center has small and large lymphs, blast cells, macrophages, and dentritic cells. Medulla contains plasma cells and large lymphs.

  b. **Spleen**
  1) Purpose: filter blood.
  2) Contains both T- and B-cells.
  c. **Mucosal-Associated Lymphoid Tissue**
  1) Found in submucosa in GI tract, respiratory tract, and urogenital tract.
  2) These surfaces interact with environment and can begin the immune response early.
  d. **Lymphoid Circulation**
  1) Lymphs migrate from one secondary lymph organ to another.

III. MAJOR HISTOCOMPATIBILITY COMPLEX (MHC)

A. MHC are cell surface markers that allow immune cells to distinguish "self" from "not self."

B. 3 classes of MHC products

key concepts

Analyze the major histocompatibility complex structure and know why these antigens are important.

  1. **Class I products:** HLA-A, HLA-B, HLA-C, HLA-E, HLA-F, HLA-G, HLA-H, and HLA-J which are cell surface markers.
  a. Classical Class I products (HLA-A, -B, -C) are composed of an α heavy chain and β_2 microglobulin.
  b. Class I products are found on every cell.
  2. **Class II products:** HLA-D, HLA-DR, HLA-DQ, and HLA-DP which are cell surface markers.
  a. Composed of a parallel α and a β chain that begin in the cytoplasm and end in the environment.
  b. Located on monocytes, macrophages, B-lymphocytes, activated T-lymphocytes, dendritic cells, Langerhans' cells, and some epithelial cells.
  c. These cells present antigens to helper T-cells
  3. **Class III products:** C2, C4, factor B, enzymes, tumor necrosis factor α and β, and heat shock proteins (HSP70-1 and HSP70-2)
  a. Not associated with cell membrane surfaces.
  b. Proteins that generate the classical pathway C3 convertase and alternate pathway C3 convertase.

C. Nomenclature

  1. HLA antigens are named according to the product expressed by the gene locus (capital letter) and the allele (number), for example, HLA-A2, where A is the locus and 2 is the allele.
  2. The gene locus designations are A, B, C, D, DR, DQ, and DP.
  3. A "w" can be used to distinguish HLA-C antigens from complement proteins, identify HLA-D loci defined by mixed lymphocyte reaction, and identify epitopes rather than alleles.

D. HLA Detection

  1. **Serologic assays** use antibody to identify the specific locus product—A, B, C, D, DR, DQ, and DP.
  2. **Complement-mediated cytotoxicity** is used to detect HLA-A, -B, -C, -DR, and -DQ.

3. **Cell-mediated assays** are used to detect HLA-Dw (one-way mixed-lymphocyte culture) and -DPw (primed lymphocyte test).

E. Inheritance of HLA
1. Haplotype: combination of HLA alleles inherited.
2. Two haplotypes (one from each parent) are a genotype.

F. Clinical Significance
1. **Transplantation:** transplants last longer if the HLA antigens from the recipient and the donor are closely matched.
2. **HLA paternity testing:** HLA loci are polymorphic and recombination is rare. HLA inheritance patterns can exclude fathers with 99 percent confidence in whites, and 98 percent confidence in blacks.
3. **HLA and disease:** not all individuals that have a particular HLA antigen have a disease, but many more people with the disease express a particular HLA antigen, for example, HLA B-27 is associated with ankylosing spondylitis.

IV. TUMOR IMMUNOLOGY
A. Definitions
1. **Neoplasia:** a normal mass of tissue that results from the uncontrolled growth of normal cells even after the growth stimuli is removed.
2. **Benign tumor:** causes clinical disease by interfering with normal cell function.
3. **Malignant tumor:** not only interferes with normal cell function but also invades normal tissues and robs the normal tissues of the nutrients needed to survive.
4. **Oncology:** study and treatment of tumors or neoplasms.

key concepts

Compare the immunology of tumors (including separate tumor markers) and how this information is used.

B. Immune Response to Tumors
1. **Tumor-associated antigens**
   a. **Tumor-specific peptides:** expression of intracellular proteins on the surface of a tumor due to interaction with MHC Class I and Class II molecules.
   b. **Virus-induced tumors:** tumors that are caused by viruses usually have viral antigens on their surface.
   c. **Genome-encoded tumor antigens:** oncogenes are formed when there is a point mutation of a proto-oncogene and/or tumor suppressor genes.
   d. **Oncofetal antigens:** unexpressed antigens that become expressed after malignant transformation—α-fetoprotein, carcinoembryonic antigen.

C. Natural Immunity to Tumors
1. **Natural immunity** occurs in individuals with macrophages, natural killer (NK) cells, killer (K) cells, lymphokine-activated killer (LAK) cells, and tumor-infiltrating lymphocytes (TIL).
   a. Macrophage-mediated cytotoxicity: the tumor killing function of activated macrophages. Occurs when macrophages come in close contact with tumor cells, then kill the tumor cells.

      b. Natural killer cells: do not have MHC Class I products expressed on their surfaces are destroyed by NK cells.

      c. LAK cells are activated by IL-2. These are thought to be unstimulated NK cells which are able to destroy cells resistant to killing by NK cells.

  2. **T-cell mediated immunity to tumors**

      a. **Cytokines involved in tumor immunity**

        1) Interleukin-1 (IL-1) activates T-cells, B-cells, and NK cells and causes a fever in the host.

        2) Tumor necrosis factor (TNFα) destroys tumor cells.

        3) INFγ is produced by activated T-cells and NK cells.

        4) IL-6 is produced by activated CD4+ T-cells and stimulates the acute phase response of the liver.

        5) Cytokines secreted by the tumor that have immunosuppressive ability are TGFβ and IL-10.

      b. Cytotoxic lymphs directly lyse tumor cells to which they have been previously exposed.

D. Tumor Markers

  1. **Glycoproteins**

      a. Derived from fetal or placental tissue and can be found in small amounts in normal serum.

      b. **Carcinoembryonic Antigen (CEA)**

        1) Used in management of gastrointestinal tumors (colon cancer), adenocarcinomas of the colon, pancreas, liver, and lung.

        2) Can also be found in inflammatory bowel disease, ulcerative colitis, Crohn's disease, multiple polyps, and tumors of the GI tract, and cigarette smokers.

        3) Highest CEA levels are found in metastatic disease—CEA elevated in serial samples.

      c. **α-Fetoprotein (AFP)**

        1) AFP levels high in fetal serum, maternal serum, and in patients with hepatomas (liver cancer), ovarian, presacal, and testicular teratoblastomas.

        2) Can also be elevated in viral hepatitis, chronic active hepatitis, cirrhosis, Crohn's disease, and ulcerative colitis.

        3) Most specific test currently available for liver carcinoma.

      d. **β-Human Chorionic Gonadotropin (β-HCG)**

        1) Found in serum and urine during pregnancy.

        2) Also found in patients with hydatiform mole, inflammatory bowel disease, duodenal ulcers, cirrhosis, seminoma, teratoma, choriocarcinoma, lung cancer, breast cancer, gastrointestinal cancer, and germ cell tumors of the testes and ovaries.

        3) Useful in diagnosis, correlating response to therapy, metastasis detection, and predicting treatment failure or relapse.

      e. **Squamous Cell Carcinoma Antigen**

        1) Subfraction of tumor antigen 4 (TA-4).

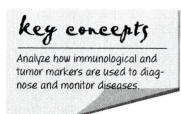

key concepts

Analyze how immunological and tumor markers are used to diagnose and monitor diseases.

2) Increased in squamous cell carcinoma of the uterus, endometrium, other genital tract cancers, head/neck cancer, lung cancer, and cervical cancer.

f. **Prostate-Specific Antigen (PSA)**

1) A glycoprotein that dissolves seminal gel formed after ejaculation.

2) Normal, prostate tissues contain PSA, but not present in blood.

3) Increased in prostate cancer, benign prostatic hypertrophy, and acute or chronic prostatitis.

4) Levels correlate with prostate size, stage of prostate cancer, and response to treatment.

5) Used to diagnosis prostate cancer in conjunction with a digital rectal exam.

g. **Mucinous glycoproteins:** found on epithelial surfaces: CA 15-3, CA 19-9, and CA 125

1) **CA 15-3**

a) Found in lactating mammary glands, lung epithelium, breast cancer, ovarian cancer, pancreatic cancer, lung cancer, stomach cancer, and liver cancer

b) Low levels found in chronic hepatitis, cirrhosis, sarcoidosis, tuberculosis, and systemic lupus erythematosis (SLE)

c) Highest levels if metastases present

d) Serial measurements predict relapses of breast cancer—monitoring breast cancer therapy

2) **CA 19-9**

a) Identical to Lewis A antigen

b) Increased in acute and chronic pancreatitis, benign liver disease, pancreatic cancer

c) Good for diagnosing colon, gastric, hepatobiliary, and pancreatic cancer

d) Decreased after surgical removal of tumor

3) **CA 125**

a) Useful in diagnosing ovarian cancer in postmenopausal women

b) Elevated in 80 percent of ovarian cancer patients

c) Also elevated in patients with endometrial cancer, metastatic breast cancer, colon, pancreatic, and lung cancers

d) Useful for monitoring treatment

2. **Hormones:** calcitonin, thyroglobulin, catecholamines, epinephrine, and norepinephrine are increased in malignancies of the gland involved.

3. **Other markers**

a. **Monoclonal immunoglobulins (M proteins)**

1) Diagnostic of multiple myeloma, Waldenström's macroglobulinemia, chronic lymphocytic leukemia, or lymphoma.

2) Immunoglobulin type determination is necessary for diagnosis and prognosis.

b. **β-2 microglobulin**
   1) Found on membrane of nucleated cells.
   2) Used to predict treatment failures and poor survival in lymphoma patients.

V. CELL-MEDIATED IMMUNE RESPONSE

A. Antigen Recognition

1. **Antigen processing**
   a. B-cells attach to antigens in their native form.
   b. T-cells recognize protein antigen that was processed by other cells.
2. **Antigen receptors**
   a. **B-cell**
      1) B-cell antigen receptor is IgG.
      2) The B-cell surface receptors have 2 identical antigen-binding pockets.
   b. **T-cell**
      1) T-cell receptor is peptide/MHC binding pocket and CD3.
      2) These receptors are active signal transductors.

B. Effector Mechanisms

1. **T-cells**
   a. T_H-Cell Activation (T-Helper)
      1) Occurs when T_H cells recognize an antigen.
      2) Requires direct cell contact, IL-1, and IL-2.
   b. **Cell-mediated immunity**
      1) Mediated by T_H lymph.
      2) Cytotoxic T-cells (T_C) destroy targets by cell contact.
      3) Cytokines activate other cells involved in the response.
      4) NK cells kill targets without being previously sensitized.
   c. **T_C -cell activity**
      1) T_C-cells kill targets without antibodies, but with direct cell contact.
      2) The T_C-cells can kill many targets in succession.
      3) T_H-cells secrete cytokines that activate T_C-cells.
      4) Main function: remove cells infected with viruses.
      5) T_C-cells are CD8 positive.
2. **B-cells**
   a. **B-cell activation** occurs when antibody binds to antigen and cytokines are present in the environment
   b. **Antibody diversity:** antibodies can be produced that recognize an unlimited number of antigens, but there are a limited number of B-cells.
3. **Antibody production**
   a. Primary and secondary antibody response
      1) **Innate or primary response:** produced when host first encounters antigen
         a) Latent phase: no antibody produced: 5–7 days. Host producing B cells to produce antibodies.

        b) IgM produced.

        c) Antibody production starts slowly, peaks, levels off, then declines.

     2) **Adaptive or secondary response:** produced after the host has already been exposed to antigen again

        a) Short latent phase (3–5 days)

        b) Higher antibody concentration

        c) IgG produced

        d) Antibodies in circulation longer than IgM

  b. **Affinity maturation:** increased affinity of antibodies from secondary response for antigen. The surface of B-cell and antibody produced by plasma cells have the same antigen specificity and affinity.

  c. **T- and B-cell interactions**

     1) Secondary response: B- and T_H-cells work together: B-cell processes the antigen, then activates the T_H-cells to produce cytokines.

     2) The synergy between the B- and T_H-cells produces increased antibodies for an extended period.

4. **Other cells**

  a. **Macrophages:** inflammatory reaction cells controlled by cytokines: cytokine production is antigen specific, but cytokine-activated macrophage activity is not antigen specific.

  b. **Natural killer cells:** activities are governed by cytokines.

  c. **Antibody-dependent cell-mediated cytolysis:** cytolytic effector cells can lyse antibody coated targets if there is direct contact.

C. Regulatory Mechanisms

1. **Antibody**

  a. The more antibody produced, the more binds with antigen and the less available for B-cell activation.

  b. Cross-linking of B-cells also leads to decreased B-cell activation.

2. Suppressor T-cells decrease B-cell activity.

VI. NONSPECIFIC IMMUNE RESPONSE

A. Nonspecific immune response: cellular mechanisms

1. **Barrier epithelial cells:** first line of defense—skin and mucous membranes

2. **Polymorphonuclear neutrophils (PMNs)**

  a. Involved in nonspecific immune response by attaching to damaged epithelium, locomotion, migration into tissues, chemotaxis, phagocytosis of target, increased metabolism, degranulation, and digestion of target

  b. **Diseases of dysfunctional PMNs**

     1) Chronic granulomatous disease

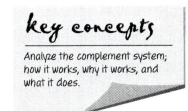

key concepts

Analyze the complement system; how it works, why it works, and what it does.

      2) G-6-PD deficiency

      3) Myeloperoxidase deficiency (MPO)

      4) Chédiak-Higashi (CD)

    3. **Eosinophils**

      a. Granules contain acid phosphatase and peroxidase.

      b. **Function hypothesized**

        1) Clearing immune complexes.

        2) Limiting inflammatory reactions.

        3) Protein in granule is toxic to parasites.

    4. **Mediator cells**

      a. Mast cells, basophils, and platelets release substances that mediate immune reactions.

      b. The mediators produce increased vascular permeability, smooth muscle contraction, and increased inflammatory response.

      c. **Mast cells** can degranulate by IgE attachment or nonimmunologic mechanisms such as surgical incisions, heat, skin or mucous membrane infections.

      d. **Basophils** function is to amplify the reactions that start with the mast cell at the site of entry of the antigen.

    5. **Mononuclear phagocyte system**

      a. **Formerly the reticuloendothelial system**

      b. Includes lymph nodes, alveolar macrophages, splenic macrophages, kidney phagocytes, Kupffer cells of the liver

B. Humoral (Chemical) Mechanisms of the Nonspecific Immune Response

    1. **Complement**

      a. 14 components involved in 3 separate pathways of activation

      b. 5 proteins unique to classical pathway: C1q, C1r, C1s, C4, and C2

      c. 3 proteins unique to alternative pathway: Factor B, Factor D, and P (properidin)

      d. 6 proteins that are common to both pathways: C3, C5, C6, C7, C8, and C9

      e. Activation of complement:

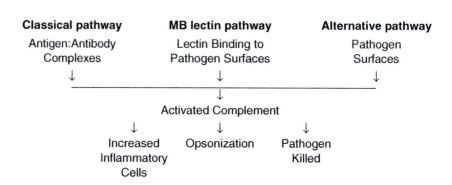

f. Classical Pathway

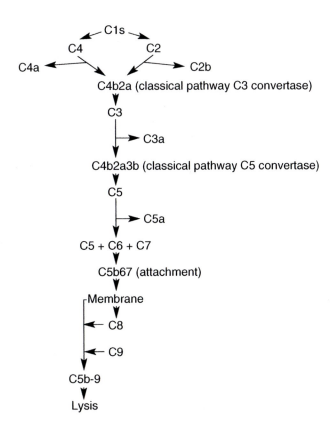

g. Alternate Pathway

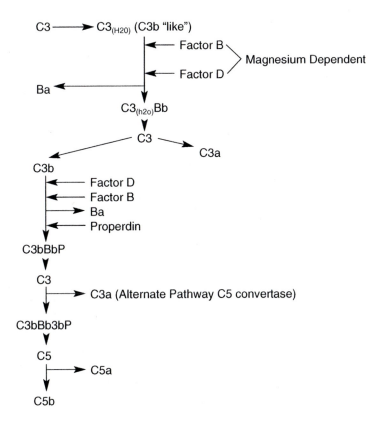

h. End product of complement

1) **Anaphylatoxins:** C4a, C3a, and C5a cause basophils and mast cells to release histamine, smooth muscle contraction, and increased vascular permeability.

2) **Immune adherence:** C3b adheres to immune complexes and surfaces of substances to facilitate clearing these molecules.

3) **Opsonization:** If C3b and IgG are attached to a particle, phagocytosis is enhanced.

4) **Chemotaxis:** C5a is an anaphylatoxin and induces the migration of neutrophils and monocytes to the site.

5) **Kinin activation:** C2b interacts with C1s to produce smooth muscle contraction, mucous gland secretion, pain, and increased vascular permeability.

6) **Cell lysis**

i. Deficiencies of complement

1) Complement can be consumed in infections and collagen vascular diseases.

2) C3 and C4 are measured to indicate consumption and follow disease states.

   a) Decreased C4, normal C3 indicate a mild consumption with classical pathway activation.

   b) Decreased C4 and decreased C3 indicate significant consumption and activation of classical pathway by antigen-antibody complexes.

   c) Total functional complement assay (CH50) is used to measure the health of the classical pathway. Used to screen for hereditary disorders.

   d) Decreased C1 (q, r, or s), C4 and C2 indicates collagen disease.

   e) Decreased C3 indicates overwhelming infection.

   f) Decreased C5, C6, and C7 indicate a *Neisseria* infection.

   g) Decreased C1INH indicates angioedema.

   h) Decreased H or I indicates a recurrent bacterial infection.

j. Control mechanisms

1) C1 inhibitor (C1INH) combines with C1r and C1s to block enzyme activities.

2) BIH (B) and C3b Inactivator (I): I inactivates C3b and C4b and H shortens half-life of C3 convertase.

3) Anaphylatoxin inactivator: this compound removes a single amino acid from C4a, C3a, and C5a, rendering them useless as anaphylatoxins.

4) Membrane attack complex (MAC) inhibitors: MAC is not formed because S protein binds to C5b-7 complex.

5) Complement receptor type I (CRI, CD35): CRI binds C3b and C4b and inhibits the amplification loop.

6) Complement receptor type II (CRII, CD21): CRII binds to C3d and this turns off complement activation.

7) Anaphylatoxin receptors: membrane receptors that affect anaphylatoxin activities of C5a.

8) Decay accelerating factor (DAF) binds to C4b2b and C3bBb to speed up dissociation.

9) Membrane cofactor protein (MCP, CD46) binds to C3b and C4b to cleave them.

10) Homologous restriction factor (HRF) binds to C8 and C9 and ultimately blocks their cell lysis ability.

11) Membrane inhibitor of reactive lysis (MIRL, CD5a) binds to C7 and C8 and prevents these components from causing cell lysis.

12) Properdin (P): an enhancer that stabilizes C3 and C5 convertases.

13) C3 nephritic factor (NF): enhances protein for disease, IgG antibody that binds to C3 convertase, and prevents activation of complement.

k. **Synthesis of complement components:** components are synthesized in the liver except C1 which is synthesized in the epithelial cells of the intestine.

2. **Acute phase response**

a. When injured, the body produces acute phase proteins

1) **C-reactive protein:** concentration increases several hundred times after injury. Can activate the classical pathway of complement. Can also bind to NK cells and monocytes, making them target tumor cells.

2) **Haptoglobin:** removes free hemoglobin from circulation.

3) **Fibrinogen:** found in increased quantities at the site of an injury; is converted to fibrin to heal the injury.

4) **α-1-antitrypsin:** a family of serine protease inhibitors synthesized in the liver. Deficiency causes premature loss of elasticity in the lung and liver damage.

5) **Ceruloplasmin:** principal copper-transportation proteins. Vital in aerobic energy production, collagen formation, and protection against superoxide ions. Deficiency is called Wilson's disease.

6) **α-2-macroglobulin:** protease inhibitor. α-2-macroglobulin and protease complexes are phagocytized by macrophages and fibroblasts.

b. **Inflammation definition:** many sequenced events that protect the host from foreign antigens, but minimize tissue damage.

1) **Increased vascular permeability:** upon injury, capillaries, arterioles, and venules are dilated to increase blood flow to the site.

a) Fluid moves from nearby cells to the space around the injury which allows the PMNs and fibrinogen to access the injury site.

b) As the fluid fills the site, the capillaries, arterioles, and venules constrict and reduce blood flow.

    c) When the blood stops flowing, the RBCs clump together and activate the coagulation cascade to form a clot.

   2) **Migration of Neutrophils**

    a) After the injury, PMNs adhere to endothelial cells.

    b) Soon the endothelial cells are covered by cells.

    c) Chemicals are released, and more PMNs are released from the storage pool, and the injury site is flooded with PMNs.

   3) **Migration of Mononuclear Cells**

    a) Migrate about 4 hours after injury.

    b) The PMNs release IL-1 which attracts monocytes, macrophages, and lymphs to the injury site.

   4) **Cellular proliferation and repair:** fibroblasts help repair damage and return the injury site to normal

VII. AUTOIMMUNE DISEASE

A. Definition—when a person produces antibodies to his/her own antigens.

B. Autoimmune Mechanisms

 1. Antibody-cell-surface component interaction

 2. Formation of autoantigen-autoantibody complexes

 3. Sensitization of T-cells

C. Beneficial Autoimmune Responses

 1. An anti-idiotype antibody can control the activity of B- and T-cells.

 2. Old red blood cells and other cells are removed from circulation.

D. Autoimmune Theories

 1. **Forbidden-clone theory:** Burnet postulated that when an error in self-recognition occurs during fetal life and lymphocytes against an autoantigen are not destroyed, then autoantibodies are produced.

 2. **Clonal anergy:** clones developed during fetal life are not stimulated by low doses of antigens. The ability to produce antibodies against higher doses of antigens is still present.

 3. **Sequestered-antigen theory:** some antigens are hidden from the immune system. Tolerance results because the immune system never "sees" these antigens. When the tissue is damaged, the hidden cells are exposed to the immune system and antibodies are produced against these "hidden cells."

 4. **Immunologic deficiency theory:** suppressor T-lymphocytes control the antibodies produced by B-cells. When the suppressor T-lymphocytes decrease activity, then antibodies against autoantigens are produced.

E. Diagnostic Tests for Non–Organ-Specific Autoimmune Diseases

 1. **Antinuclear antibodies (ANA)**

  a. Associated with systemic lupus erythematosus (SLE), mixed connective tissue disease (MCTD), and rheumatoid arthritis (RA)

---

key concepts

Describe the mechanism for autoimmune diseases and specific diseases: systemic lupus erythematosus, rheumatoid arthritis, Sjögren's syndrome, scleroderma, autoimmune hemolytic anemia, Hashimoto's disease, Graves' disease, myasthenia gravis, multiple sclerosis, diabetes mellitus, and Goodpasture's syndrome.

b. Techniques used to detect ANA: agglutination, indirect immunofluorescence, light microscopy, fluorescence immunoassay, and enzyme immunoassay
c. Interpretation of results:
  1) **Diffuse or homogenous:** evenly stains the nuclei and is associated with DNA.
  2) **Peripheral:** stains around the edge of the nuclei and is associated with native DNA.
  3) **Speckled:** stains as numerous evenly distributed speckles within the nuclei and is associated with extractable nuclear antigens.
  4) **Nucleolar:** stains 2 or 3 large fluorescent areas within the nucleus and is associated with nucleolar RNA.
  5) **Centromere:** stains as a discrete speckled pattern as the centromere fluoresces.
  6) **Spindle fiber:** only the spindle fiber fluoresces.
d. Nuclear antigens and disease association
  1) ds: DNA-SLE
  2) Histone: CLE or drug-induced SLE
  3) Sm: diagnostic for SLE
  4) Nuclear RNP: SLE, scleroderma, crest, mixed connective tissue disease
  5) SS-A: SS, SLE
  6) SS-B: SS, SLE
  7) Scl-70: scleroderma, crest
  8) Centromere: scleroderma, crest
  9) Jo-1: MYO
  10) Nucleolar: SLE

2. **Rheumatoid factor (RF)**
  a. RF is an anti-antibody: an antibody that reacts with another antibody.
  b. Two agglutination methods are available: latex agglutination and hemagglutination.
    1) **Latex agglutination:** patient serum is inactivated, then mixed with IgG-coated latex particles.
    2) **Hemagglutination:** sheep blood cells are coated with hemolysin, then mixed with patient sera. If RF is present, macroscopic agglutination will occur.

3. **Cryoglobulins**
  a. Proteins that reversibly precipitate at 4°C.
  b. **Type I cryoglobulins** are monoclonal immunoglobulins; Type II are monoclonal immunoglobulins made in response to a polyclonal immunoglobulin, and Type III are polyclonal antibodies.
  c. **Type I** and **II** cryoglobulins are associated with monoclonal gammopathies.
  d. **Type II** and **III** are circulating immune complexes.
  e. **Symptoms:** Raynaud's phenomenon, vascular purpura, bleeding tendencies, cold-induced urticaria, pain, and cyanosis.

F. Non–Organ-Specific Autoimmune Diseases

1. **Systemic lupus erythematosus (SLE)**
   a. Chronic, noninfectious, inflammatory disease involving many organs.
   b. Disease is 9 times more likely to occur in women than men and in African Americans than Caucasians.
   c. Immune complex disease where tissue injury is caused by immune complexes deposited in the tissues. There is depressed suppressor T-lymphocyte function allowing production of antibodies against "self"—especially DNA.
   d. Correlation between SLE and HLA DR3.
   e. Severity of the disease varies from person to person.
   f. Symptoms: fever, weight loss, malaise, weakness, arthritis, skin lesions, photosensitivity, butterfly rash (malar rash), renal disease, pleurisy, pericarditis, seizures, psychosis, ocular changes, pancreatitis, and small-vessel vasculitis.
   g. Hematology findings include a normochromic, normocytic anemia with leukopenia and thrombocytopenia.

2. **Rheumatoid arthritis**
   a. Chronic noninfectious systemic inflammatory disease that primarily affects the joints.
   b. Women are affected 2 to 3 times more often than men.
   c. The disease starts when lymphocytes are stimulated to produce IgG or IgM antibodies against IgG antibodies (anti-antibodies) in the synovium. Immune complexes form, which activates complement. The inflammatory response proceeds and the synovium is damaged from the response—immune complexes, neutrophils and macrophages migrate to the joint.
   d. **Symptoms** include fatigue, weight loss, weakness, mild fever, anorexia, morning stiffness, joint pain (that improves during the day), vasculitis, rheumatoid nodules, and Sjogren's syndrome.
   e. **Laboratory results:** normochromic, normocytic anemia and thrombocytosis, elevated ESR, positive CRP, positive RF, cryoglobulins, and even positive ANAs. Synovial fluid is cloudy, cell count between 5000 and 20,000/μL, elevated protein, poor mucin clot development, decreased complement, and positive RF.

3. **Sjögren's syndrome**
   a. An inflammation of salivary and lacrimal glands causing dryness of mouth and eyes.
   b. Laboratory findings: polyclonal hypergammaglobulinemia, positive RF, positive ANA (speckled or diffuse pattern), autoantibodies against the salivary glands, positive SS-B, SS-A, and rhematoid arthritis nuclear antigen.

4. **Progressive systemic sclerosis (scleroderma)**
   a. A systemic disease where fibrosis and degenerative changes occur in the skin, synovium, and internal organs.
   b. **CREST:** a milder syndrome of scleroderma characterized by calcinosis, Raynaud's phenomena, esophageal dysmotility, sclerodactyly, and telangiectases.

  c. **Laboratory results:** polyclonal hypergammaglobulinemia, positive ANA (speckled or nucleolar pattern), Scl-70 positive, or a positive centromere antibody (in CREST).

5. **Polymyositis-dermatomyositis**
  a. Acute or chronic inflammatory changes in muscle and skin.
  b. Laboratory results: polyclonal hypergammaglobulinemia, rheumatoid factor, antinuclear antibody (PM-1 or Jo-1), myoglobinemia, increased ESR, elevated CK, and elevated urine creatine.

6. **Autoimmune hemolytic anemia (AIHA)**
  a. Increased rate of RBC destruction.
  b. Results in a normocytic, normochromic anemia.
  c. Autoantibody is directed against RBC antigens.
  d. Laboratory tests: positive direct antiglobulin test (DAT).

G. Organ versus Non-Organ Specificity

1. Organ-specific autoimmune disease: antibody-antigen reactions take place in only one organ.

2. **Autoimmune thyroiditis**
  a. **Hashimoto's (chronic lymphocytic thyroiditis)**
   1) Humoral and cellular immunity are activated and destruction of normal thyroid tissue leads to hypothyroidism, loss of thyroid function, and low levels of thyroid hormones in the blood.
   2) Thyroid antibodies detected include antithyroglobulin, antithyroid peroxidase (microsomal antigen), and second colloid antigen (CA-2).
  b. **Graves' disease**
   1) Hyperplasia and diffuse goiter caused by an overstimulated thyroid gland.
   2) Thyrotoxicosis results from overstimulation; both free and total T_3 and T_4 are elevated, and TSH is decreased.
   3) Common findings: exophthalmos (bulging eyes) and infiltrative dermopathy.
   4) An autoantibody reacts with thyroid receptor on cells and are considered anti-idiotype antibodies.

3. **Autoimmune chronic hepatitis (AI-CAH)**
  a. Lymphocytes and plasma cells infiltrate the liver.
  b. A polyclonal increase in immunoglobulins occurs due to decreased number and function of suppressor T-cells.
  c. Called lupoid chronic active hepatitis because antinuclear antibodies are present.
  d. Smooth-muscle antibodies are also present in a high titer.

4. **Primary biliary cirrhosis**
  a. Most patients have high titers of mitochondrial antibodies.
  b. Affects small intrahepatic bile ducts leading to liver failure
  c. The disease also produces circulating immune complexes that lead to arthritis, arteritis, and glomerulonephritis

5. **Myasthenia gravis**
  a. Neuromuscular disease where the nerve muscles do not function normally.

    b. Most patients exhibit antibodies to acetylcholine receptors.

    c. Other symptoms include thymic hyperplasia, thymoma, and smooth-muscle antibodies.

    d. Thymus removal is treatment, and many patients do much better after removal.

6. **Multiple sclerosis (MS)**

    a. Considered a chronic progressive inflammatory disease where demyelinization of the nerves occurs.

    b. Active lesions (plaques) contain suppressor T-cells, helper T-cells, and macrophages

    c. Most MS patients have increased IgG concentrations in their CSF.

    d. The IgG index differentiates true increases due to production rather than increases in permeability of the blood-brain barrier.

$$\text{IgG index} = \frac{\text{IgG}_{CSF}/\text{albumin}_{CSF}}{\text{IgG}_{serum}/\text{albumin}_{serum}}$$

    e. Normal range for IgG index is 0.0–0.77.

    f. Oligoclonal bands in CSF on high-resolution electrophoresis is also indicative of MS, but patients with other conditions (SLE, viral meningitis, neurosyphilus, etc.) can cause oligoclonal bands in CSF.

7. **Diabetes mellitus**

    a. Islet cell antibodies produce insulin-dependent or Type I diabetes mellitus.

    b. Mechanism of disease: autoantibodies cause marked atrophy and fibrosis of the islet cells. This, in turn, causes insulin deficiency.

    c. Viruses can be the trigger for the autoantibodies because after outbreaks of mumps, measles, rubella, Coxsackie B virus, and infectious mononucleosis, new cases of Type I diabetes appear in communities.

    d. MHC Class II antigens (HLA-DQ3.2) increase the risk of developing diabetes, whereas HLA-DQ1.2 decreases the risk of developing diabetes.

8. **Chronic atrophic gastritis with pernicious anemia**

    a. Stomach atrophy can be caused by antibodies directed against the chief and parietal cells. This atrophy results in reduced hydrochloric acid, pepsinogens, and intrinsic factor production.

    b. Most pernicious anemia patients have parietal cell and intrinsic factor antibodies.

9. **Idiopathic adrenal failure:** antibodies directed against the mitochondrial cells of the adrenal cortex leads to Addison's disease.

10. **Goodpasture's syndrome:** Complement activation causes pulmonary hemorrhage and glomerulonephritis

11. **Autoimmune bullous skin diseases**

12. **Spermatozoa antibody-mediated infertility**

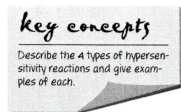

key concepts

Describe the 4 types of hypersensitivity reactions and give examples of each.

VIII.   **HYPERSENSITIVTY**

  A. Type I Hypersensitivity

    1. **Type I: immediate hypersensitivity** because it occurs within minutes of contact with an antigen or allergen. Basophils and

macrophages are sensitized by IgE which causes release of amines from those cells that causes allergic symptoms.

a. **Allergy:** magnitude of allergic response depends on where allergen enters the body. People that exhibit symptoms are predisposed to Type I hypersensitivity and produce increased amounts of IgE.

1) **Allergens and disease**

a) Individuals can be exposed to allergens through the upper respiratory tract, absorption from the intestinal tract, and direct skin contact.

b) Allergic reactions occur in tissues with many mast cells—skin, nasal membranes, tongue, lungs, and gastrointestinal tract.

c) Allergens contacting the nasal mucosa cause runny nose, itching eyes and nose, sneezing, and nasal congestion. Eosinophil levels in blood and nasal secretions may be elevated, and IgE may be normal or elevated.

d) Allergens contacting the bronchus cause asthma. Serum IgE levels are usually increased.

e) Atopic dermatitis can occur with allergic rhinitis, intrinsic asthma, eosinophilia, and very high levels of IgE.

f) Food allergies are the least common form of predisposition to Type I hypersensitivity. Symptoms include nausea, vomiting, cramps, abdominal pain, and diarrhea within 2 hours of ingestion.

g) Anaphylaxis is the systemic form of Type I immediate hypersensitivity. Can be life threatening when it causes shock or edema of the upper respiratory track. Substances that can precipitate this condition include peanuts, seafood, egg albumin, honeybee, wasp, or hornet stings, vaccines, penicillin, or sulfonamides.

b. **Laboratory evaluation of allergies**

1) **Total serum IgE levels:** methods used include competitive radioimmunosorbent test (RIST), noncompetitive RIST, double-antibody radioimmunoassay (RIA), and sandwich enzyme-linked immunosorbent assay (ELISA).

2) **Allergen-specific IgE: radioallergosorbent test (RAST)** is used to detect IgE for specific allergens.

c. **Treatment:** allergen avoidance, drug therapy, and immunotherapy.

d. **Mechanism of amine release**

1) Cells involved are basophils and mast cells.

2) IgE antibodies attach to the surface of these cells. A second exposure to the allergen causes release of vasoactive amines. These amines cause a generalized allergic response

e. **Histamine**

1) Causes contraction of bronchioles and smooth muscle of blood vessels.

2) Increases capillary permeability.

3) Increases mucus gland secretion in the airway.

4) Duration of activity is 10 minutes.
   f. **Eosinophil chemotactic factor of anaphylaxis:** stimulates eosinophils to migrate to site of an antibody-antigen reaction.
   g. **Prostaglandin D+2** causes vasodilation and increases vascular permeability. Half-life is approximately 1 hour.
   h. **Leukotrines** C_4, D_4, and E_4 cause erythema and wheal formation. 30 to 1000 times the ability of histamine to cause bronchospasms. Also stimulate mucus secretion by airways.

B. Type II Hypersensitivity
1. **IgG or IgM antibodies** directed against cell surface markers.
2. **Antibody-mediated tissue damage:** antibody-sensitized cells are cleared more quickly by phagocytic cells.
3. **Complement-mediated cell lysis:** antibody-antigen complex activates the complement pathway to cause cell lysis. Transfusions are the best example of this type of hypersensitivity.
4. **Damage to tissue cells:** antibody production against tissue cells causes inflammation which, in turn, causes damage to innocent tissue cells. For example, Goodpasture's syndrome where antibodies to basement membranes cause renal tissue damage.

C. Type III Hypersensitivity
1. Antibody-antigen complexes are deposited on tissues causing inflammation.
2. **Circulating immune complexes:** large immune complexes are rapidly cleared by mononuclear phagocytes, but the smaller immune complexes stay in circulation longer and can be deposited on tissue cells.
3. Two tissues where immune complexes are deposited include the heart valves and renal glomeruli
4. Examples:
   a. **Arthus reaction:** an antigen is injected intradermally to an individual.
   b. **Immune complex disorders (serum sickness):** patients develop antibodies against heterologous serum proteins and develop a disorder.
   c. **Glomerulonephritis** immune complexes deposit on renal glomeruli causing inflammation of the kidney and possibly renal failure.
   d. **Vasculitis:** inflammation of the vessel walls.

D. Type IV Hypersensitivity (Delayed Hypersensitivity)
1. Caused by soluble factors or lymphokines released by T-lymphs—antibody and complement are not involved in this reaction.
2. **Mechanism**
   a. Lymphokines are produced by T-lymphs.
   b. These chemicals attract macrophages that become activated.
   c. As more and more macrophages pool at the site, ulceration and necrosis occur approximately 24 to 48 hours after exposure to antigen.

3. Examples:

    a. Tuberculin-type hypersensitivity: subcutaneous injection of TB antigen in an individual. Swelling and redness occur at the site within 24 to 72 hours.

    b. Contact sensitivity (contact dermatitis): poison ivy and poison oak cause systemic sensitization to an antigen. Edema in the skin with the formation of microvesicles results.

    c. Granulomatous hypersensitivity occurs when bacteria remain in macrophages and are not destroyed. Occurs in tuberculosis, leprosy, and sarcoidosis.

IX. IMMUNE DEFICIENCY

A. Primary Immune Deficiencies

1. **Humoral immune deficiencies**

    a. **Bruton's X-linked agammaglobulinemia**

        1) A deficiency of all classes of immunoglobulins after 6 months of age.

        2) Recurrent, life-threatening infections occur with *Streptococcus pneumoniae* and *Haemophilus influenzae*, resulting in pneumonia, sinusitis, bronchitis, otitis, furunculosis, meningitis, and septicemia.

        3) B-cells are markedly decreased or absent.

    b. **Selective IgA deficiency**

        1) Symptom: tiny amounts or absence of serum and secretory IgA.

        2) Usually caused by a genetic defect or by drugs (phenytoin and penicillin).

        3) Anaphylaxis may result if IgA is administered to someone with this deficiency, i.e., blood transfusion.

    c. **Common variable immunodeficiency (CVID)**

        1) Late onset disorders with both autosomal dominant, recessive, and X-linked inheritance. May also show no inheritance pattern

        2) Shows marked decrease in serum immunoglobulin concentrations and infections with *Streptococcus pneumoniae* and *Haemophilus influenzae*.

        3) Occurs between 15 and 35 years of age.

        4) Patients have decreased B-cells.

        5) 8 percent of these patients develop malignancy—leukemia, lymphoma, and epithelial cell tumors.

    d. **Hyper-IgM syndrome (HIM)**

        1) Serum IgM is increased, IgG is markedly increased, and IgA is absent.

        2) Pyogenic infections (*S. pneumoniae, H. influenzae)* and opportunistic infections.

        3) Prone to autoimmune diseases (autoimmune hemolytic anemia, thrombocytopenia purpura, and neutropenia).

2. **Cellular immune deficiencies**

    a. **Thymic hypoplasia (DiGeorge syndrome)**

        1) Main symptom: hypocalcemic tetany after birth due to underdevelopment of the parathyroids and thymus.

key concepts

Compare and contrast immune deficiencies and explain the disease mechanism and laboratory findings for the most common deficiencies.

2) Associated abnormalities: wide-set eyes, antimongoloid eye slant, low-set and notched ears, small jaw, short philtrum of the upper lip, mandibular hypoplasia, and cardiac and aortic arch anomalies (tetralogy of Fallot).

3) No T-lymphocytes in blood, very susceptible to opportunistic infections.

4) Prone to develop graft-versus-host disease from lymphocytes in nonirradiated blood.

b. **Nezelof syndrome (cellular immunodeficiency with normal or increased immunoglobulins)**

1) Profound T-cell dysfunction with abnormal immunoglobulin synthesis.

2) Children have chronic pulmonary infections, failure to thrive, oral or cutaneous candidiasis, chronic diarrhea, recurrent skin infections, gram negative sepsis, urinary tract infections, and severe progressive varicella.

3. **Combined humoral and cellular immune deficiencies**

a. **Severe combined immune deficiency (SCID)**

1) **Autosomal recessive SCID (Swiss-type lymphopenic agammaglobulinemia) with or without adenosine deaminase deficiency**

a) Apparently normal infants begin to waste away after diarrhea and infections begin, and death is usually caused by an opportunistic infection.

b) Very low percentage of T-cells.

c) Both T- and B-cells are nonfunctional.

2) **SCID with hematopoietic hypoplasia**

3) **Combined immunodeficiency (CID)-MHC class deficiency (bare-lymphocyte syndrome)**

a) Symptoms include severe and protracted diarrhea, sclerosing cholangitis, upper respiratory tract infections, pneumonia, and failure to thrive.

b) MHC Class II deficiencies demonstrate hypogammaglobulinemia and no delayed hypersensitivity reactions.

c) MHC Class I deficiency demonstrate recurrent and severe bacterial pulmonary infections starting in late childhood.

b. **Partial combined immune deficiency**

1) **Wiskott-Aldrich syndrome**

a) Patients demonstrate eczema, thrombocytopenic purpura, and increased risk of infection.

b) Early on, pneumonia, meningitis, otitis, and sepsis followed by infection with *Pneumocystis carinii* and herpes viruses. Death occurs as few patients survive past the teenage years.

2) **Ataxia-telangiectasia**

a) Autosomal recessive disorder that presents with ataxia, telangiectasia, recurrent sinopulmonary infections, a high incidence of malignancy, and variable immune defects.

b) Defects are in the B-cells and helper T-cells.

    c. **Phagocytic deficiencies**
      1) **Leukocyte-adhesion defect (LAD)**
        a) Leukocytes cannot adhere to endothelial surfaces or cell membranes.
        b) Patients are unable to form pus.
      2) **Chronic granulomatous disease (CGD)**
        a) Phagocytes are unable to kill ingested bacteria due to an inability to produce oxygen radical and hydrogen peroxides (toxic superoxides).
        b) Symptoms include pneumonia, lymphadenitis, abscesses in the skin, liver, and other organs.
    d. **Complement deficiencies**
      1) **Hereditary angioedema (HAE)**
        a) Deficiency or dysfunction of C1 inhibitor.
        b) Symptoms: swelling or edema in the face and upper respiratory airway, abdomen, and intestines.

B. Secondary Immune Deficiencies

1. **Transient hypogammaglobulinemia of infancy:** decline in serum immunoglobulins during the first few months of life. Person eventually produces normal amounts of immunoglobulins.
2. **Malignancy**
    a. Cancers can exert a suppressive effect on the immune system.
      1) T-cell function defects cause Hodgkin's disease.
      2) Impairment of antibody production is found in lymphomas, chronic lymphocytic leukemia, and multiple myeloma.
3. **Viral Disease**
    a. Certain viruses impair the function of the immune system
      1) HIV-1
      2) Epstein-Barr
      3) CMV
      4) Herpes family of viruses

X. HYPERGAMMAGLOBULINEMIA

A. Polyclonal hypergammaglobulinemia—when tremendous amounts of several classes of immunoglobulins to several specific antigens are produced resulting in a broad spike in the gamma protein region on a serum protein electrophoresis.

1. **Infectious diseases:** chronic antigenic stimulation from infectious organisms creates this condition.
2. **Inflammatory process:** many acute-phase proteins are produced during inflammation and reveal themselves as a broadening of the alpha-2 peak in a serum protein electrophoresis.
3. **Liver disease:** due to a polyclonal increase in the gamma region and also an increase in IgA, the depression between the gamma region and the beta region is absent. As a result, the beta and gamma region form only one peak on serum protein electrophoresis; (**beta-gamma bridging**) consistent with cirrhosis.

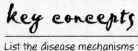

key concepts

List the disease mechanisms that produce hypergammaglobulinemia and the laboratory findings in the disease.

\ **B. Monoclonal hypergammaglobulinemia**—a malignant transformation of one clone of B-cells to produce the same exact antibodies. This causes a narrow peak on the serum protein electrophoresis scan.

1. **Multiple myeloma**
   a. Lymphoproliferative disease where a single B-cell clone produces a high concentration of one type of immunoglobulin.
   b. 50 percent of multiple myeloma patients have Bence Jones protein in their urine. This can be nephrotoxic and can result in kidney damage and ultimately failure.
   c. Symptoms: weakness, anorexia, weight loss, skeletal destruction, pain, anemia, renal insufficiency, and recurrent bacterial infections.
   d. Laboratory results: monoclonal gammopathy and plasma cell infiltrate in bone marrow.

2. **Waldenström's macroglobulinemia**
   a. Uncontrolled proliferation of a clone of B-cells that synthesize a homogenous IgM.
   b. Symptoms: weakness, fatigability, headache, weight loss, and hyperviscosity syndrome.
   c. Hyperviscosity causes congestive heart failure, headache, dizziness, partial or total loss of vision, bleeding, and anemia.
   d. Laboratory results: a spike in the beta or gamma region on serum protein electrophoresis, increased plasma viscosity, and abnormal accumulation of lymphoid cells in the bone marrow and tissues.

3. **Heavy-chain diseases**
   a. Rare lymphoproliferative disorders presenting with fragments of heavy immunoglobulin chains, but no light chains.
   b. **Alpha-heavy chain disease**
      1) Most common.
      2) Symptoms: diarrhea, abdominal pain, and malabsorption.
   c. **Gamma-heavy chain disease:** symptoms: fever, malaise, weight loss, peculiar edema, and erythema of palate and uvula, generalized lymphadenopathy, and hepatosplenomegaly.
   d. **Mu-heavy chain disease**
      1) Hepatosplenomegaly and lymphadenopathy.
      2) Plasma cells have vacuoles and are present in high numbers in the peripheral blood.

4. **Primary amyloidosis**
   a. Accumulation of a complex extracellular proteinaceous substance with a fibrillar component.
   b. The fibril called amyloid A is an immunoglobulin fragment that is produced by a specific clone of B-cells.
   c. Laboratory results: frequent abnormalities of serum immunoglobulins, hypogammaglobulinemia.

5. **Monoclonal gammopathy of undetermined significance (MGUS) – (Benign monoclonal gammopathy):** Monoclonal protein present in serum or urine with no other symptoms

XI. TRANSPLANT IMMUNOLOGY

A. Types of Grafts

1. **Autograft:** transfer of tissue from one site to another within an individual
2. **Isograft:** transfer of tissue between genetically identical individuals
3. **Allograft:** transfer of tissue between two individuals of the same species

B. Graft Acceptance and Rejection

1. Graft acceptance is when revascularization and healing lead to a repaired site in about 2 weeks.
2. 2 types of graft rejection
   a. **First-set rejection:** first time a graft is encountered and rejected (the immune system attacks and ultimately destroys the "non-self tissue." Occurs 10 to 14 days after transplantation.
   b. **Second-set rejection:** the second time the same set of "non-self" tissue is encountered and rejected within 6 days.

C. Clinical Indications of Graft Rejection

1. **Hyperacute rejection** occurs within 24 hours of transplantation.
   a. Caused by a preexisting antibody to antigens on the grafted tissue.
   b. ABO antibodies and MHC Class I antibodies cause hyperacute rejection.
   c. Crossmatches are performed on tissue transplants because alloimmunization can lead to alloantibody production and hyperacute rejection of a transplanted tissue.
   d. In this crossmatch, serum of the recipient is mixed with mononuclear donor cells, and the mixture is monitored for cytotoxicity.
2. **Acute rejection** occurs within weeks of transplantation.
3. **Chronic rejection** occurs months to years after transplantation.

D. Tissue Typing

1. **Transplantation antigens** are major histocompatibility complex (MHC): HLA system.
2. The donor and recipient must be typed and matched for ABO and HLA antigens.
3. HLA-identical donors have lowest rate of rejection.
4. HLA antigens involved in matching of organs: 2 HLA-A, 2 HLA-B, and 2 HLA-DR antigens are matched.

E. Immunosupression

1. All allogenic transplants require immunosuppression if the organ is to survive.
2. These drugs prevent the recipient from rejecting the graft, but maintain enough immune system function to avoid recurrent infections.
   a. Azathrioprine, cyclophosphamide, and methotrexate interfere with nucleic acid metabolism of the mononuclear immune cells.

      b. Corticosteroids are anti-inflammatory drugs that decrease the number of circulating lymphocytes.

      c. Cyclosporin A prevents helper T-cell activation.

      d. Antilymphocyte serum contains antibodies to kill lymphocytes in the recipient.

3. Irradiation of the recipient will reduce numbers of lymphocytes prior to transplantation and new lymphocytes are more tolerant of graft

F. Transplantation

1. Types of transplants now performed

    a. Kidney

    b. Cornea

    c. Heart

    d. Lung

    e. Liver

    f. Bone marrow

    g. Pancreas

    h. Peripheral blood stem cells

2. **Complications of Transplantation**

    a. Contracting a bacterial, fungal, viral, or parasitic infection.

    b. Chemotherapy or radiation therapy may also be toxic to organs.

    c. Graft-versus-host disease (GVHD) can occur when new lymphocytes in a bone marrow transplant are released into the peripheral blood.

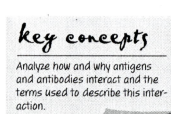

key concepts

Analyze how and why antigens and antibodies interact and the terms used to describe this interaction.

XII. ANTIGEN-ANTIBODY INTERACTION

A. Antigen-Antibody interaction

1. **Forces that participate in antibody-antigen interaction:**

    a. Electrostatic force or ionic bonding

      1) Positively charged portions of one molecule are attracted to negatively charged portions of another molecule.

      2) This bonding is affected by the pH and ionic strength of the environment

      3) Electrostatic force increases as the two molecules get closer together.

    b. Hydrogen bonding

      1) When two electronegative atoms form hydrogen bond

      2) A weak bond, but it contributes greatly to the antigen-antibody interaction

      3) Maximum binding strength occurs below 37°C.

    c. Hydrophobic bonding

      1) This is the attraction between nonpolar groups

      2) The groups tend to aggregate to reduce surface area and this increases the strength of the bond

    d. Van der Waals force

      1) A weak, attractive force between an electron orbital of one atom and the nucleus of another atom

2. **Antibody affinity**

    a. Antibody and antigen binding is governed by the law of mass action. The law of mass action states that this reaction is in equilibrium—as many antibodies are attaching to the antigen as are unattaching themselves from the antigen.

b. The affinity constant describes whether the antigen-antibody complex is highly complimentary and therefore would bind readily, or not very complimentary and therefore would not bind readily.

3. **Avidity**

a. The affinity for multivalent antigens and multiple antibodies to combine.

b. This is more than the cumulative affinity constants for all antigen-antibody pairs.

4. **Specificity and Cross Reactivity**

a. **Specificity** refers to the antibody's greatest affinity for a particular antigen.

b. **Cross reactivity** is when the antigen combines with another antigen that is structurally similar to antigen that the antibody has the greatest affinity for, i.e., heterophile antibodies in infectious mononucleosis.

B. Assays Using Antibody-Antigen Interactions

1. **Assays that use antibody-antigen reactions are called immunoassays**.

2. Examples

a. **Precipitation reactions:** soluble antigen and soluble antibody react: double gel diffusion, radial immunodiffusion, immunoelectrophoresis, immunofixation, nephelometry, turbidimetry

b. **Agglutination reaction:** soluble antibody reacting with solid antigen or soluble antigen reacting with solid antibody: latex particles, red blood cells, dye, or liposomes

c. **Labeled immunoassays:** a label that produces a measurable end product and is attached to an antibody or antigen: fluorochromes, enzymes, radionucleotides, or chemiluminescent molecules

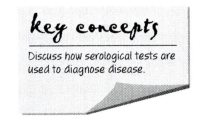

key concepts

Discuss how serological tests are used to diagnose disease.

XIII. PRECIPITATION REACTIONS

A. Precipitation—soluble antigen and antibody combine to form a solid

1. **Zone of equivalence:** maximum precipitation occurs when the concentration of the antigen and antibody are about equal.

2. **Prozone:** excess amount of antibody present and the antigen and antibody do not clump together to form solids—the complexes remain soluble.

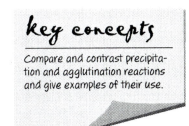

key concepts

Compare and contrast precipitation and agglutination reactions and give examples of their use.

B. Types of Precipitation Reactions

1. **Fluid-phase precipitation:** passive diffusion of soluble antigen and antibody

a. Procedure: in a capillary tube, soluble antigen solution is placed over a soluble antibody solution. The antigen and antibody diffuse toward one another. When the two meet, they form a precipitate that is directly proportional to the concentration of the antigen and the antibody.

2. **Precipitation reactions in gel**
   a. Antigen and antibody diffuse through the gel and form precipitates in the agarose gel.
   b. Molecular size determines the speed of travel through the gel.
   c. **Double immunodiffusion (Ouchterlony technique)**
      1) Involves using soluble antigen and soluble antibody and allowing diffusion of both into the agarose gel. When optimum concentrations are met for both the antibody and the antigen, a precipitate line forms in the gel.
      2) Can be used to determine if a specific antibody is present in serum
      3) Serial dilutions can determine the concentration of the antibody present.
      4) Common errors include overfilling of wells, irregular well punching, uneven incubation area, gel drying, increased room temperature, and antigen or antibody contamination by bacteria or fungi.
   d. **Countercurrent immunoelectrophoresis (CIEP)**
      1) On a gel plate, antigen is added to one well and antibody is added to the other well. An electric current speeds up the movement of the antigen and antibody towards each other resulting in precipitation.
      2) Used to detect autoantibodies, antibodies to infectious agents, and particular microbial antigens.
   e. **Immunofixation electrophoresis (IFE)**
      1) Serum, urine, or CSF is electrophoresed. Antisera contained in a cellulose acetate strip is then placed on top of the electrophoresis gel. The antibodies diffuse into the electrophoresis gel and combine with the antigens, forming a precipitate.
      2) **Immunofixation electrophoresis:** detect the presence of an immunoglobulin in serum or urine.
   f. **Rocket technique (also called Laurel technique)**
      1) Used to quantitate antigens other than immunoglobulins.
      2) Antisera is a part of the gel; antigens are electrophoresed. The antibody and antigen combine to form precipitates in the shape of a rocket.
      3) The distance the antigen travels is directly proportional to the antigen concentration.

XIV. AGGLUTINATION
A. General Information
1. **Definition:** occurs when particles in suspension clump together due to antibody-antigen interaction.
2. Excess antibody can cause prozone as described for precipitation.
3. Antibody-antigen interaction and clumping occur more quickly in agglutination than in precipitation.
4. IgM and IgG antibodies participate in agglutination reactions, with IgM agglutination occurring more quickly.

5. **Comparison of agglutination and precipitation**
   a. Agglutination uses a solid antigen, whereas precipitation uses soluble antigens.
   b. Agglutination and precipitation reactions use antigens with at least 2 antigenic determinants.
   c. In agglutination and precipitation, antigen excess can result in a postzone reaction, whereas antibody excess can result in a prozone reaction.
   d. Agglutination reactions take minutes to hours whereas precipitation reactions may take hours to days.
   e. Methods that utilize agglutination reactions are qualitative or semiquantitative, whereas precipitation methods give qualitative, semiquantitative, or quantitative results.

B. Classification of Agglutination Reactions

1. **Direct agglutination:** this method uses naturally occurring antigens to demonstrate agglutination. For example, red blood cells can be used.
2. **Viral hemagglutination:** this is a naturally occurring process where a virus will agglutinate red blood cells by binding to surface receptors.
3. **Passive and Reverse Passive Agglutination**
   a. **Passive agglutination:** a technique where soluble antigen is attached to a particle; causing agglutination instead of precipitation.
   b. **Reverse passive agglutination:** a technique where the antibody is attached to a particle; demonstrating the presence of soluble antigen.
   c. Particles used are latex, charcoal, gelatin, resin beads, and red blood cells.
   d. **Sources of error** for these reactions include prozone, and cross reactivity.
4. **Column Agglutination Technology (CAT)**
   a. The antigen and antibody are placed above a column of glass bead microparticles or in a gel.
   b. The tubes are centrifuged.
   c. If the red blood cells are at the bottom of the tube, no agglutination has occurred.
   d. If the red blood cells are in the middle of the tube, agglutination has occurred. The agglutination reaction can be semiquantitated.
5. **Complement fixation**
   a. **Principle**
      1) An antigen-antibody reaction that initiates complement to bind to the immune complex.
      2) Hemolysis is a negative reaction, and no hemolysis is a positive reaction.
      3) When the antibody and antigen combine in this technique, the complement present in the system also combines with

the antigen-antibody complexes and no free complement is available to cause lysis of the sensitized indicator red blood cells.

4) When there is free complement, it attaches to the sensitized indicator RBCs and causes lysis.

b. Used to detect antibodies to viruses, *Rickettsia*, and fungi, i.e., Rocky Mountain spotted fever, herpes simplex, and influenza.

c. Serial dilutions (titration) can be performed to make the results semiquantitative.

d. **Polyethylene glycol (PEG)** enhances the rate of antibody uptake.

e. **Polybrene** brings the cells closer together so that the antigens and antibodies can bind and form lattices.

f. **Antihuman globulin (AHG)** used to detect sensitized RBCs. This reagent binds to the antibodies on RBCs and forms a lattice, hence agglutination.

XV. IMMUNOFLUORESCENCE

A. **Definition**—antibodies labeled with a fluorescent dye used to detect an antibody or antigen.

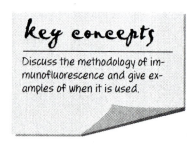

key concepts

Discuss the methodology of immunofluorescence and give examples of when it is used.

B. **Methods**

1. **Direct immunofluorescence:** conjugated reagent antibody reacts with the antigen to form an antigen-antibody complex.

2. **Indirect immunofluorescent assays:** antigen reacts with unlabeled antibody forming an antigen-antibody complex which is then complexed with a labeled antibody, creating an antibody-antigen-antibody "sandwich."

3. **Biotin-avidin immunofluorescence:** an indirect assay where the detection system is modified by using a biotin-labeled antibody followed by avidin-labeled fluorochrome. This extra step increases the specificity and sensitivity of the assay.

C. **Common Fluorochromes Used in Assays**

1. Fluorescein isothiocyanate
2. R-phycoerythrin
3. Quantum red
4. Tetramethyl rhodamine isothiocyanate
5. Texas red
6. Phycocyanin
7. Allophycocyanin
8. Acridine orange
9. Propidium iodide

D. **Applications**

1. **Antinuclear antibodies (ANA):** antibodies to nuclear antigens are present in many systemic diseases: systemic lupus erythematosis, mixed connective tissue disease, and rheumatoid arthritis. This test is used for diagnosing, developing a prognosis, and monitoring treatment.

a. Indirect immunofluorescence is used for ANA screening.

      b. Procedure: rodent liver or tissue culture cells are incubated with patient serum. Tissue is washed, then incubated with antihuman immunoglobulin conjugated with fluorescein. Slide is washed again, then viewed using a fluorescent microscope.

  2. Direct immunofluorescence on a skin biopsy indicates Bullous pemphigoid, pemphigus vulgaris, or dermatitis herpetiformis.

  3. **Indirect immunofluorescence**

      a. Smooth muscle antibody indicates autoimmune chronic active hepatitis.

      b. Mitochondrial antibody indicates primary biliary cirrhosis.

      c. Thyroglobulin antibody indicates Hashimoto's thyroiditis and Graves' disease.

      d. Thyroid peroxidase antibody indicates Hashimoto's thyroiditis and Graves' disease.

      e. Parietal cell antibody indicates chronic atrophic gastritis with pernicious anemia.

XVI. CELLULAR ASSAYS

A. Lymphocyte Subsets

  1. **T-cell subsets**

      a. Classical test: E-rosette assay.

      b. Monoclonal antibodies are now used in conjunction with flow cytometry to identify CD7, CD2, CD5, CD1, CD4, and CD8.

  2. **B-Cell subsets**

      a. Classical test: labeled antibody to surface membrane immunoglobin.

      b. Monoclonal antibodies are now used in conjunction with flow cytometry to identify CD19 or CD20.

  3. Lymphocyte Phenotyping in HIV Infection

      a. HIV kills circulating T-helper cells and the viral receptor for infection is CD4.

      b. CD4 and CD8 markers are monitored during treatment. Physicians look at the absolute CD4 count to make sure it is above 200/μL. If it falls below 200/μL, the patient is susceptible to opportunistic infections.

  4. **Other cells identified by flow cytometry and monoclonal antibodies:**

      a. CD16 on NK cells, macrophages, and neutrophils

      b. CD34 on immature cells

      c. HLA-DR on B cells, monocytes, myeloid, and erythroid precursors

      d. Glycophorin A on erythroid cells

      e. CD14 on myelomonocytic cells

      f. CD45 on all blood cells except red blood cells

      g. CD41 on platelets and megakaryocytes

B. Assays to Assess Cell Function

  1. **Lymphocyte transformation**

      a. Cells are challenged with 3 antigens.

      b. The cells are observed as they transform.

key concepts

Discuss the methodology of cellular assays and give examples of when it is used.

c. Normal cells are stimulated by all antigens, while the patient's cells are observed for normal stimulation.

2. **Mixed-lymphocyte culture**
   a. Used to detect HLA-Dw on the surface of cells to ensure compatibility of donor cells with recipient cells.
   b. This is critical for bone marrow transplants.

3. **Cytotoxicity:** extremely difficult, used to determine HLA-A and HLA-B antigens.

4. **Measurement of immune activation**
   a. **Definition:** all the events that lead to an immune response.
   b. Measurement includes a white blood count with differential, immunoglobulin levels, and complement levels.
   c. Signs of immune activation in the patient include swollen lymph nodes, fever, and malaise.
   d. Cytokines are beginning to be measured to detect immune disorders (IL-2).

5. **Neutrophil function assays**
   a. Dysfunctional neutrophils cannot kill bacteria, so patients develop recurring bacterial infections. The most common disease is chronic granulomatous disease.
   b. Nitroblue tetrazolium (NBT) test: normal neutrophils reduce this dye to formazan, which appears as dark blue granules. Dysfunctional neutrophils are unable to reduce this dye.
   c. Other dysfunctional neutrophils exhibit defects in chemotaxis. A stimulant is added to patient neutrophils, and the amount of movement among cells is measured.

XVII. INFECTIOUS DISEASE SEROLOGY
A. Infectious Disease Definitions

1. **Infection:** when a microorganism invades a host and multiplies enough to disrupt normal function by causing signs and symptoms of disease.

2. **Pathogenicity:** ability of an organism to cause disease.

3. **Incubation period:** time between the infection and signs and symptoms of disease.

4. **Prodromal phase:** time immediately before the onset of acute disease (1 to 2 days).

5. **Acute phase:** most severe signs and symptoms of disease occur.

6. **Acute titer:** antibody level drawn when symptoms of disease appear.

7. **Convalescent phase:** signs and symptoms are receding and person is returning to normal health.

8. **Convalescent titers:** antibody level drawn 2 weeks after symptoms appear.

XVIII. STREPTOCOCCAL SEROLOGY
A. Organism

1. Gram positive cocci that occur in chains.

2. Cause: pharyngitis, pyoderma, puerperal sepsis, and acute endocarditis. Also produce toxins that result in scarlet fever.

3. **Poststreptococcal sequelae**
   a. Antibody-antigen complexes can lead to rheumatic fever and glomerulonephritis. Usually diagnosed by the antistreptolysin O (ASO), streptozyme, antihyaluronidase (AHT) or anti-DNase B tests.
   b. **Rheumatic Fever**
      1) **Symptoms:** carditis, chorea, and/or erythema marginatum
      2) Occurs 3 to 4 weeks after infection with group A beta-hemolytic streptococcus
      3) Most common between 5 and 15 years of age
   c. **Glomerulonephritis**
      1) **Symptoms:** proteinuria, hematuria, hypertension, impaired renal function, and edema.
      2) Occurs 10 days after a throat infection or 18–21 days after a skin infection.
      3) **Mechanism:** circulating antigen-antibody complexes are deposited on the glomerular basement membranes where complement is activated and damage to the membranes results. Platelet aggregation and fibrin and fibrinogen build up to cause capillary obstruction and impaired renal function.

B. **Diagnostic Tests**
   1. Culture results producing a beta-hemolytic Group A strep are most reliable, but the actively growing organism is no longer producing infection and may not be found.
   2. **ASO Titer**
      a. Streptolysin O is produced by most beta-hemolytic Group A strep.
      b. Streptolysin O begins rising 1 week after infection and peaks 3–6 weeks after infection.
      c. Principle: neutralization assay.
      d. Results: titer is the last tube with no hemolysis. The reciprocal of the original serum dilution are the Todd units: i.e. 1:8 = 8 Todd units.
      e. Interpretation: a fourfold increase in titer between acute and convalescent tubes indicates a recent Group A strep infection.
   3. **ASO Rapid Latex Agglutination Test**
      a. **Principle:** latex particles are coated with Streptolysin O agglutinate when mixed with a patient's serum containing ASO antibody.
      b. **Interpretation:** positive result is >200 U/mL of ASO.
   4. **Streptozyme**
      a. Screening test produced by Wampole Laboratories, Cranbury, New Jersey, which detects 5 antibodies—DNase B, hyaluronidase, NADase, streptokinase, and Streptolysin O.
      b. **Principle:** passive hemagglutination.
      c. **Interpretation:** cells will agglutinate when antibodies are in the patient's serum.
   5. **Antihyaluronidase test**
      a. **Principle:** neutralization assay.

      b. **Results:** titer is reciprocal of the highest dilution with definite clot formation.

      c. **Interpretation:** a fourfold rise between acute and convalescent serums is indicative of an infection.

6. **Antideoxyribonuclease B test**

      a. Peaks at 4–6 weeks after Group A strep infection and lasts for months.

      b. **Principle:** neutralization test. Anti-DNase-B neutralizes DNA in the DNA-methyl green complex, resulting in a loss of color.

      c. **Results:** color graded from 0–4+ (colorless to green).

      d. **Interpretation:** test acute and convalescent paired sera. Four-fold rise from acute to convalescent sera is diagnostic of a recent Group A strep infection.

XIX. SYPHILIS

A. *Treponema pallidum:* spirochete, causative agent of syphilis.

B. Epidemiology: transmitted by sexual contact, direct contact, and through the placenta.

C. Disease stages

1. **Incubation:** *Treponema palladium* enters the body and filters into the blood system to be disseminated to all organs. This occurs up to 33 hours postinfection. Lasts 9–10 days. Asymptomatic phase.

2. **Primary syphilis**

      a. Initial lesion is painless (nonbleeding, painless ulcer) called a **chancre**.

      b. Chancre appears 2–3 weeks after initial infection.

      c. Within one week after chancre appears, lymph nodes enlarge.

      d. Antibodies are produced 1–4 weeks after chancre appears.

      e. Darkfield analysis of lesion demonstrates spirochetes.

3. **Secondary syphilis**

      a. Symptoms include skin rash, low-grade fever, malaise, pharyngitis, weight loss, arthralgia, and lymphadenopathy.

      b. Spirochetes are throughout the body at this stage.

      c. Mucus patches develop on mucus membranes.

      d. Serological tests: positive.

4. **Latency**

      a. Stage of syphilis with no signs or symptoms.

      b. Nontreponemal and treponemal tests are positive.

      c. Early latency: 1 in 4 relapse into secondary syphilis.

      d. Late latency: patient resistant to reinfection and relapses.

5. **Tertiary syphilis**

      a. Produces symptoms 2–40 years after initial infection.

      b. **Gummas** (syphilis lesions) are found throughout the body.

      c. Syphilitic aortitis, aortic valve insufficiency, and thoracic aneurysm possible.

      d. Neurosyphilis: causes blindness and insanity.

6. **Congenital syphilis**

      a. *Treponema pallidum* crosses the placenta during all stages of the disease

      b. Infection of the fetus causes late abortion, stillbirth, neonatal death, neonatal disease, or latent infection.

key concepts

Discuss the stages of disease that syphilis produces and the test (and test methodology) used to diagnose this disease.

    c. The outcome depends on the stage of the mother's disease—primary or secondary syphilis causing the worst outcome.

    d. If the mother receives treatment during the first 4 months of pregnancy, congenital syphilis is avoided.

    e. Congenital syphilis presents in the neonate as sniffles, diffuse maculopapular desquamatous rash (particularly around mouth and on palms and soles), hemolytic anemia, jaundice, hepatosplenomegaly, and bone involvement.

  7. Diagnosis: detection of spirochetes in lesion, signs and symptoms of disease stage, and positive syphilis serologies.

  8. Treatment: drug of choice is penicillin. Alternative drug is doxycycline.

D. Direct detection

1. Definitive diagnosis of syphilis is detection of *Treponema pallidum* from lesion, CSF, umbilical cord, nasal discharge, or skin lesions—depending on the stage of the disease.

2. *Treponema pallidum* is detected using darkfield microscopy.

3. DFA-TP (Direct Fluorescent Antigen—*Treponema pallidum*): developed to detect *Treponema pallidum* from lesions with increased sensitivity and specificity over VDRL.

E. Serological tests

1. **General principles**

    a. *Treponema pallidum* infection causes the host to produce reagin and specific treponemal antibodies.

    b. The tests that detect the nonspecific antibodies (reagin) are used for screening only because this antibody will cross react with similar antigens present in systemic lupus erythamatosis, autoimmune disease, pregnancy, drug addicts, and some chronic infections (biological false positives).

    c. The percent of false positives in this test is high (30–40%) so every positive must be confirmed using a test that can detect antibodies specifically directed at *Treponema pallidum*.

2. **VDRL (veneral disease research laboratory) test**

    a. This test measures the antibody a patient has formed toward VDRL antigen—cardiolipin, cholesterol, and lecithin.

    b. Results are reported as NR (nonreactive), WR (weak reactive), and R (reactive).

    c. VDRL is positive 1–3 weeks after the chancre appears.

    d. Mainly used on CSF now.

3. Unheated serum reagin test (USR): modified VDRL test where choline-chloride EDTA is added to VDRL antigen. The addition of this compound allows serum that has not been heat inactivated to be used.

4. **Rapid plasma reagin (RPR) test**

    a. Macroscopic flocculation.

    b. Uses modified VDRL antigen with charcoal particles for visualization.

    c. Can be qualitative or quantitative. Dilutions are made to quantitate the amount of antibody present.

5. ***Treponema pallidum* immobilization test (TPI):** test principle is to measure the ability of antibody and complement in patient serum to immobilize live treponemas.

6. **Fluorescent treponemal antibody absorption test (FTA-ABS)**
   a. Principle: indirect antibody test.
   b. Nichol's strain of *T. pallidum* smeared onto slides.
   c. Patient serum is heat inactivated.
   d. Nontreponemal antibody absorbed out of serum. With a sorbent of Reiter's strain of *T. pallidum*.
   e. Serum placed on antigen smears.
   f. Fluorescein-thiocyanate-labeled antihuman gamma globulin is added.
   g. Fluorescent reactions are graded 1–4+.

7. **Hemagglutination assays: MHA-TP, HATTS, TPHA**
   a. MHA-TP: microhemagglutination assay for antibody to *T. pallidum*.
   b. Hemagglutination treponemal test for syphilis (HATTS).
   c. *T. pallidum* hemagglutination assay (TPHA).

8. Enzyme-linked immunosorbent assay (ELISA) produces results similar to FTA-ABS

XX. *BORRELIA BURGDORFERI* SEROLOGY

A. Organism—spirochete that causes **Lyme disease**

B. Transmission
   1. The spirochete is transmitted to humans in the saliva of a tick (Ioxedes) that bites man.
   2. Because ticks take days to feed, if a tick is removed within 24–36 hours, infection can be prevented.

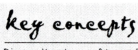

key concepts

Discuss the stages of Lyme disease and the test (and test methodology) used to diagnosis this disease.

C. Lyme Disease
   1. **Early stage**
      a. A reddened area on the skin that occurs 2–32 days after being bitten by an infected tick.
      b. Reddened area can develop into the classical target rash.
   2. **Late stage**
      a. Most common symptom is arthritis affecting knees, shoulders, and elbows.
      b. 15 percent of patients exhibit aseptic meningitis, facial nerve palsy, encephalitis, cranial neuritis, and radiculoneuritis.
      c. 8 percent of patients exhibit carditis.
      d. Chronic disease may show up as a sclerotic or atrophic skin lesion or a lymphocytoma.
   3. **Antibody response**
      a. The first antibody produced in Lyme disease is IgM which is not specific for *B. burgdorferi*.
      b. Subsequently, the IgG antibody specific to *B. burgdorferi* is produced, and the highest levels are seen in patients who develop arthritis.
      c. If a patient develops **erythema chronicum migrans** (target rash), antibodies will persist in their system for 3 years.

D. Diagnosis

1. **Organism culture:** small numbers of organisms can be cultured from skin biopsies, lymph node aspirates, synovial fluid, CSF, and blood. Requires an incubation of 12 weeks or more.

2. **Serology tests**

   a. Diagnosis can be made if a fourfold increase in titer is detected between acute serum and a specimen is taken 6 to 8 weeks later.

   b. **Immunofluorescence assay (IFA)**

      1) Procedure (*see* Section XV Immunofluorescence, B. Methods, 1. Direct immunofluorescence)

      2) **Results and interpretation**

         a) Titers of >128 for serum and >16 for CSF are positive for *B. burgdorferi* infection.

         b) Only 50 percent of early Lyme disease cases are seropositives, whereas 71 percent of late Lyme disease cases are seropositive.

         c) False positive reactions have been observed in other spirochete infections and autoimmune diseases.

   c. **Enzyme-linked immunosorbent assay (ELISA)**

      1) Results and interpretation

         a) The intensity of the color is proportional to the amount of antibody present in the specimen.

         b) Every specimen is compared with the color intensity of the low positive control.

         c) False positives occur in other spirochete infections and autoimmune disease.

   d. **Western blot**

      1) Procedure

         a) Antigens and antibodies are electrophoretically separated on a polyacrylamide gel to form bands.

         b) The bands are transferred to an inert membrane filter, then incubated with patient sera.

         c) After incubation, the membrane is washed and a labeled antihuman immunoglobulin is added.

         d) Enzyme substrate is added to detect antigen-antibody reactions.

      2) **Results and interpretation**

         a) Negative sera reaction with few, if any antigens.

         b) Positive sera react with several antigens.

3. **Detection of the organism:** this type of testing is in experimental stages and has drawbacks: false negatives in the early disease stage, inappropriate treatment leading to decreased antibody production, and false positive results from cross reactive antibodies and in endemic areas.

E. Treatment

1. Doxycycline, amoxicillin with probenicid, or cefuroxime.

2. Intravenous ceftriaxone, cefotaxime, or penicillin G is used to treat neurologic and disseminated disease.

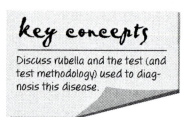

key concepts

Discuss rubella and the test (and test methodology) used to diagnosis this disease.

XXI. RUBELLA SEROLOGY

A. Virus

1. Single-stranded RNA
2. Member of the Togaviridae

B. Diseases

1. **German measles**
   a. Mild, contagious disease characterized by an erythematous maculopapular rash.
   b. May be asymptomatic.
   c. May have a 1–5 day prodromal syndrome of malaise, headache, cold symptoms, low-grade fever, and swollen lymph glands at the back of the head.
   d. This virus is spread by droplet infection through the upper respiratory tract.
   e. Complications may include arthritis, encephalitis, and thrombocytopenic purpura.

2. **Congenital rubella**
   a. Infection of the mother during pregnancy can result in abortion, stillbirth, infection of the fetus, or birth defects.
   b. Classical birth defects that occur if the mother is infected during the first 8 weeks of pregnancy include congenital heart disease, cataracts, and neurosensory deafness.
   c. Mothers infected after 20–24 weeks of pregnancy rarely give birth to babies with birth defects.
   d. Babies born with rubella syndrome exhibit thrombocytopenia, hepatitis, long-bone lesions, retinitis, encephalitis, interstitial pneumonitis, psychiatric disorders, thyroid disorders, and diabetes mellitus.

3. **Immunologic response**
   a. As the rash fades, the antibody response kicks in, and IgG and IgM antibodies can be detected.
   b. IgG antibodies offer lifetime immunity, whereas the IgM antibodies disappear at about 4–5 weeks.
   c. Reinfection can occur, but it is asymptomatic.

C. Clinical Indications

1. **Recent infections**
   a. If a person is exposed to rubella, a blood specimen should be drawn when the symptoms start, then 5 to 7 days later.
   b. If at least a fourfold rise in antibody titer is detected and clinical symptoms are present, then a diagnosis of rubella can be made.
   c. If an acute serum at the start of symptoms is not available, testing for IgG antibodies can establish a diagnosis.

2. **Congenital infections:** diagnosis can be established in an infant if IgM antibodies are present in neonates that have a low birthweight or any symptoms of congenital rubella.

3. **Immune status:** most rubella testing in the United State is done to determine a person's immune status against rubella.

D. Diagnostic Tests

1. Test methods used include latex agglutination, passive hemagglutination, ELISA, and indirect immunofluorescence.

   a. **Hemagglutination inhibition test**

     1) Principle: the rubella virus agglutinates chick red blood
   cells. Patient sera is combined with rubella antigen. If the
   patient has antibodies to the rubella antigen, an antigen-antibody complex forms and does not allow the antigen to agglutinate the indicator chick red blood cells. Agglutination
   indicates there are antibodies present.

   b. **Passive hemagglutination**

     1) Principle: human red blood cells are coated with rubella
   virus which are agglutinated by rubella antibodies, if
   present.

   c. **Immunoassays** (*see* **Chapter 4 Clinical Chemistry, Section
   XII. Immunochemical Techniques**)

E. Rubella Vaccination

1. There are 3 live, attenuated rubella vaccines available in the United
   States.
2. The rubella vaccine should be given alone at 12 months of age or in
   the MMR (mumps, measles, rubella) vaccine at 15 months of age.

XXII. EPSTEIN-BARR SEROLOGY

A. Epstein-Barr Virus

1. DNA virus.
2. Part of herpes virus group.
3. Transmission is through saliva.
4. Immunity lasts a lifetime.
5. Virus remains viable, and the infected person is a carrier for life.
6. Serological tests target the heterophile antibodies and virus specific
   antibodies.

key concepts

Analyze the disease produced by
Epstein-Barr virus and the test
(and test methodology) used to
diagnosis this disease.

B. Diseases

1. **Burkitt's lymphoma**

   a. Burkitt's lymphoma: a malignant neoplasm of β lymphocytes

     1) Found in a restricted area of Africa and New Guinea

     2) Found primarily in children

     3) In the rest of the world, infects immunocompromised people

2. **Nasopharyngeal carcinoma:** nasopharyngeal squamous cell carcinoma is caused by EBV and found mainly in southern China.

3. **Infectious mononucleosis**

   a. A disease of the reticuloendothelial system.

   b. Incubation period is 4 to 7 weeks.

   c. Onset may be acute or insidious with sore throat, fever, and
   lymphadenopathy.

   d. Common findings are hepatosplenomegaly, lymphocytosis with
   many reactive lymphs, and enlarged cervical lymph nodes.

   e. Other signs include skin rash, conjunctivitis, central nervous
   system damage.

    f. Acute phase lasts 2 weeks with long convalescence.

    g. People infected produce IgM heterophile antibodies (that come and go rapidly), have abnormal differentials, and liver function tests.

    h. Infections usually resolve in 4 to 6 weeks.

    i. Complications include becoming immunocompromised or malfunction of any organ system.

C. Laboratory Tests

1. **Heterophile antibodies**

    a. Heterophile antibodies produced in infectious mononucleosis react with red blood cells from sheep, beef, ox, and horse.

    b. **Paul-Bunnell presumptive test**

       1) **Principle:** heterophile antibodies peak around 2–3 weeks after infection. Serial dilutions of serum are incubated with a 2 percent suspension of sheep red blood cells.

       2) **Results**

         a) Titer of 28 or less is normal.

         b) Titer of >56 indicates a high concentration of heterophile antibodies are present.

       3) **Interpretation**

         a) Screening test to detect heterophile antibodies—not specific to infectious mononucleosis.

         b) False negative rate is 10–15 percent.

    c. **Davidsohn differential test**

       1) **Principle:** differentiates between 3 heterophile antibodies based on their absorption onto beef RBCs and guinea pig kidney. Infectious mononucleosis (IM) antibodies are absorbed onto beef RBCs, but not guinea pig kidney; Forssman antibodies are absorbed onto guinea pig kidney, but not beef RBCs; and serum sickness antibodies are absorbed onto both beef RBCs and guinea pig kidney.

       2) **Interpretation**

         a) The beginning titer is 56.

         b) IM reduces the guinea pig titer by sixfold or less and the beef titer by eightfold.

         c) In serum sickness, the titer is reduced by at least eightfold in both tubes.

         d) The Forsmann antibody reduces the guinea pig tube by eightfold or greater, and the beef tube is not reduced at all.

    d. **Slide red cell tests**

       1) **Principle**

         a) Differential test: patient serum is adsorbed by guinea pig antigen and beef RBC antigen, then checked for agglutination with horse RBCs.

         b) Nondifferential test: patient sera is added to horse RBCs and checked for agglutination.

         c) Latex test: bovine RBC antigens are adsorbed onto latex particles.

2) **Interpretation**
   a) Differential test: positive if there is agglutination with guinea pig suspension and no agglutination with beef RBC suspension. This test is negative if both sides show agglutination or if neither side shows agglutination.
   b) Nondifferential and latex test: if there is agglutination, the test is positive, and if there is no agglutination, the test is negative

   e. **Membrane-based enzyme immunoassay (EIA)**
   1) Procedure
      a) Ox RBC antigens are placed on a membrane in a self-contained cassette.
      b) Patient serum and reagent antibody added to a spot and diffused along membrane past antigen.
      c) Color development occurs if IM heterophile antibodies are present.
   2) Interpretation
      a) Color development means IM heterophile antibodies are present.
      b) No color indicates IM heterophile antibodies are not present.

   f. **ELISA**
   1) Beef RBC antigens are attached to solid phase
   2) Incubate with patient serum, then add detector antibody to tube which will turn a yellow color if IM heterophile antibodies are present.

2. **EBV-specific tests**
   a. **Immunofluorescent tests**
   1) Principle: antigen is fixed to slide, reacts with patient sera, and is layered with fluorescein-conjugated antihuman IgG or IgM.
   2) Able to detect anti-Viral Capsid Antigen(VCA)-IgM, anti-Viral Capside Antigen-IgG, and anti-EA-IgG, and anti-EBNA-IgG antibodies.
   3) Interpretation
      a) Highest titer is last dilution showing fluorescence.
      b) VCA antibodies peak 3–4 weeks following infection, and IgM is not detectable in 12 weeks.
   b. **Enzyme immunoassays (*see* Chapter 4 Clinical Chemistry, Section XIII, Molecular Techniques)**

XXIII. VIRAL HEPATITIS
A. Hepatitis Testing
1. Testing for antibodies and antigens in patient sera can determine the responsible virus, stage of infection, and immune status of patient.
2. Most widely used test methods are ELISA and RIA.

B. Hepatitis A (HAV)
1. Member of Picornaviridae family

key concepts

Discuss the hepatitis viruses, explain the diseases produced by each virus, and know when antibodies and antigens rise and fall in hepatitis B.

2. **Epidemiology**
   a. Transmission by **fecal-oral route.**
   b. Epidemics occur through fecal contamination of food, water, or milk.

3. **Clinical symptoms**
   a. May be asymptomatic or symptomatic.
   b. Incubation period is 10–50 days.
   c. Symptomatic Infections
      1) Patient may become jaundiced or may not become jaundiced.
      2) Symptoms include fever, anorexia, vomiting, fatigue, and malaise.
      3) AST and especially ALT levels are increased and peak before jaundice occurs.
      4) Jaundice begins with right upper quadrant pain, tea-colored urine, and pale-colored stools.
      5) Other laboratory findings include hyperbilirubinemia and decreased albumin levels.
      6) Recovery occurs in 2 to 4 weeks.
      7) Mortality rate is 0.1 percent.
      8) Chronic disease rarely occurs.
      9) Vaccine developed in 1995, recommended for health care workers, travelers, drug abusers, and children.
   d. **Laboratory tests**
      1) Paired sera (acute collected at onset of symptoms and again 3–4 weeks later) run to detect an increase in anti-HAV antibodies. A fourfold increase to IgM and total (IgM and IgG) is considered diagnostic.
      2) Anti-HAV antibodies are present at onset of symptoms and for years afterward.

C. Hepatitis B

1. **Hepatitis B virus**
   a. Double-stranded DNA.
   b. Belongs to Hepadnaviridae family.
   c. Dane particle—complete HBV virus that causes infection.

2. **Epidemiology**
   a. 3 transmission routes: perenteral, perinatal, and sexual.
   b. The virus is transmitted through mucous membranes or wounds coming in contact with infected blood and body fluids or parenterally. Parenteral infection occurs through transfusion of contaminated blood products, hemodialysis, intravenous drug use, contaminated needle sticks, tattooing, acupuncture, ear piercing, or insect vectors.
   c. Groups at high risk for getting infected with HBV include intravenous drug users, homosexual men, hemodialysis patients, and health care workers.

3. **Symptoms**
   a. Incubation period of 50–180 days.
   b. Fever, anorexia, vomiting, fatigue, malaise, jaundice, and arthralgia are main symptoms. Symptoms come on abruptly.

      c. Long clinical course: acute infection can last up to 6 months. Most patients recover within 6 months.

      d. Can turn into a chronic infection where the patient remains HBsAg positive forever.

      e. If chronic infections are active, severe damage to the liver occurs, which can result in liver cancer.

      f. All chronic carriers shed infectious virus.

  4. **Laboratory tests**

      a. First marker that appears at the end of the incubation stage is HBsAg. The concentration of the surface antigen continues to rise and peaks about midway through the acute infection.

      b. Right after the HBsAg appears in the blood, HBeAg appears. HBeAg peaks at about the same time as the surface antigen, but its concentration never reaches the amount of surface antigen. HBeAg disappears about two-thirds of the way through the acute infection phase.

      c. The next marker to rise is anti-HBc which begins to rise a couple weeks into the acute infection. Anti-HBc peaks at the end of the acute infection stage and plateaus at that concentration forever.

      d. The same time the anti-HBc total is rising, so is the anti-HBc IgM. The anti-HBc IgM peaks a few weeks after the acute infection stage, then disappears in about 6 months during recovery.

      e. At the end of the acute infection stage, anti-HBe begins to rise and peaks about halfway through the recent acute infection stage (2–16 weeks). The concentration of this antibody decreases slightly during a person's lifetime, but never disappears.

      f. The last marker to appear is the anti-HBs. This appears at the end of the recent acute infection stage and the beginning of the recovery stage. Its concentration peaks, then plateaus during recovery, and never disappears.

D. Hepatitis C

  1. **Hepatitis C virus**

      a. Single-stranded RNA virus.

      b. Related to the pestivirus and flavivirus groups.

  2. **Epidemiology**

      a. Parenteral transmission is most common.

      b. Sexual and perinatal transmission of the virus is uncommon.

  3. **Symptoms**

      a. Causes either acute or chronic disease.

      b. Incubation period 2 to 26 weeks.

      c. Acute infections are asymptomatic or mild—nausea, vomiting, abdominal pain, fatigue, malaise, and jaundice.

      d. 50 to 80 percent of cases become chronic with 25 percent leading to cirrhosis.

      e. 20 percent of cirrhosis cases lead to cancer.

  4. **Laboratory Tests**

      a. Anti-HCV is diagnostic of HCV infection.

      b. Anti-HCV IgM does not distinguish between acute and chronic disease because both antibodies are retained in a patient for years.

      c. ELISA tests have false positive tests, so the best test to use for diagnosis is an immunoblot assay.

E. Delta Hepatitis

1. **Hepatitis D Virus**
   a. Single-stranded RNA.
   b. Requires help from HBV to replicate and infect hosts.

2. **Epidemiology**
   a. Occurs worldwide.
   b. Transmission is linked to HBV virus–parenteral and transmucousal routes.

3. **Symptoms**
   a. Coinfection: occurs in conjunction with HBV infection.
   b. Superinfection of chronic HBV infection can occur and progress to chronic HDV infection.
   c. Patients with chronic HDV infection have poor prognoses due to severe liver damage, inflammation, and cirrhosis.
   d. Vaccination against HBV is also effective against HDV.

4. **Laboratory Tests**
   a. Only HBsAg positive patients are tested for HDV.
   b. HDV-Ag is first marker to appear about 1–4 days before symptoms start.
   c. IgM anti-HDV appears next followed by low levels of IgG anti-HDV.
   d. The switch to high levels of IgG anti-HDV indicates chronic HDV infection

F. Hepatitis E

1. **Hepatitis E Virus**
   a. Single-stranded RNA virus.

2. **Epidemiology**
   a. Hepatitis E is a disease of underdeveloped countries.
   b. Transmission by the fecal-oral route.

3. **Symptoms**
   a. Acute, self-limiting disease.
   b. Anorexia, malaise, nausea, and vomiting.
   c. Incubation period of 15–64 days.

4. **Laboratory tests:** usually not performed. Diagnosis dependent on travel history, symptoms, and exclusion of other hepatitis infections.

G. Non-A-E Hepatitis

1. Hepatitis caused by viruses other than A–E fall in this category.
2. Sequelae include liver failure, aplastic anemia, and fatal liver disease.

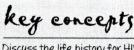

key concepts

Discuss the life history for HIV disease, how the virus is detected, and how transmission can be prevented.

XXIV. HUMAN IMMUNODEFICIENCY VIRUS SEROLOGY

A. Human Immunodeficiency Virus (HIV)

1. Retrovirus known as human immunodeficiency virus.
2. Retrovirus called lentivirus.

3. HIV-1 causes AIDS (acquired immunodeficiency syndrome), found here in United States.
4. HIV-2 immunodeficiency syndrome, found in West Africa.

B. HIV Life Cycle
1. HIV binds to CD4 molecule on helper T-lymphocytes, B-cells, monocytes, and macrophages.
2. HIV then penetrates the cell and exposes the viral RNA.
3. The RNA is transcribed to DNA then enters the cell's DNA.
4. The viral RNA and proteins go into the host cell cytoplasm where they form viruses, and leave the host cell through budding.
5. This process kills the CD4 cell and leads to a diminishing number of helper T-cells. The immune deficiency worsens as more viruses are produced and invade CD4 cells.

C. Immune Response and HIV
1. **Serologic effects**
   a. Increased α-interferon
   b. Increased α_1-thymosin
   c. Increased β_2-microglobulin
   d. Increased serum and urine neopterin
2. **Effect on T-cells**
   a. Depletion of CD4 lymphs
   b. Increased, normal, or decreased suppressor CD8 lymphs
   c. The ratio of CD4 to CD8 cells reduced from 2:1 (normal) to 0.5:1
   d. Decreased delayed type hypersensitivity
   e. Decreased production of interleukin-2
3. **Effect on B-cells**
   a. Polyclonal hypergammaglobulinemia
   b. Inability to produce a serologic response to a new antigen
   c. Increased numbers of spontaneous immunoglobulin secreting cells
4. **Effect on immune cells**
   a. Decreased natural killer cell activity
   b. Defective chemotaxis in monocytes and macrophages
   c. Enhanced release of interleukin-1 and cachectin by monocytes

D. Epidemiology
1. HIV-1: Number one cause of death for people between 20 and 35 years of age.
2. HIV-1: Transmitted by unprotected sex, contaminated blood or blood products, contaminated needles, or perinatal.
3. HIV-1: Isolated in the following: mononuclear cells, plasma, semen, cervical/vaginal secretions, saliva, tears, urine, breast milk, CSF, lymph nodes, brain, and bone marrow.
4. HIV-2: transmitted through blood products, sexual contact, or from mothers to infants.

E. Symptoms

1. Initially infected persons will be asymptomatic.
2. Symptomatic infection (also called AIDS-related complex [ARC]) includes fatigue, fever, sore throat, and lymphadenopathy.
3. Final stage includes severe T-cell depletion resulting in opportunistic infections and cancers (AIDS), e.g., candidiasis, cryptococcus, cytomegalovirus, Herpes simplex, Kaposi's sarcoma, *Pneumocystis carinii* pneumonia
4. CD4+ T-cell counts are used to monitor the severity of the disease.

F. Therapy

1. Zidovudine (AZT).
2. Inhibitors of reverse transcriptase—ddI and ddC.
3. Protease inhibitors—saquinavir, ritonavir, and norvir.

G. Laboratory Tests

1. ELISA tests are used to detect antibodies to HIV and HIV antigen. Repeatedly positive samples must be confirmed by a Western blot test.
2. Genetic probes can detect latent or actively replicating HIV viruses
3. PCR assays detect nucleic acid gene sequences in HIV-1 and HIV-2.
4. Rapid slide agglutination tests have been developed.
5. Western blot assay is the confirmatory test for HIV. Two of the three bands must appear for a western blot to be considered positive: p24, gp41, or gp120/160.
6. The indirect immunofluorescence assay is used to detect HIV antigen in infected cells. This can also be used as a confirmatory test.

XXV. MORE INFECTIOUS DISEASE SEROLOGIES

A. Rickettsia

1. **Spotted Fever Group**

   a. **Rocky Mountain spotted fever** is caused by *Rickettsia rickettsii.*

      1) **Incubation** period is up to 14 days.
      2) High fever, chills, myalgia, rash on the wrists, ankles, palms, soles, and forearms is characteristic. Rash later spreads to axilla, buttocks, trunk, neck, and face.
      3) Spread by ticks.
      4) Most common test for diagnosis is immunofluorescence antibody test.
      5) Treatment is large doses of tetracycline until the patient improves and becomes afebrile.

2. **Typhus group**

   a. **Epidemic typhus** is produced by *R. prowazekii.*

      1) Carried by lice and is found in South America and Africa.
      2) Symptoms include headache, chills, fever, followed by a skin rash several days later.
      3) Fatal in up to 40 percent of infected patients.

   b. **Endemic (murine) typhus** is caused by *R. typhi.*

      1) **Flea Borne**

key concepts

Discuss the disease and tests used to diagnose Rocky Mountain spotted fever, typhus group diseases, mycoplasma diseases, Legionnaire's disease, fungal infections, ehrlichiosis, babesiosis, chlamydia infections, leptospirosis, amebiasis, toxoplasma infections, cytomegalovirus infections, and human T-cell leukemia virus.

  c. **Scrub typhus** is caused by *R. tsutsugamushi.*
    1) Carried by **chiggers.**
    2) Common in Asia, Australia, and the Pacific Islands.
  3. **Q fever is caused by** *Coxiella burnetii.*
    a. Transmitted by an **arthropod.**
    b. Symptoms: cough, chest infiltrates, and hepatitis.

B. Mycoplasma
  1. *Mycoplasma pneumonia* causes a mild pneumonia.
  2. Diagnosis is made by finding cold agglutinins in infected patients' sera.
  3. Treatment includes tetracycline and the macrolides.

C. Legionella
  1. *Legionella pneumonia* causes fulminant pneumonia with fever and flulike symptoms.
  2. Diagnosis: an indirect immunofluorescent test for the organism.
  3. Treatment: erythromycin; immunocompromised patients receive rifampin.

D. Fungi
  1. Antibodies to fungi can be useful in diagnosing infections.
  2. Fungi that can be detected by serological tests include *Aspergillus fumigatus*, histoplasma, *Blastomyces*, cryptococcus, cocciodiodes, and candida.
  3. Diagnosed: detecting IgG antibodies by double diffusion.
  4. Treated with antifungal drugs such as diflucan, nizoral, etc.

E. Toxoplasma
  1. *Toxoplasma gondii:* parasitic infection that can kill immunocompromised patients.
  2. ELISA tests are available to detect antibodies.
  3. Can be carried by cats.
  4. Treated with pyrimethamine and trisulapyrimidines.

F. Cytomegalovirus (CMV)
  1. Generally causes asymptomatic infection.
  2. Produces fulminant disease in immunocompromised patients.
  3. Antibodies are detected using ELISA tests.
  4. Treatment is gancyclovir.

G. Human T-Cell Leukemia Virus I (HTLV-I)
  1. Retrovirus that infects T-helper cells.
  2. Usually asymptomatic, but can cause T-cell leukemia and tropical spastic paraparesis.
  3. Common in the Caribbean and Japan.
  4. HTLV-I antibodies can be detected by ELISA tests.

H. Leptospirosis
  1. *Leptospira interrogans* is the main pathogen for humans and animals.

    2. Symptoms: chills, fever, severe headaches, rash, aseptic meningitis, and hepatic and renal damage.

    3. Diagnosis: microagglutination test (MAT) or EIA.

    4. Treatment: penicillin G is treatment of choice, and amoxicillin is used to treat severe disease.

I. Ehrlichiosis

    1. A new tick-borne disease caused by an obligate intracellular bacterium—*Ehrlichia chaffeensis* or *Ehrlichia sennetsu*.

    2. Symptoms: fever, malaise, myalgia, headache, rigors, diaphoresis, nausea, vomiting, cough, arthralgias, rash, and confusion.

    3. Testing: EIA, indirect fluorescent antigen tests (IFA), and Western blot.

    4. Treatment: tetracycline or doxycycline.

J. Chlamydia

    1. Obligate intracellular parasites: *Chlamydia psittaci* and *Chlamydia pneumoniae* are human pathogens. *Chlamydia trachomatis* is a sexually transmitted disease and will not be covered here.

    2. Cause pneumonia.

    3. Testing: identified using complement fixation tests.

    4. Treatment: tetracycline.

K. Amebiasis

    1. Causative agent: *Entamoeba histolytica*.

    2. Symptoms: amebic colitis, abdominal cramping, bloody diarrhea, and liver abscesses.

    3. Testing: EIA and IFA techniques.

    4. Treatment: metronidazole plus iodoquinol.

L. Babesiosis

    1. A tick-borne disease caused by *Babesia microti*.

    2. Symptoms: low grade fever, malaise, fatigue, headache, rigor, nausea, vomiting, and musculoskeletal problems. Patients can also present with jaundice, hepatomegaly, splenomegaly, hemolytic anemia, hemoglobinuria, thrombocytopenia, and increased liver enzymes.

    3. Testing: IFA, EIA, and Western Blot tests.

    4. Treatment: clindamycin and quinidine.

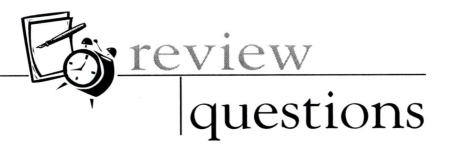

review | questions

DIRECTIONS Each of the questions or incomplete statements below is followed by suggested answers or completions. Select the **one answer** that is best in each case.

---

1. Immunology includes all the following EXCEPT:
   a. antigen synthesis
   b. inflammation
   c. phagocytosis
   d. antibody synthesis

2. The 5 classes of antibodies are
   a. IgM, IgF, IgG, IgE, IgC
   b. IgF, IgG, IgM, IgR, IgS
   c. IgG, IgM, IgF, IgE, IgH
   d. IgG, IgM, IgE, IgD, IgA

3. In the peripheral blood, these cells are monocytes; in the tissues they are called
   a. monophage
   b. macrophages
   c. eosinophil
   d. basophil

4. The following cytokines have antiviral properties EXCEPT:
   a. interferon α
   b. interferon β
   c. interleukin 1
   d. interferon γ

5. Secondary lymph organs include all the following EXCEPT:
   a. thymus
   b. spleen
   c. lymph nodes
   d. lymphoid tissues

6. Clinical significance of major histocompatibility antigens include all the following EXCEPT:
   a. blood grouping
   b. transplantation
   c. paternity testing
   d. disease-association

7. All the following cytokines are involved in tumor immunology EXCEPT:
   a. tissue necrosis factor-α
   b. interferon α
   c. interferon γ
   d. interleukin 1

8. Tumor markers include all the following EXCEPT:
   a. CEA
   b. AFP
   c. HCG
   d. TSH

9. Cell-mediated immunity is mediated by
   a. T-natural killer cells
   b. B-cells
   c. T-helper cells
   d. T-cytokine cells

10. IgG antibodies are produced as a _____ response.
    a. primary
    b. tertiary
    c. secondary
    d. lymphocyte

11. The largest portion of the nonspecific immune response is the
    a. complement cascade
    b. B-lymphocytes
    c. eosinophils
    d. natural killer cells

12. Autoimmune diseases include all the following EXCEPT:
    a. Goodpasture's syndrome
    b. diabetes insipidus
    c. SLE
    d. myasthenia gravis

13. Type I hypersensitivity is
    a. complement-mediated cell lysis
    b. activated macrophages
    c. immune-complex deposition
    d. immediate, an allergic reaction

14. ANA is used to diagnose all the following EXCEPT:
    a. Hashimoto's disease
    b. SLE
    c. RA
    d. MCTD

15. SCID is
    a. immunodeficiency with decreased B-cells, dysfunctional T-cells, and leukocytopenia.
    b. immunodeficiency with decreased lymphocytes and decreased leukocytes.
    c. immunodeficiency with lymphocytopenia and leukocytosis.
    d. immunodeficiency with decreased T-cells, dysfunctional T- and B-cells, and lymphopenia.

16. Multiple myeloma is a
    a. lymphoproliferative disease where a single T-cell clone produces decreased antibodies.
    b. lymphoproliferative disease where a single B-cell clone produces increased antibodies.
    c. lymphoproliferative disease where a single B-cell clone produces decreased antibodies.
    d. lymphoproliferative disease where a single T-cell clone produces increased antibodies.

17. All the following transplants are performed EXCEPT:
    a. pancreas
    b. liver
    c. muscle
    d. bone marrow

18. Immunoelectrophoresis is used to
    a. identify monoclonal proteins.
    b. identify polyclonal proteins.
    c. quantitate serum proteins.
    d. identify serum proteins.

19. Direct immunofluorescence is where
    a. conjugated reagent antigen reacts with antibodies to form antigen-antibody complexes.
    b. antigens react with unlabeled antibody forming antigen-antibody complexes that attach to labeled antibodies.
    c. a dye is attached to a molecule and it reacts with the complex to produce a color.
    d. conjugated reagent antibody reacts with antigen to form antigen-antibody complexes.

20. Nitroblue tetrazolium test looks for
    a. dysfunctional lymphs
    b. dysfunctional T-lymphs
    c. dysfunctional B-lymphs
    d. dysfunctional neutrophils

21. Natural history of an infectious disease contains all these phases EXCEPT:
    a. infection
    b. primary response
    c. prodromal
    d. acute

22. Streptococcal antibodies can be diagnosed with all the following tests EXCEPT:
    a. antistreptolysin O
    b. antihyaluronidase
    c. anti-RNA A
    d. anti-DNase B

23. Disease stages of syphilis include all the following EXCEPT:
    a. quarternary
    b. primary
    c. latency
    d. tertiary

24. This test is a macroscopic flocculation test and uses modified VDRL antigen with charcoal particles to diagnose syphilis
    a. VDRL
    b. MHA-TP
    c. FTA-ABS
    d. RPR

25. This disease initially produces a classical target rash (erytherma chronicum migrans) and needs a serological test to confirm this diagnosis
    a. Rocky Mountain spotted fever
    b. Lyme disease
    c. Q fever
    d. syphilis

26. This virus produces an erythematous maculopapular rash, low-grade fever, and swollen glands at the back of the head.
    a. Rocky Mountain spotted fever
    b. rubella
    c. Q fever
    d. typhus

27. This virus produces all the following diseases EXCEPT:
    a. infectious mononucleosis
    b. Burkitt's lymphoma
    c. jaundice
    d. nasopharyngeal carcinoma

28. Hepatitis A is transmitted by
    a. fecal-oral route
    b. blood and body fluids
    c. kissing
    d. tsetse fly

29. All the following are routes for hepatitis B transmission EXCEPT:
    a. food or water
    b. transfusion of contaminated blood products
    c. hemodialysis
    d. tattooing

30. All the following are true about hepatitis C EXCEPT:
    a. 50 – 80 percent of cases become chronic
    b. leads to cirrhosis
    c. spread by fecal-oral route
    d. leads to cancer

31. Patients with hepatitis D virus have a poor prognosis due to
    a. virus configuration
    b. genetic predisposition
    c. coinfection
    d. severe liver damage

32. This hepatitis is a disease of underdeveloped countries
    a. E
    b. B
    c. C
    d. D

33. This virus causes destruction of its CD4 cells
    a. HTLV-1
    b. HIV
    c. HBV
    d. HCV

34. HIV has the following effects on immune cells EXCEPT:
    a. decreased NK–cell activity
    b. immobilization of B-cells
    c. defective chemotaxis in monocytes and macrophages
    d. enhanced release of IL-1

35. Symptomatic infection with HIV is ARC and has the following symptoms EXCEPT:
    a. fatigue
    b. lymphadenopathy
    c. fever
    d. maculopapular rash

36. This disease is spread by ticks and produces the following symptoms—high fever, chills, myalgia, and rash on the wrists, ankles, palms, soles, and forearms.
    a. Rocky Mountain spotted fever
    b. Lyme disease
    c. typhus
    d. Q fever

37. This disease is cause by *R. tsutsugamushi* and spread by chiggers
    a. Q fever
    b. Rocky Mountain spotted fever
    c. scrub typhus
    d. Lyme disease

38. This disease is diagnosed by finding cold ag-
    glutinins in a patient's serum.
    a. pneumonia caused by CMV
    b. pneumonia caused by HIV
    c. pneumonia caused by AIDS
    d. pneumonia caused by mycoplasma pneu-
       monia

39. This virus is common in the Caribbean and
    Japan and is a retrovirus that infects T-helper
    cells.
    a. HIV-1
    b. HIV-2
    c. human T-cell leukemia virus 1
    d. typhus

40. Antibodies to this fungus can be detected in
    serum
    a. *Toxoplasma gondii*
    b. *Pneumocystis carinii*
    c. *Aspergillus fumigatus*
    d. *Mycoplasma pneumoniae*

6 Immunohematology

contents

➤ KEY CONCEPTS

1. Discuss the role of the blood bank in transfusing blood to patients.
2. Analyze the role of pretransfusion testing in making blood safe for patients.

I. IMMUNOHEMATOLOGY

A. **Definition**—the study of blood group antigens and antibodies, HLA antigens and antibodies, pretransfusion testing, identification of unexpected alloantibodies, immune hemolysis, autoantibodies, and drugs, blood collection, blood components, cryopreservation of blood, transfusion-transmitted viruses, tissue banking and organ transplantation, blood transfusion practice, safety, quality assessment, records, blood inventory management, and blood usage review.

B. **Immunity**
1. **Acquired immunity** is a **specific response** where antibodies specific **to** a particular antigen are produced. **B-lymphs and plasma cells** produce **antibodies.**
2. **Innate immunity** is a **nonspecific reaction** from the immune system that attacks all invaders and includes the skin, nasal mucosa, normal flora, and chemicals.

C. **Antigen Characteristics**
1. **Antigens** are substances that combine with an antibody. An **antigen** that causes a **specific immune response** is an **immunogen. Immunogens** are made of protein, carbohydrates, and combinations of both. Present on WBCs and RBCs. Some immunogens produced a greater response than others.
2. There are **23 RBC antigen systems** containing over 200 RBC antigens. RBC antigens are inherited and are composed of proteins, glycoproteins, and glycolipids.
3. **Human leukocyte antigens (HLA)**
   a. Present on **leukocytes and tissue cells.**
   b. Genes that encode the **HLA antigens** are part of the **Major Histocompatibility Complex (MHC) system.**
   c. MHC is on chromosome 6 and is divided into **Class I, II, III:**
      1) **Class I** includes A, B, and C loci
      2) **Class II** includes DR, DP, and DQ.
      3) **Class III** includes complement proteins.
   d. Immune response to HLA causes fever and chills

key concepts

Compare and contrast the differences between antibodies and antigens and the characteristics of each.

      e. **HLA** must be matched for **organ, tissue, bone marrow,** and **stem cell** transplant donors and recipients. If not matched, then a severe graft versus host disease results.

      f. HLA test applications include paternity testing, organ and tissue transplantation, bone marrow and stem cell transplantation, and platelet matching.

  4. **Platelet antigens**

      a. Membranes have **protein antigens.**

      b. **Platelet antigens** less frequent in population due to less antigen variability.

      c. **Diseases:** neonatal alloimmune thrombocytopenia and post-transfusion purpura.

D. Antibody Characteristics

  1. **Molecular structure**

      a. Each molecule has 2 heavy chains and 2 light chains.

      b. **The heavy chain is responsible for the immunoglobulin group specificity.**

      c. Antibody binding site is found in the variable region of the light chain.

  2. **IgM antibodies**

      a. **5 basic** immunoglobulin units

      b. Can directly bind with RBCs and produce agglutination

      c. Activate complement

      d. Cannot cross the placenta

  3. **IgG antibodies**

      a. Immunoglobulin unit

      b. Cannot visibly agglutinate RBCs

      c. Can activate complement (2 molecules necessary)

      d. Can cross the placenta

E. Antigen-Antibody Interactions

  1. Follows the Law of Mass Action

  2. **Reversible**

  3. Antigen-antibody complex formed

  4. Properties that influence antigen-antibody interactions

      a. Fit of antigen into antibody binding site

      b. Size of antigen

      c. Shape of antigen

      d. Charge of antigen

  5. **Antigen-antibody complexes** held together by electrostatic charges, hydrogen bonding, hydrophobic bonding, and Van der Waals forces

F. Antigen-Antibody Reactions In Vivo

  1. **Transfusions** can lead to antigen-antibody complex formation in vivo if wrong type of blood is transfused.

  2. Transfusion of foreign antigens (RBC, HLA, platelet) into a donor can cause an immune response and antibody formation in the donor (alloantibodies).

3. Antigen-antibody complexes are removed by the reticuloendotheial system: spleen, liver, and lymph nodes.

G. Antigen-Antibody Reaction In Vitro

1. Reactions detected by **agglutination or hemolysis.**
2. Some antigen-antibody complexes require 2 stages for detection—**sensitization** and **lattice** formation.
   a. **Sensitization:** antibody attaches to antigen but does not produce agglutination or hemolysis.
      1) **Factors Affecting First Stage of Agglutination**
         a) **Serum to cell ratio:** amount of antibody compared to the number of cells in solution. Increased amount of serum equals an increase in the number of antibodies in the solution.
         b) **Reaction temperature:** temperature where the antibody reacts best—most clinically important antibodies react best at 37°C.
         c) **Incubation time:** the time allowed for the antibody to attach to the antigen. This reaction occurs by chance. Times will vary according to the antibody and media used in vitro (i.e., albumin, low ionic strength saline [LISS]).
         d) **pH:** optimal pH for in vitro reactions is 7.
   b. Lattice formation-random collisions of antibody-coated RBCs links antibodies together to form visual lattice.
      1) Factors affecting visual agglutination
         a) **Zeta potential:** force around an RBC, in normal saline (net negative charge), that repels other RBCs in solution. This inhibits charge agglutination.
3. **Antigen and Antibody Agglutination**
   a. **Zone of equivalence:** when antigen and antibody concentrations produce maximum agglutination.
   b. **Prozone:** antibody excess.
   c. **Antigen excess:** too much antigen compared with antibody concentrations.
4. **Grading Agglutination Reactions**
   a. To standardize the strength of agglutination reactions:
      1) **4+ RBC button** is solid with a clear supernatant
      2) **3+ RBC button** breaks into several large clumps, clear supernatant.
      3) **2+ RBC button** breaks into many medium-sized clumps, clear supernatant
      4) **1+ RBC button** breaks into many medium and small-sized clumps, background has many free RBCs
      5) **+^{w} RBC button** breaks into many clumps, barely or not visible macroscopically, many RBCs in the background (use microscope to see clumps)
      6) **0 = no agglutinated RBCs**
5. **Hemolysis:** another indication of antibody-antigen reactions. Caused by complement activation. The supernatant appears red with a smaller or nonexistent RBC button.

II. GENETICS

A. Definitions

1. **Chromosomes:** structures that carry genetic information encoded on double stranded DNA.
2. **Mitosis:** a process of cell division that results in the same number of chromosomes in the new and old cells.
3. **Meiosis:** a process of cell division that occurs in gametes that results in one half the chromosomes in each new cell.
4. **Blood group systems:** groups of related RBC antigens that are inherited according to Mendelian genetics.
5. **Phenotype:** physical observable expression of inherited traits; detectable products.
6. **Genotype:** inherited genes; actual genetic makeup.
7. **Pedigree chart:** a visual map that displays a family history and can display inheritance patterns for individual traits.
8. **Gene:** the smallest unit of inheritance
9. **Genetic locus:** site on the chromosome where specific genes are located.
10. **Alleles:** alternative forms of a gene.
11. **Antithetical:** opposite form of a gene—different allele.
12. **Polymorphic:** having 2 or more possible alleles at a locus.
13. **Codominant:** equal expression of both alleles in phenotype.
14. **Recessive:** same allele must be inherited from both parents to be expressed—homozygous.
15. **Dominant:** only 1 allele must be inherited for it to be expressed; gene product always present.
16. **Autosomal:** genes expressed with equal frequency in males and females, on non sex chromosome.
17. **Sex-linked dominant:** no father to son transmission; will be expressed if passed from father to daughter.
18. **Sex-linked recessive:** males inherit from carrier mothers, traits exhibited exclusively in males, i.e., hemophilia A.

key concepts

Discuss how blood groups are inherited.

B. Mendelian Inheritance Principles

1. **Law of Independent Segregation:** traits are **passed on** from 1 generation to the next in a predictable manner.
2. **Law of Independent Assortment:** traits that are inherited from different chromosomes are **expressed separately** and **discretely.**
3. **Inheritance patterns:** the inheritance of blood group antigens (A, B, O) can be predicted using a **Punnett square.** Punnett squares have the one person's genotype on the top and the other person's genotype on the side.

Punnet Square

	A	B
B	AB	BO
O	AO	OO

4. Each square represents a possible genotype for an offspring. An offspring from these parents would have a 25 percent chance of inheriting any 1 of the 4 possible variants. Punnett squares are useful for understanding inheritance of blood groups and ramifications of **heterozygosity** or **homozygosity.**

5. **Homozygous:** an individual inherits identical genes.

6. **Heterozygous:** an individual inherits different alleles.

7. **Dosage effect:** agglutination reactions are generally stronger in homozygous cells and slightly weaker in heterozygous cells.

8. **Cis:** genes inherited on the same chromosome

9. **Trans:** genes inherited on separate chromosomes. Genes inherited in the trans formation can weaken the trait's expression.

10. **Linkage and Haplotypes**
    a. **Linked genes:** genes that are close together on a chromosome and inherited as 1 unit. The Law of Independent Assortment does not hold with linked genes.
    b. **Haplotypes:** linked genes.
    c. **Amorphs:** genes that do not produce a detectable product.

11. **Population genetics:** statistical calculation that determines the prevalence of antigens in specific populations.
    a. **Phenotype calculations:** determines the frequency of an antigen in a population.
    b. If a patient has **multiple antibodies,** to **determine the percentage of compatible units, the frequency for each antibody must be multiplied.**

       For example,

50% E positive	50% E negative = 0.50
60% M positive	40% M negative = 0.40
80% c positive	20% c negative = 0.20

       percentage of compatible units $= 0.50 \times 0.40 \times 0.20 = 0.04$ or 4% of units

12. **Paternity testing: RBC antigens and HLA antigens follow Mendelian genetics** principles and can be used to determine the parents of offspring. Blood groups with the greatest number of alleles are used. The more alleles, the less likely to find 2 identical individuals. Paternity works on the principle of excluding falsely accused individuals using statistics.

III. ABO AND H BLOOD GROUP SYSTEMS AND SECRETOR STATUS

A. Landsteiner's rule—if an individual **has the antigen,** that individual will **not have the antibody.** This is a universal law with few exceptions.

B. ABO antigens—found on **RBCs, lymphs, platelets, tissue cells, bone marrow,** and **organs.** These antigens can be secreted by tissue cells if the appropriate genes are present.

1. ABO antigens are **glycolipid** or **glycoprotein.**

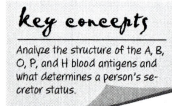

key concepts

Analyze the structure of the A, B, O, P, and H blood antigens and what determines a person's secretor status.

2. ABO antigens are developed in utero at 5–6 weeks of gestation.
3. **Full expression of ABO antigens occurs between 2–4 years of age.**
4. Frequencies:

	Frequency (%)		
Type	*Whites*	*Blacks*	*Asians*
O	45	49	40
A	40	27	28
B	11	20	27
AB	4	4	5

C. Inheritance and Development of A, B, and H Antigens

1. The **H antigen** is the building block for the **A and B antigens.** There are only two alleles in the H gene: H and h. **H is found in 99.99 percent of the world's population,** and h is a rare amorph.
2. The **H antigen acts as the acceptor molecule** for the 2 sugars that make up the A and B antigens.
3. The **A blood type** is the H antigen with **N-acetylgalactosamine** attached.
4. The **B blood type** is the H antigen with **D-galactose** attached.
5. The **O blood type** is the H antigen with **no additional sugar** attached.

D. ABO Subgroups

1. **Subgroups are not different antigens, only a different amount of the antigen expressed on the RBCs. The exception to this rule is subgroup A_1—A_1** has both A and A_1 antigens on the RBC surface.
2. **Blood group A has 2 major subgroups: A_1 and A_2.** 80 percent of group A people are A_1, and 20 percent of group A people are A_2.
3. People with subgroups of the A antigen can produce antibodies against A_1 and other subgroups.
4. Subgroups of A include **A_1, A_2, A_{int}, A_3, A_x, A_m, A_{ind}, A_{el}, and A_{bantu}.**
5. **Subgroups of A can be detected by Anti-A, B.** This is produced by people with an O blood type. Anti-A, B will agglutinate A subgroups because it has specificity for both A and B antigens, but cannot be separated into Anti-A and Anti-B. *Dolichos biflorus* lectin is active against A_1, but not the other A subgroups.
6. Subgroup A_3 produces a mixed field reaction with polycolonal Anti-A and polyclonal Anti-A, B. This is characteristic of A_3.
7. Subgroup A_x will not agglutinate or agglutinate weakly with polyclonal Anti-A. Polyclonal Anti-A, B will agglutinate more strongly with A_x cells.
8. A_{el} subgroup does not agglutinate with polyclonal Anti-A, monoclonal Anti-A, or polyclonal Anti-A, B. Complex techniques are needed for A_{el} identification.
9. B subgroups are rare and can be detected by weak agglutination with polyclonal or monoclonal Anti-B.

10. If weak subgroups are not detected, there is no harm in a person with the subgroup receiving type O blood. However, if the person with the subgroup donates blood which is transfused to a group O patient, it may cause intravascular hemolysis.

E. **A and B are codominant traits**—they express themselves over O. O is a morph with no detectable product.

F. **Anti-A and Anti-B occur in all humans as a result of naturally occurring substances that resemble A and B antigens**—humans produce antibodies to these substances.

G. **Anti-A and Anti-B are IgM antibodies**—this means they activate complement and cause hemolysis and visible RBC agglutination at room temperature.

H. Routine ABO grouping
   1. **Forward type:** patient RBCs mixed with Anti-A and Anti-B.
   2. **Reverse type:** patient's serum mixed with known A_1 and B RBCs.
   3. **ABO discrepancies occur when the front and reverse groupings do not agree.**
      a. Problems with front type (extra antigen present, weak antigens) could be caused by acquired B phenotype, polyagglutination, rouleaux, ABO subgroups, transfusion of nontype specific blood, bone marrow, or stem-cell transplants.
      b. Problems with reverse type (unexpected antibodies or weak/missing anibodies) could be caused by A subgroups with Anti-A_1, cold alloantibodies, cold autoantibodies, rouleaux, newborn, or elderly patient.

I. Bombay Phenotype
   1. Person inherits **hh genotype.**
   2. **Types as an O (front and reverse),** but has an anti-H capable of activating complement and causing a hemolytic transfusion reaction.
   3. **These people can only be transfused with Bombay type blood.** Many times collected as autologous or from siblings who are also Bombay, and frozen.

J. Secretor Status
   1. Two alleles: **Se** and **se.**
   2. People who inherit Se are secretors.
   3. A and B antigens are found in saliva, urine, tears, bile, amniotic fluid, breast milk, exudate, and digestive fluids of secretors (Se).

IV. Rh AND LW BLOOD GROUPS
A. Rh Blood Group System
   1. **Controlled by 2 genes RHD and RHCE.** RHD controls D expression, **NO d allele.** RHCE controls C, c, E, e expression.
   2. Rh antigens are proteins.
   3. Rh Terminology

Rosenfield	Weiner	Fisher-Race
Rh1	Rh_0	D
Rh2	rh′	C
Rh3	rh″	E

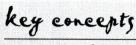

key concepts

Discuss the Fisher-Race, Weiner, and Rosenfield nomenclature for the Rh blood system, the weak D concept, and the characteristics of Rh antibodies.

Rh4	hr′	c
Rh5	hr″	e
Rh6	hr	c
Rh7		Ce
Rh8	rh^{wl}	C^w
Rh9		C^x
Rh10		ce^s
Rh12	rh^G	G

4. **Phenotype:** RBC antigens identified with specific antisera; **genotype:** the genes present on a person's chromosomes.
5. **Rh System Antigens**
   a. **D antigen:** most immunogenic of Rh antigens (old name was Rh Factor).
   b. **Weak D (D^u)**
      1) Occurs when D is weakly expressed. Must be detected by an IAT (indirect antiglobulin test).
      2) **Genetic cause:** weaker expression cDe haplotype and the IAT are needed to detect this weakly expressed D.
      3) **Position effect** occurs when the C antigen is inherited *trans* to the D antigen. This weak D is detected without doing an IAT.
      4) **Partial D:** when only part of the D antigen is inherited. There are 9 phenotypes of this type of D. These are usually detected because the antigen reacts strongly with monoclonal reagents. A partial D is suspected when a seemingly D positive person makes anti-D after transfusion with D positive blood.
      5) **Weakly reactive D means a person is D positive.** AABB standards state that all Rh negative donor units are tested for weak D and positive units identified as D positive. However, weak D recipients are transfused with D negative donors.
   c. **Other Rh System Antigens**
      1) **f or ce:** rare, if blood is c or e negative, then f negative.
      2) **Ce or rh$_i$:** C and e inherited as a haplotype made by D positive patients who make anti-C.
      3) **C^w:** low frequency antigen
      4) **C^x:** rare
      5) **V or Ce^s:** 30% prevalence in African-Americans
      6) **G or rh^G:** appears to be anti-D and anti-C
      7) **Rh29 or total Rh:** anti-total Rh made by Rh$_{null}$ people
      8) **Rh:17 or Hr$_o$:** made by individuals who have D deletion
      9) **hr^s, hr^B:** antibody found when e+ person makes apparent anti-e
   d. **Unusual phenotypes**
      1) **D deletion:** no reaction when tested with anti-E, anti-e, anti-C, and anti-c. **Written as -D-.**
      2) **Rh$_{null}$ phenotype:** appears to have no Rh antigens. The membranes of their RBCs are abnormal and the RBCs have a shortened life span. This can also be produced from inheriting a regulator gene.

3) **Rh$_{mod}$ phenotype**: this is like the Rh$_{null}$ phenotype because the RBCs lack most of the Rh antigens. This phenotype alters the RBC membrane and causes a hemolytic anemia.

6. **Rh Antibodies**
   a. Produced in humans through pregnancy or transfusions.
   b. IgG antibody.
   c. Optimal temperature: 37°C.
   d. Reactive phase: AHG.
   e. Agglutination enhancement occurs with LISS, enzymes, and polyethylene glycol (PEG).
   f. Stronger reactivity of antibody from homozygous individuals is shown with anti-C, anti-c, anti-E, and anti-e (dosage).
   g. C and e and E and c are usually found together.
   h. These antibodies produce **hemolytic transfusion reactions (HTR).** Antibodies may not be detected, but the person should always receive antigen negative blood if they have a history of Rh antibodies.
   i. Anti-D produces **hemolytic disease of the newborn (HDN).** Anti-D can cross the placenta. Rh immune globulin after delivery (within 72 hours) can protect a woman from making anti-D. Anti-C, anti-c, anti-E, and anti-e can also cause hemolytic disease of the newborn.

B. **LW Blood Group System**
   1. This system is serologically related to Rh, but not genetically.
   2. Possible phenotypes: LW (a+b−), LW(a+b+), LW(a−b+), LW(a−b−).

V. OTHER BLOOD GROUP SYSTEMS

A. **Kell Blood Group System**
   1. Abbreviation: **K.**
   2. Antibody class: **IgG.**
   3. Optimal reaction temperature: **37°C.**
   4. Reactive phase: **AHG.**
   5. Enzyme treatment: **no effect.**
   6. Antigens: K (Kell), k (Cellano)(rare), Kp^a, Kp^b (rare), Kp^c, Js^a, Js^b (rare), Cote (K11), Wk^a, and Ku.
   7. High frequency antigens include K12, K13, K16, K18, K19, K20, and K22.
   8. Low frequency antigens include U1^a, K23, K25 (VLAN).
   9. **K is very immunogenic.** It can cause hemolytic transfusion reactions (HTR) and hemolytic disease of the newborn (HDN).
   10. Kell$_{null}$: RBCs that lack the Kell antigens, but have the K$_x$ antigen.
   11. Alleles include K and k, Kp^a and Kp^b, Js^a and Js^b, KEL11 and KEL17.

B. **K$_x$ Blood Group System**
   1. The K$_x$ antigen is in the K$_x$ system. This antigen is inherited independently from the Kell antigens, but it is biochemically similar to the Kell antigens. K$_{null}$ individuals have increased amounts of K$_x$.

2. **McLeod Phenotype**
   a. XK1 gene is not inherited, and there is decreased expression of Kell antigens.
   b. These individuals have decreased RBC survival and RBC morphologic and functional abnormalities.

C. Duffy Blood Group System

1. Abbreviation: **Fy.**
2. Antibody class: **IgG.**
3. Optimal reaction temperature: **37°C.**
4. Reactive phase: **AHG.**
5. Enzyme treatment: **destroys antigens.**
6. Alleles: Fy^a and Fy^b, Fy^x.
7. Antigens: Fy^a, Fy^b, Fy3, Fy4, Fy5, Fy6.
8. Four phenotypes: Fy (a+b−); Fy (a−b+); Fy (a+b+); Fy (a−b−).
9. **Characteristics**
   a. Does not bind complement.
   b. Weak antibodies react stronger with homozygous cells.
   c. Anti-Fy^a and anti-Fy^b can cause HR and HDN.
   d. The Fy a-b- phenotype is more resistant to malarial infection.

D. Kidd Blood Group System

1. Abbreviation: **Jk.**
2. Antibody class: **IgG.**
3. Optimal reaction temperature: **37°C.**
4. Reactive phase: **AHG.**
5. Enzyme treatment: **enhance (increase agglutination).**
6. Antigens: Jk^a, Jk^b, Jk^3.
7. Four phenotypes: Jk (a+b−); Jk (a−b+); Jk (a+b+); Jk (a−b−).
8. Alleles: Jk^a codes for Jk^a and Jk^3, Jk^b codes for Jk^b and Jk^3.
9. **Dosage effect:** weak antibodies agglutinate homozygous cells more strongly than heterozygous cells.
10. These antibodies bind complement.
11. These antibodies are associated with HTR and mild HDN.
12. **The antibodies deteriorate in storage and can cause delayed HTR (DHTR).**

E. Lutheran Blood Group System

1. Abbreviation: **Lu.**
2. Antibody class: **IgG/IgM.**
3. Optimal reaction temperature: **37°C and 4°C.**
4. Reactive phases: **room temperature and AHG.**
5. Enzyme treatment: **variable effect.**
6. Alleles: Lu^a, Lu^b.
7. Antigens: 18 total including Au^a and Au^b.
8. **Anti-Lu^a** can be present without prior transfusion or pregnancy. Can be IgG/IgM. Best reactions are at room temperature with a characteristic mixed field agglutination. **NO clinical significance.**

9. **Anti-Lu^b:** rare, IgG, mixed field agglutination in AHG and associated with hemolytic transfusion reactions and mild hemolytic disease of the newborn.

F. Lewis Blood Group System

1. Abbreviation: **Le.**
2. **Clinically significant: no.**
3. Antibody class: **IgM.**
4. Optimal reaction temperature: **37°C and 4°C.**
5. Reaction phase: room temperature, **37°C, and AHG.**
6. Enzyme treatment: **enhanced agglutination.**
7. Produced by tissue cells and secreted into fluids. The antigens are adsorbed onto the RBC membranes.
8. May take 6 years to fully develop these antigens.
9. **Genetics: if Le gene inherited, Le^a adsorbed onto RBCs—Le (a+b−).** Le^a is the only antigen that can be secreted by a nonsecretor.
10. **If Se gene is also inherited, Le^b adsorbed onto the RBC—Le (a−b+)**
11. Bombay phenotypes are Le^a positive.
12. Cells type as Le (a+b+); Le (a+b−); Le (a−b+); Le (a−b−).
13. Lewis antibodies are sometimes formed during pregnancy but weaken and disappear after delivery.

G. Ii Blood Group System

1. Abbreviation: **I.**
2. Clinically significant: **no.**
3. Antibody class: **IgM.**
4. Optimal temperature: **4°C.**
5. Reaction phases: **immediate spin and 37°C.**
6. Enzyme treatment: **Enhanced agglutination.**
7. Can be a bothersome antibody. May mask the reactions of a clinically significant alloantibody. May need to prewarm cell suspension and reagent to find clinically significant alloantibodies.
8. Strong anti-I is associated with *Mycoplamsa pneumoniae* infection.

H. P Blood Group System

1. Abbreviation: **P_1.**
2. **Not clinically significant.**
3. Antibody class: **IgM.**
4. Optimal temperature: **4°C.**
5. Reaction phases: **immediate spin, 37°C and AHG.**
6. Enzyme treatment: **enhanced agglutination.**
7. Alleles: P^{1k}, P^k, and p; and P^2 and $P^{2.0}$.
8. Phenotypes: P_1, P_2, p, P_{1k}, P_{2k}, and Luke.
9. P_1 phenotype: P_1 and pantigens; P_2 phenotype: pantigen.
10. P_1 antigens can be detected in hydatid cyst fluid.
11. Autoanti-P is **Donath-Landsteiner antibody.** Naturally occurring and cold-reacting antibody associated with paroxysmal cold hemoglobinuria. It binds to the antigen on the patients' RBCs in the cold

and fixes complement. The RBCs are hemolyzed when the temperature reaches 37°C.

12. **Patients with autoanti-P may require a blood warmer for transfusion.**

13. Anti-PP$_1$P^k is found in P$_{null}$ people. Clinically significant. Need compatible blood from other P$_{null}$ people.

I. MNS Blood Group System

1. **M and N Antigens**
   a. Abbreviation: MNS.
   b. Clinically significant: **NO.**
   c. Antibody class: **IgM.**
   d. Optimal temperature: **4°C or 37°C.**
   e. Optimal reaction is **IS, 37°C, or AHG.**
   f. Enzyme treatment: **destroys antigens.**
   g. Antigens are M and N: associated with glycophorin A.

2. **S and s**
   a. Abbreviation: MNS.
   b. Antibody class: **IgG.**
   c. Clinically significant: **YES**
   d. Optimal temperature: **37°C.**
   e. Optimal reaction phase: **AHG.**
   f. Enzyme treatment: **variable effect.**
   g. Antigens: S, s, and U: associated with glycophorin B.

3. **Anti-M**
   a. Clinically significant if **IgG,** IgM antibody is not clinically significant.
   b. Demonstrates dosage effect.

4. Anti-N is very rare.

5. Anti-S, Anti-s, and Anti-U
   a. **Clinically significant, causing HTR and HDN.**
   b. Anti-U is rare and occurs in S-s- people.

J. Miscellaneous Blood Group Antigens

1. **Deigo (DI) system** antigens: Di^a, Di^b, Wr^a, Wr^b, Wd^a, Rb^a, WARR; Di^b and Wr^b are high incidence.

2. **Cartwright (Yt) system** antigens: Yt^a and Yt^b and Yt^a are high incidence.

3. **Xg system** antigen: Xg^a.

4. **Scianna system** antigens: SC:1, SC:2, and SC:3; SC:1 and SC:3 are high incidence antigens.

5. **Dombrock antigens:** Do^a, Do^b, Gy^a, Hy, and Jo^a; Gy^a Hy and Jo^a are high incidence antigens.

6. **Colton antigens:** Co^a, Co^b and Co^3; Co^a is a high incidence antigen.

7. **Chido/Rogers antigens:** Ch and Ra are both high incidence antigens.

8. **Girlich antigens:** Ge2, Ge3, Ge4, Wb, Ls^a, An^a, and Dah; Ge2, Ge3, and Ge4 are high incidence antigens.

9. **Cromer antigens:** Cr^a, Tc^a, Tc^b, Tc^c, Dr^a and Es^a, and IFC; Cr^a, Tc^a, Dr^a, Es^a, and IFC are high incidence antigens.

10. **Knops antigens:** Kn^a, Kn^b, McC^a, Sl^a, and Yk^a; Kn^a, McC^a, Sl^a, and Yk^b are high incidence antigens.
11. **Cost antigens:** Cs^a and Cs^b; Cs^a is a high incidence antigen.
12. **Vel system** antigen is Vel, and it is a high incidence antigen.
13. **JMH system** antigen is JMH, and it is a high incidence antigen.
14. **Sd^a system** antigen is Sd^a, and it is a high incidence antigen.

VI. PRETRANSFUSION TESTING

A. Compatibility Testing

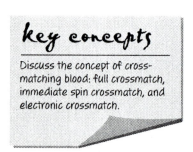

key concepts

Discuss the concept of cross-matching blood: full crossmatch, immediate spin crossmatch, and electronic crossmatch.

1. Entails crossmatching, recipient identification, specimen collection and handling, antibody screen, antibody identification, review of patient's blood bank records, ABO/Rh confirmation on donor units, screening donor units for antigens that recipients have antibodies to, and the actual transfusion.
2. Definitions
   a. **Major crossmatch:** testing donor cells with recipient serum—carried through all phases and check cells.
   b. **Compatible crossmatch:** no agglutination or hemolysis.
   c. **Incompatible crossmatch:** agglutination or hemolysis.
   d. **Immediate spin crossmatch:** only room temperature; immediate spin is done with donor cells and recipient serum. This ensures the ABO compatability of donor and recipient matches.
   e. **Electronic crossmatch:** donor ABO/Rh and patient ABO/Rh are checked and entered into a validated blood bank computer system. The recipient's transfusion history is researched through the computer also. If the patient has not been transfused in the last 2 months and the patient's antibody screen is negative, blood for the patient is issued without any additional testing.
3. **Purpose of Crossmatch**
   a. Prevent transfusion of incompatible red blood cells.
   b. Maximize RBC life after transfusion.
4. **Limitation of Crossmatches**
   a. Does not guarantee a successful transfusion.
   b. Does not detect transfusion transmitted bacteria, viruses, or parasites.
   c. Does not detect allergic reactions.
   d. Does not detect WBC antigens.
   e. Will not prevent antibody production to foreign antigens present on donor's RBCs.
   f. Does not detect delayed transfusion reactions.
5. **Procedure**
   a. Blood sample: acceptable tubes: plain red top, yellow top (acid citrate dextrose or ACD, Formula B), EDTA, blue top (citrate).
      1) Hemolyzed specimens are not acceptable.
      2) Specimens must be 72 hours old or less for patients transfused or pregnant within the last 3 months.
      3) AABB states that the following information must be on the tube:

        a) Patient first and last name, and it must match name on armband.

        b) Unique identifying number on patient and tube.

        c) Date of collection.

        d) Signature or initials of phlebotomist.

    4) The patient must be able to state his/her name before drawing the tube. Information on the tube must match information on the requisition.

6. **AABB requires comparison of current blood bank workup with other blood bank tests performed on the same patient within 12 months** (including blood type, typing problems, allo or autoantibodies, transfusion reactions, or special requirements).

7. AABB states that the ABO will be repeated on all units received into the blood bank, and Rh is tested on all Rh negative units.

8. AABB Standards for Crossmatches

    a. **Patient's serum and donor cells taken from a segment on the bag of the unit to be transfused.**

    b. **Immediate spin crossmatch:** use when recipients have no history of alloantibodies and current antibody screen is negative. The donor cells and recipient serum or plasma are added to a tube. This tube is spun and the reaction is graded. If negative, the recipient is transfused with this unit of blood. If positive, the crossmatch must be carried out as an antiglobulin crossmatch: immediate spin, 37°C incubation, and AHG phases.

    c. **Antiglobulin crossmatch:** a history of an alloantibody or the detection of one in the current antibody screen warrants an antiglobulin crossmatch. AHG crossmatch involves immediate spin phase, addition of potentiator, 37°C incubation phase, 3 washes, antiglobulin phase, and finally check cells.

    d. **Electronic crossmatch:** ABB standards require

        1) Validated computer system

        2) Validated studies submitted to FDA

        3) 2 identical ABO typings on recipient

        4) ABO on current sample

        5) ABO typing by 2 techs or on 2 samples

        6) Computer has donor unit information—product name, ABO and Rh, unique number, interpretation of ABO confirmation test

        7) Computer system contains recipient ABO & Rh

        8) Computer alert for ABO incompatibilities

        9) Method to verify the correct entry of all data

        10) Advantages: increased time efficiency, decreased volume of sample for large crossmatches

        11) Better inventory management

9. Tagging, Inspecting, and Issuing Blood Products

    a. **Every unit to be transfused is tagged.** The tag must contain the patient's full name, unique identification numbers, name of product, donor number, expiration date, ABO and Rh of unit, crossmatch interpretation, and identification of person doing testing or selecting unit.

b. **Inspecting the unit:** each unit must be inspected for expiration date, ABO and Rh, discoloration, clots, and bacterial contamination before release for transfusion.

c. **Issuing:** person taking the unit should have a request form that has the patient's full name, unique number, and product needed. Need to check the unit tag with this form and the persons issuing and receiving the unit and must record initials or signature date and time. If RBCs are not stored in a monitored refrigerator or transfused within 30 minutes of issue, the unit must be destroyed.

10. **Incompatible Crossmatches**

a. Causes for an incompatible immediate-spin crossmatch: wrong patient identification, wrong sample identification, cold alloantibody, presence of anti-A_1, or a cold autoantibody.

b. Causes for an incompatible AHG crossmatch: alloantibody, autoantibody, or high-titer low-avidity antibody.

11. **Emergency Release of Uncrossmatched Blood**

a. Emergency release must be signed by physician requesting blood.

b. Unit must be tagged just like when performing a crossmatch. Note the blood is an emergency release and not crossmatched.

c. Must have full patient name and unique identification number, donor unit number, ABO and Rh, and expiration date on tag, requisition, and blood bank records.

d. Segments are removed from the unit before issuing so that the blood can be crossmatched after the release of the unit.

e. Name of the person issuing the unit must be on the requisition and blood bank records.

12. **Massive Transfusion**

a. Definition: total blood volume replacement within 24 hours (approximately 10 – 12 units).

b. Each facility has a policy on when a new recipient sample is needed and if crossmatching is necessary.

13. Surgery blood order list: procedures that are performed according to the surgery a patient is having. Choices include type and screen, crossmatch for 2 units, crossmatch for 4 units, or crossmatch for 6 units.

14. **Crossmatching Autologous Units**

a. Blood is donated by recipient for use in or after surgery.

b. Must be transfused for intended patient—cannot be given to anyone else.

c. Not tested for infectious diseases.

d. Immediate spin crossmatch performed before issuing blood for transfusion.

15. **Crossmatching Infants Less Than 4 Months Old**

a. Newborns develop antibodies at 4 to 6 months of age. Pretransfusion testing is only ABO and Rh.

    b. Antibody screen from an infant or mother yields maternal antibodies. If alloantibodies are detected, units negative for the corresponding antigens are transfused.

16. **Pretransfusion testing for fresh frozen plasma (FFP), platelets, cryoprecipitate, platelet pheresis, and granulocyte concentrates is ABO.** These products are ABO-type specific.

VII. BLOOD BANK REAGENTS

A. Principle of Blood Bank Tests

$$Ag + Ab \leftrightarrow Ag\text{-}Ab \text{ reaction}$$

B. Routine Blood Bank Testing Procedures

1. **ABO/Rh Typing**
   a. Detects A, B, and D antigens
   b. Source of antigen: patient RBCs (forward type), reagent RBCs (reverse grouping)
   c. Source of antibody: commercial anti-A, anti-B, and anti-D (forward type); patient's serum (reverse grouping)

2. **Antibody Screen**
   a. Detects specific antibodies to RBC antigens
   b. Source of antigens: commercial screening cells
   c. Source of antibodies: patient serum

3. **Antibody Identification**
   a. Identifies antibody to RBC antigens
   b. Source of antigens: commercial antibody panel cells (10–16 cells)
   c. Source of antibodies: patient serum

4. **Crossmatch**
   a. Determines compatability of donor RBCs in patient blood
   b. Source of antigen: donor cells
   c. Source of antibody: recipient serum

C. Types of Blood Bank Reagents

1. **Reagent RBCs** possess known antigens and are treated to prolong their life span.
2. **Antisera** contain antibodies against specific RBC antigens.
3. **Antiglobulin reagents** contain poly- or monospecific antibodies against human antibodies.
4. **Enhancers:** solutions that enhance the formation of antigen-antibody complexes.

D. Regulation of Reagent Production

1. Blood bank reagents are licensed by the Center for Biologics Evaluation and Research of the FDA.
2. FDA specifies potency and specificity of reagents before production.

E. Reagent Antisera

1. **Polyclonal:** many B-cell clones produce antibodies against antigens.
2. **Monoclonal:** a single B-cell clone produces antibody against an antigen.

a. Advantages: endless production, exactly the same reagent in each batch, no human/animal sources, no contamination.

b. Disadvantages: single-specificity may not react with all portions of RBC antigen.

3. **ABO Antisera**

a. Anti-A and Anti-B are used to determine if patient is A, B, AB, or O.

Reactions:

	Anti-A	Anti-B
Type A	+	0
Type B	0	+
Type AB	+	+
Type O	0	0

b. Anti-A has blue dye added.

c. Anti-B has yellow dye added.

d. Patient cells are added to antisera.

e. Agglutination read at immediate spin. These antibodies are IgM and react best at room temperature or 4°C.

4. **D Typing**

a. Important antigens to detect because antibody-antigen reactions in vivo cause HTR and HDN.

b. 2 types of reagents:

1) **High protein:** older reagent. Need to run an Rh control with this reagent because the protein in the diluent may cause false positive reactions in patients with autoantibodies or abnormal serum proteins.

2) **Low-protein monoclonal:** Rh control is usually not required. Only need to do one when patient has abnormal serum proteins.

5. **Antiglobulin Reagents**

a. **Polyspecific:** detects both anti-IgG and anti-C3. Used often in direct antiglobulin tests.

b. **Monoclonal:** may be used to differentiate between antibodies to IgG and C3.

6. **Reagent RBCs**

a. **Check cells:** AABB Standards for Blood Banks and Transfusion Services require a control to ensure antiglobulin reagent reactivity in each negative antiglobulin test tube. Check cells are prepared by attaching an IgG antibody to RBCs (sensitized RBCs).

b. **A₁ and B cells for reverse grouping:** used to confirm front typing results. These cells detect ABO antibodies. Rule of thumb: If the patient's RBCs have an antigen, they DO NOT have the antibody.

c. **Antibody screening cells:** used to detect antibodies present in a patient's serum. Antibodies must be detected before patients are transfused to prevent hemolytic transfusion reactions and/or death. Each set of cells has 2 or 3 bottles of cells and each bottle contains antigenically different RBCs. The antigens in each bottle are known and printed on an antigram included with each set.

d. **Antibody panel cells:** antibody identification procedures use panel of RBCs whose antigen are known. The panel consists of 10 to 20 vials of these RBCs. Every panel has an antigenic profile that lists all of the known antigens on each vial of RBCs.

e. **Lectins** bind to the carbohydrate portion of RBC antigens. They can be used to identify RBC antigens.

Common lectins	Antigen specificity
Dolichos biflorus	A_1
Ulex europaeus	H
Vicia graminea	N
Iberis amara	M

f. **Other Methods for Antigen-Antibody Reaction Detection**

1) **Gel technology:** uses dextran acrylamide gel combined with reagents or diluent. Anti-IgG cards are used for DATs and IATs.

2) **Microplate methods:** The traditional tube method is adapted to the microtiter plate where smaller volumes of serum and cells are used, and it is read on an automated photometric instrument. The cell buttons are resuspended by tapping the sides of the plate.

3) **Solid-Phase Adherence Methods**
   a) RBC screening cells are bound to surface of microtiter plates.
   b) Add patient serum.
   c) RBCs capture IgGs.
   d) Plates washed.
   e) Indicator cells (anti-IgG coated RBCs) are in contact with bound antibody.
   f) Negative = RBC button, positive = RBCs (indicator cells) on sides and bottom of wells.

4) **The Indirect Antiglobulin Test (IAT)**
   a) **Purpose is to detect in vitro sensitization of RBCs.**
   b) In this procedure, RBCs are mixed with patient serum, then incubated at body temperature to allow IgG antibodies to attach to the RBCs. The solution is then washed to remove unbound proteins. **AHG is added to detect in vitro sensitization of RBCs. This is a 2-stage procedure.**
   c) **False positive tests** result when RBCs are agglutinated before the washing step (cold agglutinin); dirty glassware, over centrifugation.
   d) **False negative tests** result with poor washing of RBCs, testing is delayed, loss of reagent activity, no AHG added, or an improper RBC suspension is used.

5) **Antibody Enhancers**
   a) **Definition:** reagents added to the in vitro test to enhance antigen-antibody complex formation.

b) **Low-ionic strength solution (LISS)** increases antibody uptake of antigen.

c) **Bovine albumin (22% OR 30%)** allows sensitized cells to come close together to form agglutination lattices.

d) **Polyethylene glycol additive (PEG)** concentrates antibodies and creates a low ionic solution to allow greater antibody uptake.

e) **Proteolytic enzymes:** papain, ficin, and bromelin are used. This reduces the zeta potential and increases agglutination. Antibodies that are enhanced include Rh, Kidd, and Le blood group systems. The following antigens are destroyed by enzymes M, N, S, Xg^a, Fy^a and Fy^b.

VIII. IDENTIFICATION OF UNEXPECTED ALLOANTIBODIES

A. Detection of Atypical and Unexpected Antibodies

1. Antibodies other than ABO in a person's blood.

2. **Antibody screen (indirect antiglobulin test):** Looking for Antibodies

   a. **Purpose:** to detect antibodies in patients requiring transfusions, pregnant women, blood and blood product donors, and patients with suspected transfusion reactions.

   b. **Screening cells:** 2–3 different type O cells with known antigens included in an antigram. Looking for antibodies.

   c. **Procedure**

      1) Incubate known RBCs with patient's serum.
      2) Add potentiator and incubate at 37°C.
      3) Spin and read results.
      4) Wash 3 times with saline.
      5) Add AHG, spin, then read results.
      6) Read all negative results macroscopically (some facilities read all negative results microscopically).
      7) Add check cells to negative tubes.
      8) Spin and read agglutination reactions.

   d. **Results:** any agglutination indicates an atypical or unexpected antibody

   e. **Autocontrol:** patient's serum and patient's RBCs. Used to detect autoantibodies. Performed in conjunction with the antibody screen and is tested in all phases.

   f. **Potentiators are used to enhance antibody detection.**

   g. **Patient history:** a patient's history should be researched at that institution before transfusing the patient.

3. **Antibody Identification**

   a. **Antibody panel: type O cells with known antigens.** Usually 10–20 bottles of different cells with known antigens.

   b. **Purpose:** to identify alloantibodies detected in patient's serum.

4. **Panel Interpretation**

   a. **Autocontrol** determines if antibody is autoantibody or alloantibody.

key concepts

Analyze why the indirect antiglobulin test is performed and what it detects; how to identify antibodies using antibody identification panels; how to interpret multiple antibodies from a single antibody identification panel; and adsorption and elution procedures.

b. **Phases:** the reaction phase of the antibody is important. Will determine IgG or IgM—warm or cold. Room temperature reactions usually indicate a cold antibody.

c. **Reaction Strength**

   1) Single strength reactions usually indicate 1 antibody.

   2) Various strength reactions usually indicate more than 1 antibody or dosage.

d. **Ruling Out**

   1) Negative reaction = 0 = no antibody or if that cell is heterozygous, antibody may be showing dosage.

   2) Positive reaction = NEVER rule out! Always use this in identification.

e. **Matching the Document**

   1) Single antibody: if there is only one antibody, the reactions will match those on the antigram

   2) Multiple antibodies: if there is more than one antibody, the reactions are difficult to match a pattern on the antigram.

f. **Rule of Thumb**

   1) Are there 3 cells with positive reactions from the panel cells?

   2) Are there 3 cells with negative reactions from the panel cells?

   3) If yes, then there is a 95 percent probability that the antibody is correctly identified.

g. **Phenotype Patient**

   1) If the patient is negative for the antigen, an antibody is possible.

   2) If the patient is positive for the antigen, an antibody is not possible.

5. **Multiple Antibody Resolution**

a. May need to perform more tests to identify antibodies.

b. Selected cells can be used to complete identification: use rule of three. Can use individual cells from a panel.

c. **Additional Techniques**

   1) 1-stage enzyme: incubate patient's serum, papain, and RBCs

   2) 2-stage enzyme: pretreat panel or screening cells with enzymes, wash, then do IAT without additional enhancements.

d. When running the IAT only read agglutination in the AHG phase.

B. Antibodies to High-Frequency Antigens

1. Definition: antibodies produced against antigens that occur in at least 98 percent of the population.

2. When interpreting panels, you know you have an antibody to a high frequency antigen when:

a. The autocontrol is negative.

b. Reactions are occurring in AHG

c. Reaction strength in panel cells is the same.

3. Next, you must determine which cells to rule out.

4. Additional testing: under the **rule of three,** you must have at least 3 positive and 3 negative cells. You can choose cells from other panels that will produce negative reactions.

5. **Clues for High-Frequency Antibody Identification**

   a. I, H, P, P_1, PP_1, and P^k produce room temperature reactions.

   b. Lu^a, Ch, Rg, Cs^a, Kn^a, McC^a, Sl^a, and JMH produce weak reactions at AHG.

6. **High Titer-Low Avidity (HTLV) Antibodies (weakly reactive antibodies)**

   a. Weak AHG reaction

   b. Variable reactions in panel cells

   c. Inconsistent reactions

   d. Nonreactive in autocontrol

   e. Not clinically significant

   f. Reactions not stronger when potentiators are used

C. Antibodies to Low Frequency Antigens

1. If the antibody screen is negative and the crossmatch is positive, suspect antibodies to low frequency antigens.

2. Low frequency antigens are Lu^a, C^w, Kp^a, Wr^a, V, Bg^a, VS, Co^b.

3. Usually a crossmatch will be negative

4. If the antibody is found in a pregnant woman, test the father with the mother's serum to determine if the fetus is in danger of hemolytic disease of the newborn.

D. Enhancing Weak IgG Antibodies

1. If weak reactions are encountered that don't fit the pattern of a known antigen, repeat panel using different potentiators, increase incubation time, and/or increase serum to cell ratio.

E. Alloantibodies

1. Cold antibodies react at 4°C, and room temperature is usually not clinically significant. These antibodies can hide a clinically significant alloantibody. Prewarmed techniques or adsorption of cold antibody can help detect any alloantibodies present. If the cold antibody reacts at 37°C, it may be clinically significant.

F. Autoantibodies

1. Can be detected by a positive DAT or positive autocontrol.

2. Can be produced in response to drug effects, cold autoimmune disease, pneumonia, warm autoimmune disease, transfusion reaction, hemolytic disease of the newborn, infectious mononucleosis, etc.

G. Cold Panels

1. Cold panels are done to identify "cold" antibodies.

2. Antibody panels are performed with the incubation at 4°C instead of 37°C.

3. Because most cold autoantibodies are either anti-I, anti-H, or anti-IH, an abbreviated or "mini" cold panel can be performed:

   a. Select cells for panel: use screening cells (type O), an autocontrol, cord blood or i positive cells from a commercial panel, and type specific cells for the patient (e.g., A cells for type A, B cells for type B).

b. Add 2 drops of patient serum to cells and incubate at 4°C for 20 minutes.

c. Shake and grade reactions after incubation.

d. Interpretation:

	Screening Cell 1	Screening Cell 2	Autocontrol	Cord	Type Specific
Anti-I	3+	3+	3+	0	4+
Anti-IH	3+	3+	3+	1+	2+
Anti-H	3+	3+	2+	0	2+

H. Avoiding Cold Antibodies

1. Use IgG anti-human globulin.
2. Skip the immediate spin or room temperature phase.
3. Use 22 percent albumin instead of LISS.
4. **Use Prewarmed Technique**
   a. Put 1 drop of panel cells and autocontrol cells into tube and incubate at 37°C for 10 minutes.
   b. Simultaneously warm patient serum at 37°C for 10 minutes.
   c. Add prewarmed serum to prewarmed panel cells and incubate at 37°C for 30 minutes.
   d. Wash 3 times in saline prewarmed to 37°C.
   e. Add AHG, spin, read, and grade reactions.
   f. Interpret reactions.
   g. Add check cells to negative tubes.

I. Adsorption Techniques

1. If patient was not transfused in last 3 months, do an autoadsorption.
2. If patient was transfused, use panel cells for adsorption.
3. **Cold Autoadsorption**
   a. Incubate patient serum and cells at 4°C for 30–60 minutes.
   b. Remove serum and use serum for panel to test for alloantibody.
4. **Warm Autoadsorption**
   a. Incubate patient serum and cells at 37°C for 30–60 minutes.
   b. Remove serum and use serum in panel to test for alloantibody.

J. Elution

1. IgG that attaches to RBCs in vivo can be removed by elution (in vitro).
2. **3 Types of Elution Techniques**
   a. **Intact RBC antibody removal (RES)** uses buffers to remove the antibody from the RBC without destroying the RBC.
   b. **Digitonin** releases the antibody by destroying the RBCs.
   c. **Lui freeze-thaw** used to remove IgM antibodies (usually A or B) present on newborn RBCs.
3. Once antibody releases, the last wash and the eluate supernatant are tested on a panel.
4. The last wash panel should be negative, and the eluate supernatant should reveal alloantibodies.

IX. DIRECT ANTIGLOBULIN TESTING
A. Direct Antiglobulin Test (DAT)
1. RBCs may combine with antibodies without agglutinating.
2. **Antihuman globulin** is an in vitro reagent produced to agglutinate RBCs with antibodies attached to them (sensitized RBCs)
3. Direct Antiglobulin Test (DAT)
   a. **Ordered to detect IgG or complement proteins attached to RBCs** in autoimmune hemolytic anemia, hemolytic disease of the newborn, a drug-related mechanism, or a transfusion reaction.
   b. Indicates **immune-mediated** in vivo RBC destruction (antibodies attached to RBCs **in vivo**)
   c. **Procedure**
      1) Patient's RBCs washed 3 times with normal saline to remove unbound proteins.
      2) Antihuman globulin (AHG) is added after washing.
      3) Agglutination indicates that the patient has antibodies or complement proteins attached to RBCs.
   d. **Specimen of choice:** EDTA because EDTA negates the in vitro activation of complement.

X. HEMOLYTIC DISEASES OF THE NEWBORN
A. Etiology
1. Hemolytic disease of the newborn or **erythroblastosis fetalis** IgG antibodies cross the placenta and destroy the baby's RBCs when RBCs contain antigen specific for the antibody. Hemoglobin from lysed RBCs is metabolized into indirect bilirubin. The mother secretes the bilirubin with no problems. The fetus becomes anemic as RBC destruction continues. Cardiac failure and/or hydrops fetalis will result from anemia. After delivery, the bilirubin that was metabolized by the mother now accumulates in the baby's liver. The infant is unable to metabolize and excrete the bilirubin because its liver is not functioning at full capacity. The buildup of bilirubin is called jaundice and can cause deafness, mental retardation, **kernicterus** (brain damage), or death.

B. Rh Hemolytic Disease of the Newborn
1. Most severe.
2. D negative mom develops antibodies during first pregnancy with D positive baby. Antibodies attack second baby or donor RBCs if D positive.
3. Lab results: positive DAT, increased bilirubin.
4. Exchange transfusion may be needed to avoid kernicterus.
5. Rh immune globulin provides D antibodies so mother does not produce them. Fetal RBCs are destroyed before the mother's immune system recognizes the D antigen as foreign. The mother is not alloimmunized and does not produce her own antibodies against D.

C. ABO Hemolytic Disease
1. Most common form of HDN, A or B babies born to O mothers—mild disease.

2. Usually not treated by transfusion.
3. Infants are treated by phototherapy to break down excess bilirubin.

D. Antibody Titration

1. Used to predict severity of HDN.
2. Titer needs to be determined ASAP in pregnancy.
3. Repeat titers on positive mothers at 16 and 22 weeks, then every 1–4 weeks until delivery.
4. A twofold rise in titer indicates a serious situation and invasive procedures or an exchange transfusion may be necessary.

E. Amniocentesis

1. Total bilirubin of amniotic fluid is measured by the change in absorbance of the fluid at 450 nm.

F. Laboratory Testing for Predicting Hemolytic Disease of the Newborn

1. ABO and D.
2. Antibody screen on mother—infants do not produce antibodies

G. Rhogam workup on the cord blood of infants born to D negative moms and in suspected cases of hemolytic disease of the newborn.

1. ABO
2. D
3. DAT

H. Prevention of Hemolytic Disease of the Newborn

1. Prenatal Rh immune globulin administered at 28 weeks (300 µg).
2. One vial of Rh immune globulin should be administered after abortions, ectopic pregnancies, amniocenteses, chorionic villus sampling, percutaneous umbilical blood sampling (PUBS), intrauterine transfusions, and abdominal trauma.
3. **Postpartum Administration**
   a. D negative women who deliver a D positive infant need a full dose (300 µg) within 72 hours of delivery.
   b. 1 dose (300 µg) of Rh immune globulin will neutralize up to 15 mls RBCs (30 mls whole blood) of feto-maternal hemorrhage. If the feto-maternal hemorrhage is > 15 mls RBCs, more than 1 dose is required to neutralize the RBCs.
4. **Rosette test:** a suspension of maternal RBCs (which include a few Ph-positive fetal RBCs) is incubated with anti-D. Anti-D binds to fetal RBCs. D-positive indicator cells are added that bind to the anti-D, forming a rosette around the fetal RBCs.
5. **Kleihaur-Betke acid elution** is used to determine the amount of a fetomaternal hemorrhage. Principle: fetal hemoglobin is resistant to acid elution. A blood smear from the mother is made, then dipped in an acid buffer and stained with a counterstain. The buffer lyses the mother's cells (ghost cells) and does nothing to the fetal cells. Pink fetal cells are counted. Results are reported as percent of fetal cells (# fetal cells/total cells counted). The mls of fetal blood in maternal circulation = % fetal cells × 50. Divide the number of cells by 30 to determine the number of Rh immune globulin doses needed.

I. Exchange Transfusions

1. Selection of blood for exchange transfusion
   a. Infant cells must be tested for ABO and D.
   b. Mother's blood is used for antibody screen.
   c. Units must be antigen negative for all antibodies in mother's blood.
2. FFP is used to reconstitute pRBCs to a hematocrit of approximately 40–50 percent.
3. Any blood products to be transfused must be CMV negative and irradiated.

XI. BLOOD COLLECTION

A. Donor Selection

key concepts

Discuss the rules for selecting donors, how to collect blood units, the concept of intraoperative salvage, and the concept of hemapheresis.

1. Registration questions include name, no deferred donation, full name, address, home and work phone numbers, date of birth, gender, date of last donation, written consent, social security or driver license numbers, photo identification card, race, and intended use of donation.
2. Educational material is distributed to the donor. The donor must read material and if the prospective donor shows symptoms of an infectious disease, the donor is excluded from donation.
3. **Donor history questions include:**
   a. Have you ever donated or attempted to donate blood using a different or another) name here or anywhere else? (FDA)
   b. In the past 8 weeks, have you given blood, plasma, or platelets here or anywhere else?
   c. Have you for any reason been deferred or refused as a blood donor or told not to donate blood? (FDA)
   d. Are you feeling well and healthy today?
   e. In the past 12 months, have you been under a doctor's care or had a major illness or surgery? (FDA)
   f. Have you ever had chest pain, heart disease, recent or severe respiratory disease?
   g. Have you ever had cancer, a blood disease, or a bleeding problem?
   h. Have you ever had yellow jaundice, liver disease, viral hepatitis, or a positive test for hepatitis?
   i. Have you ever had malaria, Chagas' disease, or babesiosis?
   j. Have you ever taken etretinate (Tegison) for psoriasis?
   k. In the past 3 years, have you taken acetretin (Soriatane)?
   l. In the past 3 days have you taken piroxicam (Feldene), aspirin, or anything that has aspirin in it?
   m. In the past month have you taken isotretinoin (Accutane) or finasteride (Proscar) (Propecia)?
   n. In the past 4 weeks have you taken any pills or medications?
   o. In the past 12 months, have you been given rabies shots?
   p. Female donors: In the past 6 weeks, have you been pregnant or are you pregnant now?
   q. In the past 3 years, have you been outside the United States or Canada?

r. Have you ever received human pituitary-derived growth hormone?

s. Have you received a dura mater (or brain covering) graft?

t. Have you or any of your blood relatives ever had Creutzfeldt-Jakob disease or have you ever been told that your family is at an increased risk for Creutzfeldt-Jakob disease?

u. In the past 12 months, have you had close contact with a person with yellow jaundice or viral hepatitis, or have you been given hepatitis B immune globluin (HBIG)?

v. In the past 12 months, have you taken (snorted) cocaine through your nose?

w. In the past 12 months, have you received blood or had an organ or a tissue transplant or graft?

x. In the past 12 months, have you had a tattoo applied, ear or skin piercing, acupuncture, accidental needlestick, or come in contact with someone else's blood?

y. In the past 12 months, have you had a positive test for syphilis?

z. In the past 12 months, have you had or been treated for syphilis or gonorrhea?

aa. In the past 12 months, have you given money or drugs to anyone to have sex with you?

bb. At any time since 1977, have you taken money or drugs for sex?

cc. In the past 12 months, have you had sex, even once with anyone who has taken money or drugs for sex?

dd. Have you ever used a needle, even once, to take drugs that were not prescribed for you by a doctor?

ee. In the past 12 months, have you had sex, even once, with anyone who has used a needle to take drugs not prescribed by a doctor?

ff. Male donors: Have you had sex with another male, even once, since 1977?

gg. Female donors: In the past 12 months, have you had sex with a male who has had sex with another male, even once, since 1977?

hh. Have you ever taken clotting factor concentrates for a bleeding problem such as hemophilia?

ii. In the past 12 months, have you had sex, even once, with anyone who has taken clotting factor concentrates for a bleeding problem such as hemophilia?

jj. Do you have AIDS or have you had a positive test for the AIDS virus?

kk. In the past 12 months, have you had sex, even once, with anyone who has AIDS or has had a positive test for the AIDS virus?

ll. Are you giving blood because you want to be tested for HIV or the AIDS virus?

mm. Do you understand that if you have the AIDS virus, you can give it to someone else even though you may feel well and have a negative AIDS test?

nn. Were you born in, or have you lived in, or have you traveled to any African country since 1977?

oo. When you traveled there did you receive a blood transfusion or any other medical treatment with a product made from blood?

pp. Have you had sexual contact with anyone who was born in or lived in any African country since 1977?

qq. In the past 12 months, have you been in jail or prison?

rr. Have you read and understood all the donor information presented to you, and have all your questions been answered?

4. **Donors are deferred for:**

a. Hepatitis B IgG	12 months
b. Tattoo/piercing	12 months
c. Exposure to blood	12 months
d. Sexual contact with a person at high risk for HIV	12 months
e. Imprisonment (>72hours)	12 months
f. Return from a malarial endemic area	12 months
g. Postblood transfusion	12 months
h. Rape victim	12 months
i. Accutane use	1 month
j. Propecia use	1 month
k. Malarial infection	3 years
l. Aspirin and aspirin-containing drugs	72 hours
m. Human pituitary growth hormone injection	permanent
n. Sexual contact with anyone who used a needle to take illegal drugs	permanent
o. Taken clotting factors	permanent
p. AIDS or HIV positive	permanent
q. Males having sex with other males	permanent
r. Had viral hepatitis	permanent
s. Positive HBsAg	permanent
t. Positive HBc	permanent
u. Positive HTLV	permanent
v. History of Crutzfeldt-Jakob disease	permanent
w. History of Chagas' disease or babesiosis	permanent

5. **All donors must pass a physical exam with the following criteria:**

a. Appear to be in good health.

b. 38 percent hematocrit (minimum).

c. 12.5 g/dL hemoglobin (minimum).

d. Temperature must be below 99.5°F (37.5°C).

e. Blood pressure must be below 180/100.

f. Pulse must be between 50–100 and regular.

g. Weight must be a minimum of 110 pounds.

6. **Confidential Unit Exclusion**

a. This is used to give donors a way to indicate if this unit should be used for transfusion or discarded. The most common way to accomplish this is to give the donor 2 bar coded labels: one states that the blood is OK to use and the other states the blood should not be used. The donor chooses the label and applies it to his records. Once the label is pulled from the backing, the only way of knowing which label is on the records is to scan the bar code.

7. **Informed consent:** the donor must sign a form that allows blood to be collected and used for transfusion.

B. Phlebotomy

1. **Identification** is a crucial step. The donor must be identified before phlebotomy can be done.

2. **Bag labeling:** the bag, attached satellite bags, sample tubes, and donor registration must have the same unique identification number. The labels consist of letters and bar codes.

3. **Adverse Donor Reactions**
   a. Include sweating, rapid breathing, dizziness, nausea, fainting, convulsions, and cardiac problems.
   b. For most reactions, treatment includes removing tourniquet and bag, applying cold compress to forehead, and sniffing ammonia ampules.
   c. For serious reactions such as convulsions or cardiac problems, call for help and check the patient's airway, breathing, and circulation. For convulsions, make sure the donor cannot hurt himself.

4. **Postdonation care:** After donating, donors are urged to avoid alcohol and smoking immediately, drink lots of fluid for the next 3 days, and be aware that dizziness and fainting can occur a few hours after donation.

C. Special Blood Collection

1. **Autologous donation:** a donation of blood given by a person to be used for transfusions on themselves at a later date. There are 4 types—preoperative, intraoperative hemodilution, intraoperative collection, or postoperative collection.
   a. **Advantages:** no diseases transmitted, no alloantibodies formed, no transfusion reactions possible.
   b. **Disadvantages:** high waste amount, surgery postponed, adverse donor reactions, and increased cost.

2. **Preoperative Collection**
   a. Blood is drawn and stored before surgery.
   b. Used for stable patients having a surgery that may require a transfusion.
   c. Especially good for patients with existing alloantibodies where it's hard to find compatible units.
   d. Process begins with a doctor's order.
   e. Patients must sign informed consent.
   f. Not asked detailed questions about high risk behavior.
   g. Facility makes policy regarding patients' health, age, weight, etc. Hemoglobin should not be below 11 g/dL or hematocrit below 33 percent.
   h. Blood not drawn sooner than every 72 hours and not drawn within 72 hours of surgery.

i. Patient's name, transfusion facility, unique patient identification number, and "Autologous Use Only" or "Autologous Donor" tag is on the bag.

j. ABO and D must be performed at the collecting facility.

k. If transfused outside of the facility, HBbAg, HIV antibody and antigen, HIV 1–2 antigen and antibody, hepatitis C antibody HBcAb, and RPR must be performed before shipping.

l. If donor is positive for any of the above, doctor's permission is required to use the unit, and a biohazard sticker is attached to the unit before shipping.

m. An autologous unit cannot be used for allogenic transfusion if it is not used by the donor.

3. **Intraoperative Hemodilution**

a. 1–2 units are removed at the beginning of surgery and replaced by volume expanders.

b. Units must be labeled with patient's name, unique identification number, date and time of phlebotomy, and "Autologous Use Only."

c. This blood can be stored at room temperature for up to 8 hours or 1–6°C for 24 hours.

4. **Intraoperative Collection (Intraoperative Salvage)**

a. Blood lost into the abdominal cavity is collected by a machine. It is washed and transferred back into patient. Should not be used if blood will be contaminated with bacteria.

5. **Postoperative Collection**

a. Collect from surgical drains into sterile containers.

b. Collected blood must be transfused within 6 hours.

6. **Directed Donations**

a. When patients choose their own donors.

b. All AABB donor standards apply to directed donations.

c. Policies about switching units from directed donation to general donor pool vary among institutions.

7. **Hemapheresis**

a. **Leukapheresis:** only WBCs removed from donor blood.

b. **Plateletpheresis:** only platelets removed from donor blood.

c. **Plasmapheresis:** only plasma removed from donor blood.

d. Apheresis instrument: electronic instrument that takes blood from a donor, separates the desired component, then returns the remaining components to the donor. (Takes from 20 minutes to 2 hours.)

e. All AABB standards for donation apply to apheresis donors also. However, frequency of donation and additional testing are different for the three types of apheresis:

1) Plateletpheresis: platelet count of 150,000 per μL, 48 hrs between donations

2) Leukapheresis: not more than twice a week, 24 times/year.

3) Plasmapheresis: every 8 weeks, total protein, IgG, and IgM monitored every 4 weeks.

8. **Therapeutic Phlebotomy**
   a. One unit of blood is removed from a patient in a specified time interval. This is done to treat patient symptoms in polycythemia, hemochromatosis, and porphyria.

XII. BLOOD COMPONENTS: PREPARATION, STORAGE, AND SHIPMENT

A. Definitions
1. **Whole blood:** blood collected from donors: contains all cellular and liquid elements.
2. **Components:** parts of blood used for treating patients: red blood cells (RBCs), plasma, platelets, and cryoprecipitated antihemophiliac factor
3. **Hemotherapy:** using blood or blood components to treat a disease in a patient

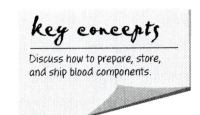

key concepts

Discuss how to prepare, store, and ship blood components.

B. Blood Collection Bag
1. A closed system. Contains needle, tubing, and up to 4 smaller bags attached to it. The entire system is sterile.
2. Standard bag = 450 mL +/− 45 mL.

C. Anticoagulant Preservative Solutions
1. **Standard volume: 63 mL**
2. If an autologous unit is drawn on a patient weighing less than 110 pounds, the anticoagulant must be reduced:

   a. Reduce Volume Factor (A) = weight of patient/110 lbs.
      A × 70 mL = amount of anticoagulant needed (B)
      70 − B = amount of coagulant to remove
      A × 500 mL = amount of blood to collect

   b. Example: 90 lb. donor.
      90 lbs./110 lbs. = 0.81 = A
      0.81 × 70 ml = 56.7 ml = B
      70 mls − 56.7 mL = 13 mL of anticoagulant to be removed from bag
      0.81 × 500 mL = 405 mL of blood to be collected

3. **Types of Anticoagulants and Preservatives**
   a. CPD: citrate-phosphate-dextrose
   b. CP2D: citrate-phosphate-2-dextrose
   c. CPDA-1: citrate-phosphate dextrose adenine-1
   d. Dextrose: sugar to support RBC life
   e. Adenine: used in ATP synthesis
   f. Citrate: chelates calcium to prevent coagulation
   g. Sodium biphosphate: buffer to prevent decreased pH

4. **Storage**
   a. Shelf life: the amount of storage blood can take that yields at least 75 percent of original RBCs still in recipient's circulation 24 hours after transfusion. Remember, blood is still "alive" when it's in a blood bag.

    b. Glucose, ATP, 2,3-DPG, and pH decrease as RBCs are stored. After cells are transfused, ATP, and 2,3-DPG levels are restored in about 24 hours.

    c. Substances that increase during storage are all metabolic end products such as potassium, hydrogen ions, etc.

5. **Additive Solutions**

    a. AS-1 contains mannitol.

    b. AS-3 contains citrate and phosphate.

    c. AS-5 contains mannitol.

    d. These must be added within 72 hours of collection.

    e. Usually added to RBCs after plasma is separated off.

    f. Extends shelf life to 42 days and reduces RBC viscosity during transfusion.

6. **Rejuvenation Solution**

    a. Contains pyruvate, inosine, phosphate, and adenine.

    b. Purpose is to restore 2,3 DPG and ATP levels before freezing or transfusing a unit.

    c. May be necessary for autologous or rare units.

    d. RBCs can be rejuvenated up to 3 days past the expiration date and can then be frozen for future use.

    e. RBCs can be rejuvenated and transfused up to 24 hours if stored at 1–6°C. The cells must be washed before transfusion to remove the inositol.

7. **Blood component preparation**

    a. Whole blood is centrifuged and can be separated into red blood cells (RBCs), platelets, fresh frozen plasma (FFP), and cryoprecipitated antihemophiliac factor.

    b. Process: whole blood bag is centrifuged; plasma separated off into platelet pack.

    c. AS-1 is put into RBC bag (if additive solution is used).

    d. RBC bag sealed and removed from system.

    e. Plasma bag centrifuged to sediment platelets.

    f. Plasma separated into FFP bag leaving platelets with a very small amount of plasma in platelet bag.

    g. Platelet bag sealed off and cut.

    h. Plasma is either frozen to make FFP or frozen and thawed to make cryoprecipitate.

8. **Storage Temperature and Expiration Dates for Components**

    a. **Whole blood:** storage: 1–6°C, expires: with CPD, CP2D anticoagulants in 21 days, with CPDA-1 anticoagulant in 35 days; with Adsol (AS-1, AS-3, or AS-5) in 42 days

    b. **RBCs:** storage: 1–6°C, expires: with CPD, CP2D anticoagulants in 21 days, with CPDA-1 in 35 days, with AS-1, AS-2, and AS-3 in 42 days

    c. **Platelets:** storage 20–24°C, expires: 5 days

    d. **FFP:** storage ≤ − 18°C, expires: 1 year; storage: −65°C, expires: 7 years

    e. **Cryoprecipitate:** storage ≤ 18°C, expires: 1 year

    f. **RBCs (frozen):** storage: ≤ −65°C, expires: 10 years

    g. **RBCs** (deglycerolized, washed): storage: 1–6°C, expires in 24 hours after thawing (deglycerization).

    h. **RBCs irradiated:** storage: 1–6°C, expires in 28 days or on originally assigned outdate—whichever comes first

    i. **Platelets (pooled):** storage 20–24°C, expires in 4 hours after pooling

    j. **Cryoprecipitate (pooled):** storage: 20–24°C, expires in 4 hours

    k. **FFP (thawed):** storage: 1–6°C, expires in 24 hours

    l. **Platelet pheresis:** storage: 20–24°C, expires in 5 days

    m. **Granulocyte pheresis:** storage: 20–24°C, expires in 24 hours

D. Storage and Transportation

1. FDA requirements and AABB standards define calibration and maintenance procedures, storage temperature limits, and monitoring parameters for equipment used to store blood products.

2. **All refrigerators, freezers, and platelet incubators must have**

    a. Recording devices that monitor the temperature at least every 4 hours

    b. Audible alarms that ensure response 24 hours a day

    c. Regular alarm checks

    d. Power failure and alarm activation emergency procedures

    e. Emergency power backups (continuous power source for alarms)

    f. Calibrated thermometers that are checked against referenced thermometers

    g. Written procedures for all of the above

3. **Transportation**

    a. Maintain temperature of 1–10°C for RBCs. Ice in plastic bags and placed on top of the units can maintain the temperature for 24 hours.

    b. RBCs are packed in cardboard boxes with a Styrofoam box inside. The ice is double-bagged and weighs approximately 9 pounds.

    c. Frozen components are shipped on dry ice. These should be well wrapped because dry ice evaporates and room in the box for movement should be allowed.

    d. Platelets are shipped at room temperature. Platelets can survive without agitation for a maximum of 24 hours.

    e. When component shipments are received, observe and record the temperature and appearance of units. If temperature is out of range, units must be evaluated before transfusion. Institutions have policies for who will determine the disposition of the units. All problems and dispositions must be documented and stored with blood bank records.

E. Administration of Blood Components

1. Positive identification of patient, sample, and crossmatched unit.

2. Only normal saline should be infused with blood components.

3. A standard 170 micron filter must be used with all blood components. Leukoreduction filters are used to reduce the number of leukocytes transfused with RBCs.

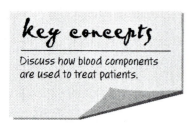

4. One blood unit transfusion should be completed within 2 hours—4 hours is the maximum transfusion time. If not, the unit should be divided and transfused as 2 units.

5. Documentation and accurate record keeping are important.

XIII. BLOOD COMPONENT THERAPY

A. Whole Blood

1. Used in actively bleeding patients, patients who have lost at least 25 percent of their blood volume, or patients requiring exchange transfusions.

2. When whole blood is not available, reconstituted whole blood (RBCs mixed with thawed type AB FFP from a different donor).

B. RBCs

1. Used in oncology patients undergoing chemotherapy or radiation therapy, trauma patients, surgery patients, dialysis patients, premature infants, and patients with sickle cell anemia.

2. Transfusing 1 unit usually increases the patient's hemoglobin approximately 1 g/dL and the hematocrit by 3 percent.

3. RBCs must be crossmatched before transfusion.

C. Leukocyte-Reduced RBCs

1. Used in chronically transfused patients.

2. The standard 170 micron filter does not remove leukocytes. A special filter is required.

3. AABB: 85% of RBCs remain and less than 5×10^6 WBCs.

D. Frozen RBCs

1. Method: RBCs are frozen by adding glycerol to prevent cell hydration and the formation of ice crystals that can cause cell lysis (40% weight per volume).

2. Unit transferred to a polyolefin or polyvinyl chloride bag, then the bag is placed in a metal or cardboard canister.

3. Initial freezing temp is −80°C, then for long-term storage at −65°C for 10 years.

E. Deglycerolized RBCs

1. Frozen RBCs are thawed, then the glycerol must be removed.

2. Deglycerolization: glycerol is drawn out of the RBCs by washing the RBCs with a series of saline solutions of decreasing osmolality.

3. Deglycerolization involves entering the bag, so the deglycerolized RBCs expire in 24 hours.

F. Washed RBCs

1. Used for patients who have a reaction to plasma proteins (reactions allergic, febrile, and anaphylactic).

2. Also used in infant or intrauterine transfusions.

3. Normal saline is used in a deglycerolizing machine. 10–20 percent of RBCs are lost in this process.

G. Irradiated RBCs

1. T-cells can cause graft vs. host disease with 90 percent of cases being fatal.

2. Gamma irradiation prevents T-cell proliferation.

3. AABB standards require irradiation of cellular components (RBCs and platelets) if a donor is a relative of intended recipient or donor unit is HLA matched for recipient.

4. Used for intrauterine transfusions, immunodeficient recipient, premature infants, chemotherapy and radiation patients, and bone marrow or progenitor cells transplant patients.

H. Platelets

1. Purpose: used to control or prevent bleeding.
2. Not indicated in patients with ITP (idiopathic thrombocytopenia).
3. Indicated in patients with chemotherapy, post–bone marrow transplant patients, or patients experiencing postoperative bleeding.
4. Transfused platelets life span: 3–4 days.
5. No crossmatch necessary, but ABO type specific preferred.

6. **Platelet Concentrates**
   a. Prepared from whole blood unit.
   b. Contain approximately 5.5×10^{10} platelets/unit.
   c. Raise platelet count by 5000 μL/unit after transfusion.

7. **Pooled Platelets**
   a. Procedure is to choose 1 platelet bag and empty content of other bags into it.
   b. Usual platelet order is 6–10 units.
   c. Opening the unit reduces the shelf life of the bag to 24 hours. Platelets should be pooled immediately before transfusion.

8. **Platelet Pheresis**
   a. HLA-matched patients that receive numerous platelet transfusions can develop antibodies to the class I HLA antigens on platelets. These patients require HLA matching before transfusion. If platelets to be transfused are not HLA matched, the platelets will not last for 5 days in the patient's circulation.
   b. Platelet pheresis packs contain 3×10^{11} platelets per unit.

9. **Leukocyte-Reduced Platelets**
   a. Filters can reduce the number of leukocytes in a bag while being transfused.
   b. Specific apheresis instruments can reduce leukocyte numbers during collection.

I. Fresh-Frozen Plasma

1. **Purpose:** to replace coagulation factors in the patient
2. Indicated in
   a. Bleeding patients who require Factors II, V, VII, X, and IX
   b. Abnormal coagulation due to massive transfusion
   c. Patients on anticoagulants who are bleeding or require surgery
   d. Treatment of TTP and hemolytic uremic syndrome
   e. Prevent or correct bleeding in patients with liver disease
   f. Antithrombin III deficiencies
   g. DIC when fibrinogen is > 100 mg/dL
3. **Thawing**
   a. Thawed at 30–37°C for 30–45 minutes before transfusion.

b. Unit should be placed in watertight container before immersing in water bath to keep ports clean and prevent contamination.

c. Water baths with agitators are preferred because the unit thaws faster.

d. FDA-approved microwaves can also be used.

4. **Solvent-Detergent-Treated Plasma**

a. Pooled plasma and solvent-detergent to lower virus transmission.

b. Indications, thawing, and expiration date after thawing are the same as for FFP.

J. Cryoprecipitated Antihemophilic Factor (Cryoprecipitate)

1. Insoluble precipitate formed when FFP is thawed between 1–6°C. Contains most coagulation factors present in FFP.

2. Used for patients with Factor XIII deficiency, fibrinogen deficiency, and as a fibrin sealant.

3. Must have at least 150 mg/dL of fibrinogen and 80 IU of Factor VIII per unit.

4. **Pooled Cryoprecipitate**

a. Like platelets, cryoprecipitate is pooled into 1 bag before transfusion.

b. Units are thawed in a similar fashion to FFP before pooling.

c. Must be given within 4 hours after pooling.

d. Formula for figuring Factor VIII in cryoprecitate:

$$\# \text{ of units } = \frac{\text{plasma volume} \times (\text{desired level } \% - \text{initial level } \%)}{80 \text{ IU / bag}}$$

e. Fibrin glue from cryoprecipitate: 1–2 units of cryoprecipitate are mixed with thrombin and applied topically to the bleeding area.

f. **Granulocyte Pheresis**

1) Granulocyte transfusions are rare and limited to septic infants.

2) The pheresis bag contains granulocytes, $> 1.0 \times 10^{10}$, platelets, and 20–50 mLs of RBCs.

3) The cells deteriorate rapidly and must be transfused within 24 hours of collection.

4) Store at 20–24°C with no agitation until transfused.

5) Crossmatching is required due to RBC contamination.

g. **Labeling**

1) Must conform with the 1985 Uniform Labeling Guideline issued by the FDA and Title 21 of the Code of Federal Regulations (CFR).

2) Current labeling requirements include proper name, unique number, amount of blood collected, amount and type of anticoagulant, volume of component, expiration date, storage temperature, ABO/D type, reference to the Circular of Information, warning regarding infectious agents, prescription requirements, donor classification, and FDA license number if applicable.

3) Other products must be labeled as follows:
   a) Irradiated components must have name of the facility performing the irradiation.
   b) Pooled components must include final volume, unique number assigned to the pool, and name of facility preparing the pooled component.
   c) Autologous units must be labeled: "For Autologous Use Only."
4) Circular of Information: guidelines that provide a description of each component, indications and contradictions for use, and information of dosage, administration, storage, side effects, and hazards.

XIV. TRANSFUSION THERAPY

A. Emergency Transfusions

1. Rapid loss of blood can result in hemorrhagic shock.
   a. Symptoms: hypotension, tachycardia, pallor, cyanosis, cold clammy skin, oliguria, decreased hematocrit, decreased central venous pressure (CVP), CNS depression, and metabolic shock.
2. **Priorities in Acute Blood Loss**
   a. Replace and maintain blood volume.
   b. Make sure oxygen carrying capacity is adequate.
   c. Maintain coagulation system integrity—especially platelets and coagulation factors.
   d. Correct metabolic imbalances.
   e. Maintain colloid osmotic pressure.
3. **Massive transfusion:** replacement of a person's entire blood volume (approximately 10 units) within 24 hours.
4. **Emergency transfusions** result from trauma (gunshot wounds, stabbings, auto accidents, etc.) or surgery.
5. **Emergency release of blood:** it is preferable to transfuse type specific blood. If time is not available to type the patient, type O, D negative blood is transfused into women of childbearing age. Type O, D positive is transfused into men. Doctor must request emergency release indicating no crossmatch is performed before the blood is transfused. The crossmatch is performed during or following the transfusion.
6. **Emergency transfusions may** also be necessary during cardiac bypass surgery when the patient is on the heart-lung machine. Coagulation factors can be used up, and too much heparin may be administered.

B. Neonatal and Pediatric Transfusions

1. **Smaller blood volume than adults.**
2. Premature infants may need transfusion to offset the effect of hemoglobin F in their system. Hemoglobin F does not give up oxygen readily.
3. **Iatrogenic blood loss** (blood taken from the neonate or infant for laboratory tests) causes the neonate or infant to develop an anemia that may be severe enough to transfuse.

key concepts

Discuss how blood transfusions can lead to transfusion reactions, the different types of transfusion reactions and how the laboratory investigates a transfusion reaction.

4. Neonates and infants do not tolerate hypothermia well, so blood warmers are used.

5. Washed or fresh blood is preferred for neonates or infants due to the liver's inability to metabolize citrate and potassium.

6. Transfusions given in small volumes in multiple packs taken from a normal size blood unit.

7. Infants don't form antibodies for the first four months, so no cross-match necessary.

8. **Transfuse CMV-negative blood and use a leukoreduction filter.**

C. Transplantation

1. **Liver transplant patients** require large amounts of blood products (approximately 20 units of RBCs, 25 units of FFP, 17 units of platelets, and 5 units of cryoprecipitate) because the liver produces many coagulation factors, and cholesterol for RBC membranes.

2. **ABO compatibility important in kidney, liver, and heart transplants.** Not important in bone, heart valves, skin, and cornea transplants.

3. **Progenitor Cell Transplants**
   a. Allogenic or autologous.
   b. Derived from bone marrow or umbilical cord blood.
   c. Transfusion support with leukocyte reduced products to prevent alloimmunization and a greater chance of rejection.
   d. Conditions treated: severe combined immunodeficiency disease, Wiskott-Aldrich syndrome, aplastic anemia, Fanconi's anemia, thalassemia, sickle cell disease, acute leukemia, CML, lymphoma, myelodysplastic/myeloproliferative disorders, multiple myeloma, neuroblastoma, breast cancer, ovarian cancer, and testicular cancer.

D. Therapeutic Hemapheresis

1. Removal of blood from a patient to improve a patient's health.

2. Conditions indicated in therapeutic phlebotomies: multiple myeloma, Waldenström's macroglobulinemia, hyperleukocytosis, thrombocytopenia, TTP/HUS, sickle cell, myasthenia gravis, acute Guillain-Barré syndrome

E. Oncology

1. Chemotherapy drugs kill all cells that are undergoing mitosis: stem cells, gastrointestinal epithelial cells, and hair follicles.

2. Action of chemotherapy drugs:
   a. Stopping DNA replication
   b. Interfering with mRNA production

F. Chronic Renal Disease

1. Dialysis patients have an increased uremic (Blood urea nitrogen-BUN) content in blood that alters the RBC shape and causes the cells to be removed from circulation from the spleen.

2. Dialysis itself mechanically destroys RBCs.

3. Nonfunctioning kidneys do not produce erythropoietin to stimulate RBC production.

4. The use of transfusions in dialysis patients has been dramatically reduced since erythropoietin therapy was initiated.

G. Sickle Cell Anemia

1. An abnormal hemoglobin causes cells to be removed from circulation, resulting in a lowered hematocrit.

2. Cells develop sharp pointed ends that cut vessels and organs as they pass through, causing bleeding.

3. Because these patients require many transfusions, phenotypically matched units are preferred.

4. Severe cases may be treated by bone marrow transplants.

H. Thalessemia

1. Caused by decreased synthesis of the α- and β-protein chains.

2. Hemolytic anemia results.

3. Support necessary.

I. Aplastic Anemia

1. Blood transfusion support is usually needed until bone marrow transplant can occur.

XV. TRANSFUSION REACTIONS

A. Types of Transfusion Reactions

1. Transfusion reactions are an adverse physiological reaction to the infusion of blood.

    a. **Hemolytic:** a reaction that destroys the transfused blood cells in vivo. Large amounts of free hemoglobin are released into the blood and can cause systemic damage.

    b. **Nonhemolytic:** febrile and allergic.

2. **Acute reactions** occur rapidly, within hours of transfusion.

3. **Delayed reactions** occur days or weeks after transfusion.

4. **Immune-mediated transfusion reactions** are due to RBC or HLA antigens and antigen-antibody reactions.

5. **Transfusion reactions** can also be caused by bacteria, viruses, or parasitic organisms.

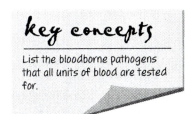

key concepts

List the bloodborne pathogens that all units of blood are tested for.

B. Hemolytic Transfusion Reactions

1. **Clinical presentation:** fever, irreversible shock, hypotension, DIC, and renal failure.

2. **Mechanism**

    a. Antibody binding to RBCs:

        1) Intravascular reaction: IgM antibodies activate the classical pathway of complement which lyses RBCs intravascularly. The lysis releases hemoglobin and RBC remnants into the blood. The excess hemoglobin binds to haptoglobin. Haptoglobin can only bind so much hemoglobin, so the excess hemoglobin is found in the blood and urine.

        2) Extravascular reaction: antibody-coated RBCs are removed from circulation by the liver and spleen. The cells lyse when

sequestered and subsequently release bilirubin into the blood. Antibodies responsible for this type of hemolysis do not activate the complement cascade or only partially activate it.

b. Anaphylatoxins: cause hypotension by triggering serotonin and histamine release.

c. Cytokine activation: sensitized RBCs are cleared from the blood by phagocytes. The phagocytes release cytokines that cause fever, hypotension, and activation of T- and B-cells.

d. Coagulation activation: antigen-antibody-complement complexes activate the clotting system and cause DIC.

e. Renal failure is caused by systemic hypotension, reactive renal vasoconstriction, and intravascular thrombi.

C. Acute and Delayed Hemolytic Transfusion Reactions

1. **Acute Hemolytic Transfusion Reactions**
   a. **Clinical signs/symptoms:** severe, rapid onset, fever, chills, flushing, pain at site of infusion, tachycardia, hemoglobinemia, hemoglobinuria, hypotension.
   b. **Major sequelae:** DIC, renal failure, irreversible shock, death.
   c. **Causes:** antigen-antibody reaction activates complement or coats RBCs, ABO incompatible blood, antibodies to Vel or PP_1P^k antigens.
   d. **Occurrence:** 1:25,000 transfusions, identification error in patient and specimen.
   e. **Diagnostic laboratory tests:** elevated plasma free hemoglobin, elevated bilirubin (6 hours posttransfusion,), decreased haptoglobin, and positive or negative DAT.

2. **Delayed Hemolytic Transfusion Reactions**
   a. **Delayed hemolytic transfusion reactions** are usually less severe than acute hemolytic transfusion reactions and are dependent on the concentration of antibody in the blood rather than the type of antibody.
   b. **Clinical signs:** 5–7 days posttransfusion, fever, mild jaundice.
   c. **Major sequelae:** none.
   d. **Causes:** alloantibodies to Rh, Duffy, and Kidd antigens; patient with low concentration of alloantibody causes anamnestic response when reexposed to RBC antigen.
   e. **Occurrence:** 1:2,500 transfusions.
   f. **Diagnostic laboratory tests:** positive DAT, positive posttransfusion antibody screen, decreased hemoglobin and hematocrit.

D. Causes of Nonimmune Mediated Mechanisms of RBC Destruction

1. Transfusion of hemolyzed units.
2. Malfunctioning or unregulated blood warming units.
3. Improper thawing and deglycerolization of a frozen RBC unit.
4. Physical destruction by needles, valves, or equipment.
5. RBC defects.

E. Immune-Mediated Nonhemolytic Transfusion Reaction

1. **Clinical Signs**
   a. Fever-temperature increase 1°C over baseline temperature 8–24 hours posttransfusion.
   b. Nausea, vomiting, headache, and back pain.
2. **Causes:** HLA antibody to donor antigens and cytokines in blood products containing WBCS and platelets.
3. **Occurrence**
   a. Common in patients with multiple pregnancies and transfusions
   b. Multiple exposures to HLA antigens
   c. Common in women
   d. 1:200 donor units transfused

F. Allergic Transfusion Reactions

1. **Urticarial Reactions**
   a. Clinical signs: wheals, hives, itching
   b. Sequelae: none
   c. Causes: antibodies to foreign proteins
   d. Occurs in 1–3 percent of recipients
2. **Anaphylactic Reactions**
   a. Clinical signs: rapid onset, severe wheezing and cough, and bronchospasms
   b. Sequelae: syncope, shock, death
   c. Causes: genetic IgA deficiency
   d. Occurs very rarely

G. Transfusion-Associated Graft versus Host Disease

1. Clinical signs: 3–30 days posttransfusion, fever, erythematous maculopapular rash, abnormal liver function.
2. Sequelae: sepsis, hemorrhage, 90 percent mortality rate.
3. Cause: transfused T-cells react against recipients.
4. Occurs rarely.

H. Bacterial Contamination of Blood Products

1. Bacterial contamination usually occurs during phlebotomy or during thawing of frozen blood components.
2. Bacteria (*Yersinia enterocolitica*—most common) live and multiply in bag in storage.
3. Bacterial endotoxins can be present in the unit of blood and cause symptoms similar to hemolytic transfusion reactions.
4. 2 percent of units are contaminated.
5. Workup blood cultures drawn from patient and gram stain and culture of the unit.
6. Person issuing unit needs to check for discoloration, clots, cloudiness, or hemolysis.

I. Circulatory Overload

1. Too much blood in a patient's vascular system caused by transfusing a unit too fast—especially in children and elderly patients.
2. Symptoms: dyspnea, severe headache, peripheral edema, and signs of congestive heart failure occurring after transfusion. Can be fatal.

J. Other Complications

1. **Hemosiderosis** occurs in chronically transfused patients—especially those with hemolytic anemias.
2. **Citrate overload:** massive transfusions introduce large amounts of citrate into the body. Citrate binds ionized calcium, but can be negated by calcium chloride or calcium gluconate injections.

K. Suspected Transfusion Reaction Workups

1. Transfusionist checks and rechecks all paperwork requisition and blood bag tag before beginning the transfusion to ensure there were no clerical errors made.
2. Vital signs (blood pressure, temperature, respiration, and pulse) are taken before beginning and every 15 minutes until the transfusion is completed.
3. If a reaction is suspected:
   a. Stop the transfusion.
   b. Notify the physician and the laboratory.
   c. Physician evaluates the patient.
   d. Draw EDTA, red top tubes, and first voided urine collected and send to laboratory according to institutional policy.
4. **Laboratory Responsibilities**
   a. Check all samples, requisition, histories, and bags for identical patient identification. Clerical errors are responsible for most transfusion reactions.
   b. Spin down tubes and check for hemolysis.
   c. Perform DAT.
   d. Additional tests performed should be in accordance with institutional policy. Repeat ABO and D on pretransfusion patient sample, posttransfusion patient sample, segments from the bag; repeat antibody screen and crossmatch on old and new patient samples. Other tests include hemoglobin, hematocrit, haptoglobin, urine hemoglobin, and bilirubin.

L. Transfusion Reaction Workup Records

1. In blood bank indefinitely.
2. Bacterial contamination and transmitted diseases are reported to blood collection facility.
3. Fatalities are reported to FDA's Office of Compliance, Center for Biologics Evaluation and Research, within 24 hours.

XVI. TRANSFUSION-TRANSMITTED DISEASES

A. Donor Infectious Disease Testing (Test and Date Started Testing)

1. HBsAg (before 1980)
2. HBcAb (1986)
3. HCV antibody (1990)
4. ALT (1986)
5. Anti-HIV 1/2 (HIV-1: 1985; HIV-2: 1992)
6. HIV-1 p24 ag (1996)
7. Anti-HTLV-I/II (1997)
8. Syphilis (RPR)

key concepts

Discuss the federal regulations guiding blood banks, know the record keeping practices in blood banks, and the safety guidelines that are adhered to in blood banks.

9. CMV: optional, usually done on blood earmarked for premature infants, intrauterine transfusion, and compromised recipients

10. Chagas' disease (optional, done only in endemic areas)

B. Look-Back Studies

1. FDA requires notification of patients that received untested units (that subsequently tested positive for HIV-1/2 or HIV p24 ag, or anti-HCV)
   a. Identify all donors positive for HCV since March 1992.
   b. Identify all blood products provided by donors.
   c. Notify facility.
   d. Trace to patients and notify patients of potential exposure.

XVII. SAFETY AND QUALITY CONTROL

A. FDA Regulations

1. Good Manufacturing Processes
   a. Write standard operating procedures.
   b. Follow standard operating procedures.
   c. Record and document all work.
   d. Qualify personnel by training and education.
   e. Design and build proper facilities and equipment.
   f. Clean by following a housekeeping schedule.
   g. Validate equipment, personnel, processes, etc.
   h. Perform preventive maintenance on facilities and equipment.
   i. Control for quality.
   j. Audit for compliance with all of the above.

B. Records

1. **Good Recordkeeping**
   a. Use permanent ink on documents.
   b. Record data on proper form.
   c. **NO white out**—cross out mistake and have person making correction date and initial it.
   d. **No ditto marks used.**
   e. **Record "broken, closed, or not in use" when appropriate**

2. Retention **(Indefinite)**
   a. Donor's identification information, medical history, physical exam, consent, and interpretations for disease markers.
   b. Blood and components from outside source, including numeric or alphanumeric identification on old unit and identification of the collecting facility. However, the information from an intermediate facility may be used if the intermediate facility retains the unit number and identification number of the collecting facility.
   c. Identification of facilities that carry out any part of the preparations of blood components, and the functions they perform.
   d. Final disposition of each unit of blood or blood component.
   e. Notification to donors of permanent deferral.
   f. Records of prospective donors who have been placed on surveillance or indefinitely deferred for the protection of the potential recipient.

key concepts

Discuss the role of blood usage review in inventory management and accreditation.

      g. Notification to transfusing facilities of previous receipt of units from donors subsequently found to be confirmed positive for HIV and human T-cell lymphotropic virus type 1 (HTLV).

      h. Difficulty in blood typing, clinically significant antibodies, and adverse reactions to transfusions.

      i. Notification to recipients of potential exposure to disease transmissible by blood.

      j. Names, signatures, initials, or identification codes and inclusive dates of employment of those authorized to sign or review reports and records.

3. Retention (**Minimum of 5 Years**)

      a. Donor's ABO, D, difficulty in blood typing, severe adverse reactions to donation, and apheresis procedure clinical record.

      b. Records of blood component inspection before issue.

      c. Patient's ABO and D type, interpretation of compatibility testing, therapeutic procedures including phlebotomy, apheresis, and transfusion.

      d. All superseded procedures, manuals, and publications.

      e. Control testing of components, reagents, and equipment.

      f. Proficiency testing surveys, including dates, performed tests, observed results, interpretations, identification of personnel carrying out the tests, and any appropriate corrective actions taken.

      g. Documentation of staff qualifications, training, and competency testing.

      h. Quality systems audits and internal assessment records.

C. Document Control

1. Must be complete, organized, appropriately stored, retrievable, and secure.

D. Personnel Qualifications

1. Job descriptions written with specific job duties are required.
2. Selection criteria for an employee must be developed.
3. Training: provided during new employee orientation and whenever procedures change or the employee performs poorly.
4. Competency assessment means evaluating the skill on a level of knowledge of an employee. Accomplished through observing performance, written tests, review of results, records, or worksheets, or testing unknown samples (i.e., proficiency).

E. Supplier Qualifications

1. Evaluates products and services received from a supplier to see if established criteria are met.

F. Validation

1. Validation ensures products or services will meet established criteria for a high degree of quality assurance.
2. All blood bank information systems must be validated before "being put into use."

G. Federal, State, and Local Safety Regulations

1. FDA
   a. **Biologics Control Act of 1902**
      1) Licensing of manufacturers and products
      2) Labeling
      3) Facility inspections
      4) Suspension or revoking license
      5) Penalties for violation
   b. Implemented under Public Health Services Act 42, USC section 262

2. Occupational Safety and Health Administration
   a. **Occupational Safety and Health Act**
      1) Ensures a safe and healthful workplace
      2) Act enforced by Occupational Safety and Health Administration.
   b. Employers must inform employees about OSHA regulations and post OSHA literature that informs employees about their right to know.
   c. Updates to OSHA are published annually in the CFR.

3. Centers for Disease Control (CDC)
   a. **CDC introduced universal precautions in 1987 to decrease risks of bloodborne pathogen exposure.**
   b. **In 1991, OSHA published the final standard on bloodborne pathogens. This regulations requires**
      1) Hazard-free workplace
      2) Provision of education and training to staff
      3) Evaluation of potential risks
      4) Evaluation positions for potential risks
      5) Post signs and use labels
      6) Implement universal precautions for handling biohazardous substances
      7) Provide personal protective equipment (PPE)—gloves, fluid resistant lab coats, splash shields, at no cost to the employee
      8) Provide free hepatitis B vaccine to at-risk staff
      9) Provide free hepatitis B immunoglobulin for any exposures to employee

XVIII. BLOOD USAGE REVIEW

A. **Peer review**—mandated by Joint Commission on Accreditation of Healthcare Organizations (JCAHO) Standards (for accreditation), CFR (for Medicare reimbursement), most states (for Medicaid reimbursement), CAP (for accreditation), and AABB (for accreditation)

1. **JCAHO requires the medical staff to review blood usage quarterly for:**
   a. Appropriateness of transfusions for blood and blood products
   b. Evaluation of transfusion reactions
   c. Development and implementation of policies and procedures for blood product distribution, handling, use, and administration

    d. Adequacy of transfusion services to meet the needs of patients

    e. Blood product ordering practices

2. **Hospital transfusion practice is usually monitored by the Hospital Transfusion Committee. This committee reviews:**

    a. Statistical data (retrospectively), i.e., data collected over a specified period of time

    b. Physician ordering patterns (retrospectively): data collected over a specified period of time

    c. Concurrent review

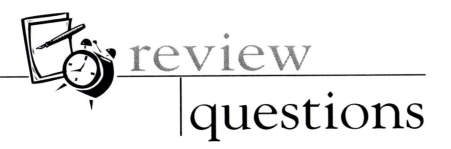
review questions

DIRECTIONS Each of the questions or incomplete statements below is followed by suggested answers or completions. Select the **one answer** that is best in each case.

1. A newborn baby has a positive direct antiglobulin test. The mother's type is O positive and the baby's type is A positive. What test would you do next?
   a. Indirect antiglobulin test
   b. Adsorption
   c. Lui Freeze-Thaw elution
   d. Digitonin elution

2. Blood components include all of the following EXCEPT:
   a. red blood cells
   b. whole blood
   c. fresh frozen plasma
   d. platelets

3. D is an _____ antibody, reacts best at _____, and is known to cause _____.
   a. IgM, 4°C, nocturnal hemoglobinuria
   b. IgM, 22°C, idiopathic thrombocytic purpura
   c. IgG, 37°C, Waldenstrom's macroglobulinemia
   d. IgG, AHG, hemolytic disease of the newborn (HDN)

4. If a father is type AO and the mother is type BO, what is the probability that they will have a type O child?
   a. 10%
   b. 25%
   c. 50%
   d. 75%

5. Anti-H will agglutinate what cells the strongest?
   a. O cells
   b. B cells
   c. A cells
   d. I cells

6. According to AABB standards, a laboratory must retest the rH of what units?
   a. Rh negative
   b. Rh positive
   c. Bombay
   d. Multiple myeloma

7. A person who visits a malaria-endemic country must wait how long before donating blood?
   a. 5 years
   b. 10 years
   c. 2 years
   d. 1 year

8. All the following are signs of a transfusion reaction EXCEPT:
   a. body temperature of recipient increases more than 2°C
   b. hives and itching
   c. pain at the infusion site
   d. tingling in fingers and toes

9. In order to prevent graft-vs-host disease with transfusions, units are irradiated. This irradiation
   a. inactivates T-cells that cause graft-vs-host disease

b. inactivates B-cells that cause graft-vs-host disease

c. inactivates macrophages that cause graft-vs-host disease

d. kills polymorphonuclear cells

10. This antibody is produced in people with pneumonia caused by *Mycoplamsa pneumonia.*
    a. anti-D
    b. anti-I
    c. anti-H
    d. anti-M

11. Give the ABO type for the following reactions, explain the cause of any discrepancy.

Anti-A	Anti-B	Anti-A$_1$	A$_1$ Cell	B cell
4+	neg	neg	neg	4+
neg	4+		4+	neg
4+	4+		3+	3+
4+	neg		1+	3+
4+	1+		neg	4+
neg	neg		neg	neg

12. Which of the following groups of antigens would always be considered as clinically significant?
    a. Le^a, MN, P$_1$, Lu^a, Lu^b
    b. D, E, Fy^a, S, A, B, K
    c. Bg, York, Rg^a, Ch^a
    d. None of the above

13. The following reactions were present for a cold panel:

Screening Cell 1	Screening Cell 2	Auto-control	Cord Cells	Type Specific Cells
3+	3+	3+	1+	2+

What antibody is most likely causing these reactions?
    a. anti-H
    b. anti-IH
    c. anti-I
    d. anti-i

14. You have a patient with an antibody identified as anti-E. This patient's cells are E positive. What type of antibody is this?
    a. alloantibody
    b. warm antibody
    c. cold antibody
    d. autoantibody

15. On the same patient as above (anti-E present, cells are E positive), you need to crossmatch 4 units of blood. You screen 4 units of blood for E, but the crossmatches of all four units are incompatible. Why?
    a. The anti-E is reacting with the donor cells.
    b. The patient is actually a Bombay person.
    c. There may be an alloantibody present.
    d. There may be a cold antibody present.

16. A cord blood types as A positive, and it has a positive direct antiglobulin test. What test would you do next?
    a. Lui freeze-thaw elution
    b. cross match
    c. phenotype
    d. indirect antiglobulin test

17. Antibody titers are used to
    a. determine if there is an antibody present in a person's serum.
    b. predict the severity of HDN.
    c. screen a unit for a particular antigen.
    d. determine if a crossmatch is necessary.

18. Donors who have been treated for malaria are deferred for
    a. 12 months
    b. 3 years
    c. forever
    d. 2 weeks

19. Once frozen, red blood cells are good for
    a. 10 years at −65°C
    b. 5 years at 2–8°C
    c. 20 years at −20°C
    d. 6 months at −10°C

20. Special blood collection methods include all of the following EXCEPT:
    a. therapeutic phlebotomy
    b. intraoperative collection
    c. hemapheresis
    d. directed donations

contents

➤ COMPREHENSIVE KEY CONCEPTS

1. List normal and pathogenic flora by body site and discuss isolation procedures, including media selection, incubation time/temperature requirements, and identifying colony morphological characteristics.

2. List key biochemical reactions of the different bacterial classes, discuss reagents, reactions, and color indicators (positive versus negative) of biochemical tests, and list positive and negative control organisms for each of the biochemical tests.

3. Summarize groups of bacteria according to Gram stain, cellular morphology, growth and media requirements, biochemical identifying characteristics, and pathology.

4. Discuss antibiotic susceptibility testing, resistance/susceptibility patterns of bacteria, classes of antibiotics, modes of action, and specific antibiotics used against specific bacteria or bacterial classes.

5. Develop flowcharts that will aid in bacterial identification.

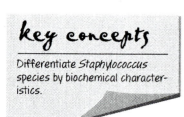

key concepts

Differentiate *Staphylococcus* species by biochemical characteristics.

I. GRAM POSITIVE COCCI (*MICROCOCCACEAE*)

A. *Staphylococcus aureus*

1. Isolated from abscesses, wound infections, and carbuncles. 30 percent of the population carries *S. aureus* as resident flora in the nose and skin.

2. Causes food poisoning (enterotoxin), pneumonia, osteomyelitis, endocarditis, and staphylococcus scalded skin syndrome.

3. Produces 6 types of enterotoxin, including toxic shock syndrome toxin (TSST-1).

4. **Identifying Characteristics**

   a. Gram positive cocci arranged in **clusters,** colonies are opaque, golden, and smooth. Grows well on most media. Beta hemolytic or BAP (blood agar plate)

   b. Penicillin resistance is due to **beta-lactamase** production.

   c. **Catalase,** and **coagulase positive**

   d. **Voges-Proskauer (V-P) positive,** and negative for L-pyrroglutamyl-aminopeptidase (PYR) and ornithine

   e. **MRSA** (methicillin resistant *S. aureus*) is resistant to most β-lactam antibiotics. Vancomycin susceptible.

   f. Facultative anaerobic.

   g. *Staphylococci* can tolerate the salt concentration of **mannitol salt agar (MSA).**

      1) *S. aureus* ferment mannitol and produce yellow colonies.

      2) Coagulase-negative *Staphylococci* do not ferment mannitol and produce red colonies.

h. **Thermonuclease test** is positive.

i. **Latex agglutination** (positive) detects protein A on surface of *S. aureus* bacteria.

B. Coagulase-Negative *Staphylococci*

1. Are very common skin bacteria, and are mostly nonpathogenic. Can cause disease in the immunosuppressed and neutropenic patients. Urinary tract infections (UTIs) and infections in catheters/shunts can be caused by this group of bacteria.

2. Gram positive cocci arranged in clusters, catalase positive, and **coagulase negative.**

3. **Colonies** appear white to gray on blood agar, nonhemolytic.

4. Species

a. *Staphylococcus epidermidis* (most common species of coagulase negative *Staphylococci*)—novobiocin susceptible

b. *Staphylococcus saprophyticus* (significant only in UTIs)—novobiocin resistant

C. *Micrococcus* species

1. Nonpathogens that may cause rare infections. Considered normal isolates of the skin and mucus membranes.

2. Arranged in tetrads and appear larger than other *Staphylococcus* species on Gram stain.

3. **Colonies** appear lemon to yellow on blood agar.

	Micrococci	Staphylococci
Acid production from glucose under anaerobic conditions	O	+
Modified oxidase test	+	O
Bacitracin (0.04 μ taxo A disk)	S	R

II. GRAM POSITIVE COCCI (*STREPTOCOCCACEAE*)

A. General Characteristics

1. **Catalase negative,** Gram positive cocci arranged in pairs and **chains.**

2. Partial ID is based on 5 percent sheep's blood agar **hemolysis,** which can be beta, alpha, or gamma.

3. **Lancefeld grouping** is based on type of cell wall antigen.

4. Diseases include pneumonia, meningitis, pharyngitis, rheumatic fever, endocarditis, and UTIs.

B. Group A *Streptococcus* (*S. pyogenes*)

1. Infections are spread by respiratory secretions, always pathogenic, and some children may carry in the respiratory tract without illness.

2. Diseases caused include **strep throat,** pharyngitis, cellulitis, **Scarlet fever,** pneumonia, otitis media, rheumatic fever, and post–*Streptococcal* glomerulonephritis.

3. Susceptible to **bacitracin (A disk),** resistant to **trimethoprim-sulfamethoxazole (SXT disk),** and diagnosed by serological latex agglutination kits.

4. **Colonies** are pinpoint (< 1mm), translucent, and will show a large zone of β **hemolysis.**

key concepts

Compare the differences in Gram-stain morphology, colonial morphology, and biochemical characteristics (catalase, etc.) of *Staphylococcus* and *Streptococcus*.

key concepts

Discuss *Streptococcus* species according to pathology, hemolytic activity, and biochemical/serological testing.

5. Some virulence factors include
   a. Erythrogenic toxin: produces the rash in Scarlet fever.
   b. Streptokinase: dissolves clots.
   c. Hyaluronic acid capsules: inhibits phagocytosis.
   d. Streptolysin O and streptolysin S: lyse erythrocytes, platelets, and neutrophils.
   e. Pyrogenic exotoxins: produce fever, respiratory distress, renal failure, and tissue necrosis.
   f. Cell Wall M: prevents phagocytosis.
   g. M Antigen and pyrogenic exotoxins: activate T-cells and systemic immunomodulators, which can produce shock and death.

C. Group B *Streptococcus (S. agalacticae)*
1. Normal flora of the GI tract of humans and animals.
2. **CAMP** and **hippurate** positive.
3. **Resistant to bacitracin and SXT.**
4. Important in **OB/GYN** patients, where 25 percent of all females will carry the bacteria as normal vaginal flora.
5. Can cause neonatal sepsis obtained during birth, neonatal meningitis, postpartum fever, osteomyelitis, and wound infections. May also cause endocarditis, pneumonia, and pyelonephritis in the immunosuppressed.
6. **Colonies** are large (> 1mm), flat, creamy, and show small zones of **β-hemolysis.** Some strains may be nonhemolytic.

D. Group D *Streptococcus*
1. *Enterococcus* **is now a genus.**
2. Alpha-hemolytic to **nonhemolytic,** and sometimes β-hemolytic; normal fecal and oral flora.
3. Diseases caused include wound infections, UTIs, and abdominal abscesses.
4. **Colonies** are gray to white, translucent, round, and convex.
5. *E. faecalis* **and** *E. faecium*
   a. Positive for **6.5 percent NaCl**
   b. Penicillin resistant
   c. **Bile-esculin** positive
   d. **PYR** positive
   e. Increasing resistance to antibiotics (especially vancomycin)
6. **Group D** *Streptococcus*, **non-Enterococcus (*S. bovis*)**
   a. Negative for **6.5% NaCl**
   b. Pencillin susceptible
   c. **Bile-esculin** positive
   d. Has been linked to colon cancer.

E. *Viridans streptococcus*
1. **α-hemolytic,** can be anaerobic or microaerophilic.
2. Normal flora of the oral, respiratory tract, and GI mucosa.
3. Major cause of bacterial endocarditis in people with damaged heart valves, also causes wound infections, and brain abscesses.
4. May enter the blood after **dental** procedures.

5. Some *Viridans streptococcus* species include ***Streptococcus mutans, S. salivarius, S. sanguis, S. mitis***.

F. *Streptococcus pneumoniae*

1. Gram positive **diplococci** that are lancet or bullet shaped, and **α-hemolytic.**
2. Normal respiratory flora but can cause:
   a. Lobar pneumonia in the elderly and alcoholics.
   b. Otitis media in infants and children.
   c. Meningitis, however, a vaccination protocol is now available that has reduced the number of new childhood meningitis cases.
   d. Community-acquired bacterial pneumonia.
3. Grows on 5 percent sheep's blood agar with 5–10 percent CO_2, at 48 hours, the central part of the colony collapses to become **concave.**
4. **Colony**
   a. **Mucoid:** produced by large amounts of capsule.
   b. **Umbilicated:** depressed centers caused by autolytic enzymes.
   c. *Note:* Colonies after 48 hours become nonviable and cannot be subcultured.
5. **Optochin (P disks)** will inhibit growth and is **bile** (10% sodium deoxycholate) soluble.
6. **Quellung reaction** swells the capsule.

III. GRAM NEGATIVE COCCI (*NEISSERIACEAE*)

A. *Neisseriaceae* Family Characteristics

1. **Oxidase positive,** normal flora of the respiratory, stomach, and urogenital systems.
2. Kidney bean-shaped, Gram negative diplococci that often appear intracellularly in neutrophils.
3. Very fastidious, grows best at 5–10 percent CO_2 at 37°C, cannot tolerate cold, therefore must bring media to room temperature before plating. Very sensitive to drying.
4. Members of the *Neisseriaceae* family include *Neisseria, Acinetobacter, Kingella,* and *Moraxella.*

B. *Neisseria gonorrhoeae*

1. Can isolate from the following sources: urethra, cervix, vagina, anal canal, oropharynx, skin lesions, joints, and blood.
   a. **Males:** causes acute urethritis which is characterized by a pus-containing urethral discharge and dysuria. Can also cause prostatitis and epididymitis.
   b. **Females:** causes cervicitis and urethral infections. Can be asymptomatic or can cause vaginal discharge, fever, acute pain, and dysuria. Can also cause pelvic inflammatory disease, gonococcal arthritis, salpingitis, endometritis, and peritonitis.
2. Neonates may be infected during vaginal delivery, resulting in **gonococcal ophthalmia neonatorum** which is a severe conjunctivitis leading to blindness. To prevent newborn conjunctivitis, antibiotic eye drops are administered (replaced silver nitrate drops).
3. *N. gonorrhoeae* is not normal flora of the body.

key concepts

State specimen sources, growth requirements, and biochemical characteristics of each *Neisseria* species.

4. Identifying biochemical tests.
   a. Catalase, oxidase, and CTA glucose—positive.
   b. CTA Maltose, DNAse, and nitrate—negative.
5. Some strains are positive for β-lactamase production.
6. Collection and culture: must culture immediately, clinical material must be free of lubricants, spermicides, and douches. **Does not grow on blood** agar, but will grow on chocolate or other selective agars. The bacteria require increased CO_2 with a humidified atmosphere.
   a. *N. gonorrhoeae* are fastidious bacteria requiring enriched medias such as chocolate, Thayer-Martin, and Martin-Lewis, New York City, or GC-Lect agar.
   b. Due to autolysis, gonococci cannot be incubated for prolonged times.
7. **Colonies** are flat, smooth, glistening gray to white.

C. *Neisseria meningitidis*

1. Causes meningococcal meningitis, and meningococcemia leading to DIC, and Waterhouse-Friderichsen syndrome.
2. Spread by respiratory droplets, and may be normal flora of the nasopharynx
3. **Will grow on blood** agar.
4. Identifying biochemical characteristics
   a. **Oxidase,** CTA glucose, CTA maltose, and catalase positive
   b. DNAse negative and **nitrate negative**
5. Specimens: CSF, sputum, blood, and nasopharyngeal swabs.
6. **Colonies** are flat, smooth, and gray to white on chocolate agar.

D. Normal Flora *Neisseria* Species

1. Many species of *Neisseria* are normal flora of the upper respiratory tract and urogenital tract.
2. Most are not fastidious and will grow on most nutrient agars.
3. In rare cases these organisms can cause meningitis, endocarditis, and other infections.
4. Species include *N. elongata, N. mucosa, N. lactamica, N. cinerea, N. polysaccharea, N. flavescens, N. subflava,* and *N. sicca.*

E. *Moraxella catarrhalis*

1. Resembles *Neisseria,* and is normal flora of the upper respiratory tract.
2. Causes otitis media, sinusitis, and respiratory tract infections.
3. Biochemical characteristics:
   a. **Oxidase,** DNase, **nitrate,** and butyrate esterase **positive.**
   b. Asaccharolytic: all carbohydrate tests are negative.
4. Old names include *N. catarrhalis* and *Branhamella catarrhalis.*
5. Will grow on most nutrient agars.

IV. GRAM NEGATIVE BACILLI (ENTEROBACTERIACEAE)
A. General Family Characteristics

1. Most medically important family of Gram negative bacilli, most are facultative anaerobes and several species show bipolar staining.
2. Major cause of nosocomial infections

3. Most are normal GI flora. (**Salmonella and Shigella are not normal GI flora.**)

4. **All enterics are glucose positive, oxidase negative, and nitrate positive.**

5. Diseases can include UTIs, gastroenteritis, septicemia, food poisoning, wound infections, peritonitis, pneumonia, and meningitis.

6. The family shows four types of serological characteristics:
   a. **O/somatic Ag** is the cell wall antigen (heat stable).
   b. **K/envelope Ag** is the capsular antigen (heat labile).
   c. **H/flagellar Ag** is the flagellar antigen (heat labile).
   d. **Vi Ag** is the capsular antigen in *S. typhi* (heat labile).

7. **Types of Enteric Media**
   a. **MacConkey** (MAC): **lactose positive** colonies are pink/red, and **lactose negative** colonies are colorless.
   b. **Bismuth sulfite agar:** *Salmonella typhi* produces black colonies; *Escherichia coli* is yellow orange.
   c. **Brilliant green agar:** *Proteus* is red/pink, *Salmonella* is red/pink, and *Shigella* will not grow on brilliant green agar.
   d. **Hektoen Enteric Agar** (HE): *E. coli* colonies are yellow/orange. *Salmonella* is blue with black centers (H_2S positive), and *Shigella* colonies are green.
   e. ***Salmonella-Shigella* Agar** (SS): *E. coli* is red, *Proteus* is colorless with black centers, *Salmonella* is colorless with black centers, and *Shigella* is colorless.
   f. **Selenite broth:** enhancement media for stool cultures, *Salmonella* growth is enhanced, whereas Gram positive and coliform (normal GI flora) bacteria are inhibited.
   g. **XLD** (xylose-lysine-deoxycholate): *E. coli* is yellow, *Proteus* is clear/yellow, *Salmonella* is red with black centers, and *Shigella* is clear.
   h. **EMB** (eosin-methylene blue): *E. coli* has a dark center and usually shows a green metallic sheen, lactose fermenters have a dark center, and lactose nonfermenters are colorless.

8. **Summary of Tests Used for Enteric Identification**
   a. **Triple sugar iron agar (TSI)** will show the pattern of glucose, lactose, and sucrose fermentation, in addition to showing H_2S production.
      1) Different TSI color combinations:
         a) Yellow (Acid) deep = glucose positive
         b) Yellow slant (acid) = lactose or sucrose positive
         c) Black deep = production of H_2S gas.
         d) Alk slant/alk deep (K/K) (red in color) = non-fermenters: not *Enterobacteriaccea*.
         e) Alk slant/acid deep (K/A) (red/yellow) = nonlactose fermenters (glucose positive).
   b. **IMViC** (indole, methyl red, Voges-Proskauer, and citrate)
      1) **Indole:** positive bacteria produce tryptophanase for the breakdown of tryptophane to pyruvic acid, ammonia, and indole.

key concepts

Describe the different enteric agars used to culture enterics and their characteristic morphology and color changes.

key concepts

List the key biochemical reaction (lactose, IMViC, etc.) of Enterobacteriaceae.

2) **Methyl red** indicates glucose fermentation. Yellow is positive, red is negative.

3) **Voges-Proskauer** shows the digestion of glucose to acetyl methylcarbinol. Red is positive, yellow is negative.

4) **Citrate** indicates when citrate is used as the sole carbon source. Blue is positive, green is negative.

c. **Deaminase reactions:** detects the ability of an organism to remove the amino group from specific amino acids.

d. **Decarboxylation reactions:** detects the ability of bacteria to remove the carboxyl group from a specific amino acid.

e. **ONPG reactions** (o-nitrophenyl-β-D-galactopyranoside): detects the presence of β-galactosidasee, an enzyme that also cleaves lactose.

f. **H_2S/:** detects enzymes that liberate sulfur from the sulfur-containing media to form H_2S. H_2S reacts with iron salt in the media to form a black precipitate composed of ferrous sulfide.

g. **Motility agar:** determines motility; indicated by growth area from the stab.

h. **Gelatin hydrolysis:** liquifaction along the growth line is a positive test.

i. **Nitrate reductase:** determines the ability of an organism to reduce nitrate to nitrite. After the addition of reagents, a pink result is positive, a colorless reaction requires the addition of zinc dust to confirm. Pink after zinc indicates a true negative. Colorless after zinc indicates a positive nitrate reductase test as nitrate was reduced to nitrite and completely reduced to nitrogen gas.

B. Genera

1. *Escherichia coli*

a. Normal gastrointestinal flora, and are very common isolates.

b. Diseases caused: UTIs, appendicitis, peritonitis, gallbladder infections, endocarditis, meningitis in newborns, gastroenteritis, and food poisoning.

c. **Identifying Characteristics**

1) **TSI:** acid slant/acid deep (late lactose fermenting *E. coli* can be K/A).

2) H_2S: negative.

3) **MacConkey:** pink/red colonies; **blood:** colonies are shiny, opaque, cream colored (2–4mm) and usually β-hemolytic.

4) **EMB:** green metallic sheen colonies with dark centers.

5) Indole, methyl red, Motility, ONPG: positive.

6) VP, citrate, urease: negative.

7) Ferments most sugars.

d. **Four Serotypes of *E. coli***

1) **Enterotoxigenic *E. coli:*** produces severe epidemic diarrhea, mainly from drinking contaminated water.

2) **Enteroinvasive *E. coli:*** causes a bloody stool by invading intestinal epithelium, also known as a shigella-like diarrhea.

3) **Enteropathogenic *E. coli:*** causes a watery diarrhea.

key concepts

List the enteric species that must be identified in stool cultures.

    4) **Enterohemorrhagic** *E. coli:* causes food poisoning ("fast-food poisoning").

e. **E. coli O157:H7** causes hemorrhagic colitis and hemolytic uremic syndrome, leading to kidney failure in young children.

    1) Acquired by eating undercooked hamburger or other contaminated foods such as apple cider, basil, sprouts, etc.

    2) Grow on **Sorbitol-MacConkey (SMAC):** agar where sorbitol replaces lactose in the medium. E. coli O157:H7 does not metabolize sorbitol, most other *E. coli* species use sorbitol. E. coli: O157:H7 colonies appear colorless on SMAC.

2. **Shigella**

  a. Causes shigellosis, which is bacterial dysentery, characterized by abdominal pain, fever, and diarrhea.

  b. Most severe in children and the elderly. Outbreaks are known to occur in day care centers and nursing homes.

  c. Very pathogenic, less than 50 bacteria can cause disease.

  d. Causes food poisoning by direct fecal contamination from infected humans.

  e. Incubation period is between 1 to 7 days.

  f. Not considered normal flora of humans.

  g. **Four Serogroups** (Based on O Antigens)

    1) *Shigella dysenteriae (A)* produces an enterotoxin, which affects the large intestines and a neurotoxin that may result in paralysis or death. *S. dysenteriae* is mannitol and ONPG negative.

    2) *Shigella flexneri (B)* produces a mild diarrhea. Mannitol positive and ONPG negative.

    3) *Shigella boydi (C)* produces a mild diarrhea. Mannitol positive and ONPG negative.

    4) *Shigella sonnei (D)* produces a mild diarrhea. Is the most common form of Shigella infection in the United States, and is mannitol and ONPG positive.

  h. **Identifying Characteristics**

    1) TSI: alk slant/acid deep (K/A).

    2) H$_2$S, VP, motility, citrate, urease, and lactose negative.

    3) Methyl red positive

3. **Klebsiella**

  a. Causes UTIs and pneumonia. Many infections are nosocomial, and diabetics and alcoholics are prone to *Klebsiella* infections.

  b. Most *Klebsiella* isolates are *Klebsiella pneumoniae*.

  c. Produces jellylike thick sputum.

  d. **Identifying Characteristics**

    1) TSI: acid slant/acid deep with gas (a/a with gas).

    2) **MacConkey** agar, colonies are **very mucoid** and pink in color.

    3) Capsulated, resistant to many antibiotics.

    4) H$_2$S, methyl red, motility, negative. Indole negative. (*K. oxytoca* is indole positive.)

    5) VP, citrate and lactose positive

4. **Enterobacter**
   a. The genus includes 12 species.
   b. Found in the soil, water, and dairy products.
   c. *Enterobacter cloacae* is the most common *Enterobacter* isolate.
   d. *Enterobacter aerogenes* is the second most common isolate.
   e. **Identifying Characteristics**
      1) TSI: acid slant/acid deep with gas (a/a with gas).
      2) H_2S, methyl red, and indole negative.
      3) VP, citrate, motility positive. Lactose positive **except** *Enterobacter taylorae.*
      4) *Enterobacter aerogenes* is arginine/lysine positive, and *E. cloacae* is arginine positive and lysine negative.

5. **Serratia**
   a. Resistant to many antibiotics.
   b. *Serratia marcescens* cause most *Serratia* infections and are very pathogenic.
   c. Causes opportunistic infections in chemotherapy and immuno-suppressed patients.
   d. **Identifying Characteristics**
      1) TSI: alk slant, acid deep (K/A).
      2) **DNAse and lipase positive** (unique in the enterics). VP and citrate positive.
      3) **H_2S and lactose, negative.**
      4) Some strain form red colonies on agar due to pigment production.

6. **Salmonella**
   a. The genus contains over 2200 serotypes; most are pathogenic to humans and animals.
   b. Serotype classification is based on the Kauffman-White system (*see* IV.A.6).
   c. Causes moderate to severe gastroenteritis.
   d. Transmitted through contaminated water and undercooked food, especially chicken.
   e. *Salmonella typhi* causes typhoid fever.
   f. Most infections are caused by *Salmonella* Subgroup I, which includes *Salmonella typhi* and *Salmonella paratyphi.*
   g. Suspect *Salmonella* infections from stool cultures showing lactose negative and H_2S positive colonies.
   h. **Identifying Characteristics**
      1) TSI: alk slant/black deep (some are acid slant/black deep.
      2) H_2S, motility, citrate, and methyl red, positive.
      3) Indole, urease, and lactose negative.
      4) **Hektoen enteric** (HE) agar: green with black centers.

7. *Proteus*
   a. *Proteus vulgaris* and *Proteus mirabilis* are the most common isolates.
   b. **Identifying Characteristics**
      1) TSI: alk slant/acid deep with gas (K/A with gas)
      2) H_2S positive.

    3) **Swarming motility** on enteric and blood agar.

    4) **Rapid urease positive.**

    5) Methyl red positive.

    6) Lactose negative.

    7) *P. mirabilis* is indole negative; *P. vulgaris* is indole positive.

    8) **IMViC**

       a) *Proteus mirabilis:* (**negative-positive-variable-variable**)

       b) Proteus vulgaris: (**positive-positive-negative-variable**)

  8. *Yersinia*

    a. Small coccobacilli

    b. Nonmotile at 37°C but motile at 25°C

    c. 3 pathogenic species of Yersinia:

      1) *Yersinia pestis:* causes the plague, endemic in the southwestern United States, infects neutrophils and macrophages.

      2) *Yersinia enterocolitica:* causes enterocolitis in humans, acquired by drinking contaminated water or by eating contaminated meat. Lactase negative, sucrose positive. Therefore, colorless on MAC, but A/A on TSI.

      3) *Yersinia pseudotuberculosis:* rare lymphadenitis in children.

  9. *Edwardsiella*

    a. *E. tarda* is the most common isolate.

    b. TSI = K/H$_2$S

    c. Indole positive, methyl red positive, citrate negative

  10. **Citrobacter.**

    a. *Citrobacter freundii* is the most common species.

    b. TSI = A/H$_2$S

    c. *C. freundii* resembles *E. coli* on MAC but can be differentiated due to H$_2$S(+) and indole (−)

    d. PAD positive—phenylalanine deaminase (PAD)

  11. *Morganella*

    a. *Morganella morganii* is the only species.

    b. **IMViC (positive-positive-negative-negative).**

    c. PAD positive

  12. *Providencia*

    a. **IMViC (positive-positive-negative-positive)**

V. HAEMOPHILUS

A. General Characteristics

1. Pleomorphic Gram negative coccobacilli ranging from very small to filamentous.

2. Nonmotile, **oxidase** and **catalase positive.**

3. Grows at 35–37°C with 5–10 percent CO$_2$, and is prone to drying and temperature changes.

4. Most species are normal respiratory flora.

5. Growth requirements include **hemin (X factor)** (blood loving) that is released from hemoglobin and/or **NAD (V factor),** which is a heat-labile compound produced by certain bacteria and yeast.

6. **Isolation:** *Haemophilus* species do not grow on **sheep's blood agar** due to NADase in the agar (NADase breaks down NAD) but will

grow on **horse/rabbit blood agar,** which contains no NADase. Chocolate agar is used for cultures. Another way of culturing *Haemophilus* is the **Staphylococcus streak method** where a single streak of *S. aureus* is streaked down a blood agar plate. *S. aureus* releases NAD. Therefore *Haemophilus* will grow near the *S. aureus* streak, forming tiny clear pinpoint colonies. This phenomenon is known as **satellitism.**

7. **Colony:** smooth, round, flat, opaque, and grayish on blood agar, produces a musty odor.

8. Three pathogenic species include:

   a. *Haemophilus influenze* "Pfeiffer's Bacillus"
      1) Includes 6 serotypes A-F, serotype B, and 8 biotypes. Biotype I causes most infections.
      2) Major historic cause of meningitis in children (***H. influenzae* type b).** Recently developed **Hib** vaccine has greatly reduced childhood meningitis.
      3) Frequent cause of respiratory infections, acute sinusitis, chronic bronchitis, and pneumonia.
      4) Must test all *H. influenza* isolates for beta-lactamase.
      5) Specimen collection: includes blood, sputum, CSF, and eye swabs.
      6) Specific antigen detection of Hib capsular antigen is by latex agglutination.

   b. *Haemophilus aegypticus* "Koch-Weeks Bacillus"
      1) Causes pink eye, very contagious conjunctivitis.
      2) Similar to *H. influenzae* with the exception of being **sucrose positive.**
      3) Recently classified as *H. influenzae* biogroup aegyptius.

   c. *Haemophilus ducreyi*
      1) Causes genital ulcers, transmitted sexually.
      2) Produces chancroids and buboes (swollen lymph nodes).
      3) Chocolate with vancomycin is used to inhibit contaminants.
      4) **Colony:** dome shaped and gray in color.
      5) Cell arrangement from chancroid specimens show railroad track patterns.

   d. **Haemophilus Identification Chart**

	X Factor	V Factor	β-hemolysis (rabbit blood)	ALA[*]
H. influenzae	+	+	−	−
H. ducreyi	+	−	−	−
H. aegyptius	+	+	−	−

[*]*aminolevulinic acid (ALA) is converted to hemin*

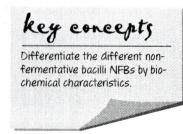

key concepts

Differentiate the different non-fermentative bacilli NFBs by biochemical characteristics.

VI. NONFERMENTATIVE GRAM NEGATIVE BACILLI/COCCOBACILLI (NFB)

A. General Characteristics

1. Found in water, soil, food, plants, and a few are normal flora of humans.

2. 20 percent of all Gram negative bacilli isolates are NFBs.

3. Do not form spores, and do not break down carbohydrates under anaerobic conditions.
4. Most species are strict aerobes.
5. General identification tests for NFB:
   a. Most are **oxidase positive.**
   b. TSI: alkaline/no change.
   c. Grows on 5 percent sheep's blood agar but varied growth on MAC.

B. *Pseudomonas aeruginosa*

1. Common clinical isolate, can infect humans, animals, plants, and fish.
2. Important pathogen in the compromised host.
3. Causes **burn wound** infections.
4. Respiratory tract infections in **cystic fibrosis** patients.
5. Causes eye (contact lens wearers) and ear infections, and is responsible for "swimmer's ear" which is an external otitis.
6. Very resistant to antibiotics, responsible for serious nosocomial infections, and is especially associated with vents, operating room equipment, whirlpools, and swimming pools.
7. **Identifying characteristics**
   a. Strict aerobe
   b. **Oxidase positive**
   c. Motile
   d. Lactose negative
   e. **Colony:** produces large, irregular mucoid colonies with a grapelike odor, and will show a metallic sheen on blood agar.
   f. **Blue/green pigment** (pyocyanin is a pigment only produced by *P. aeruginosa*) on Mueller-Hinton agar.
   g. **β-hemolytic** colonies on blood agar with a feathery edge.
   h. O-F glucose: oxidative
      1) **OF glucose test:** determines if glucose is broken down by oxidative or fermentative means. 2 tubes are used, 1 tube is closed which contains mineral oil added to the top to produce anaerobic conditions. The other tube is the open tube (aerobic) containing no mineral oil. **Oxidative positive:** open tube is yellow; closed tube is green. **Fermentative positive:** both tubes turn yellow.

C. *Stenotrophomonas maltophilia* (formerly *Pseudomonas* and *Xanthomonas*)

1. Acquired as transient flora from hospitals.
2. Causes pneumonia, UTIs, wound infections.
3. **Identifying characteristics:**
   a. Oxidase negative
   b. The only "*Pseudomonas*" that is oxidase negative, and maltose positive
   c. Resistant to most antibiotics, but is susceptible to septramethazole.

D. *Burkholderia* (formerly *Pseudomonas*) cepacia

1. **B. cepacia** causes nosocomial infections. Also important pathogen in cystic fibrosis patients.
2. Enhanced growth on *P. cepacia* (PC) agar that inhibits *P. aeruginosa*.
3. Colony: colorless or yellow on nutrient agar with a dirt odor.
4. Oxidase and lactose positive.

E. *Acinetobacter*

key concepts

Discuss the similarities and differences between *Acinetobacter* and Enterobacteriaceae.

1. Is a coccobacillusi, and is normal flora of the GI and respiratory tract.
2. Causes nosocomal infections and UTIs.
3. Looks like *Neisseria* in vaginal/cervical cultures (*Neisseria* is oxidase positive, *Acinetobacter* is **oxidase negative.**)
4. Grows on most media and may resemble enterics on MAC/EMB agar.
5. Contains 17 species.
6. **Identifying characteristics:**
   a. Nonmotile, oxidase negative.
   b. Type of hemolysis depends on species type.
   c. Resistant to penicillin,
   d. Nitrate negative, and catalase positive

F. *Eikenella corrodens*

1. Causes tooth extraction infections, human bite wound infection.
2. Normal flora of the mouth and upper respiratory tract.
3. "**Corroding bacterium**" causes pits to form on the surface of agar.
4. Requires hemin (factor X) to grow.
5. Produces a bleachlike odor.

VII. MISCELLANEOUS GRAM NEGATIVE BACILLI

A. *Francisella spp*

key concepts

Name the specialized agars used to grow *Legionella*, *Francisella tularensis*, and *Brucella*, and discuss the symptoms of the diseases they cause.

1. **Francisella tularensis** causes tularemia and is a potential agent of bioterrorism.
2. The bacteria are carried by animals in the wild, including deer, rabbits, beavers, and squirrels.
3. Humans may acquire the infection by skinning animals, animal bites, eating uncooked game, or the bite of deerflies or ticks.
4. Intracellular bacteria that resist phagocytosis.
5. **Biosafety level 3** required when handling the organism of suspect specimens.
6. Tularemia causes skin ulcers at the site of inoculation and can cause infections of the lymph nodes, eyes, lungs, and GI system.
7. **Identification**
   a. Faintly staining coccobacilli.
   b. Media of choice is **glucose-cystine blood agar.**
   c. **Colony:** small and grayish.
   d. Agglutination tests and DFA are used in identification.
   e. Strict aerobe.

B. *Brucella spp.*
1. Causes **brucellosis,** also known as **undulent fever.**
2. Is a **type 3 biohazard.**
3. Normal gastrointestinal flora of animals.
4. Usually acquire the infection by drinking contaminated milk or slaughterhouse exposure.
5. An intracellular parasite.
6. **Identification**
   a. Isolated from joint fluid, blood, and bone marrow.
   b. Grows on **Brucella, buffered charcoal-yeast extract (BCYE),** and **modified Thayer-Martin;** requires 10 percent CO_2 in humidified air, and 3–4 weeks to grow.
   c. Serology is used for presumptive identification, must culture for definitive identification.
   d. Oxidase and catalase positive.
   e. Four species that infect humans include *B. melitenis, B. abortus, B. suis,* and *B. canis*
   f. Strict aerobe.

C. *Bordetella spp.*
1. *Bordetella pertussis* causes whooping cough.
2. Inhabits the mucus membranes of the respiratory tract.
3. Infections are increasing due to the lack of immunization.
4. Grows on **Bordet-Gengou, Jones Kendrick charcoal agar,** and **Regan Lowe** agar (charcoal-horse blood agar).
5. Whooping cough (pertussis), occurs in 3 stages:
   a. Catarrhal: general flu-like symptoms
   b. Paroxysmal: repetitive coughing episodes
   c. Convalescent: recovery phase
6. Other species include:
   a. *B. parapertussis:* causes mild respiratory infections.
   b. *B. bronchiseptica:* causes wound and respiratory infections.
7. **Identification**
   a. Colonies are small and smooth, appear like **mercury droplets,** and are β hemolytic.
   b. Gram stain shows minute, poorly stained coccobacilli, single or in pairs.
   c. Most species will grow on MacConkey agar except *B. pertussis.*
   d. *B. pertussis* **is urease negative,** whereas all other species are urease positive.

D. *Actinobacillus spp.*
1. Is mostly oral flora of animals. *Actinobacillus actinomycetemcomitans* is normal oral flora of humans.
2. Infections are caused by animal bites, which can result in cellulitis. *A. actinomycetemcomitans* is associated with endocarditis and also causes gum disease.
3. Grows well on blood and chocolate agar but will not grow on MacConkey agar; produces colonies that show **starlike centers.**
4. Most species are catalase and glucose positive.

E. *Pasteurella spp.*

1. Is normal respiratory/GI flora of animals. Humans acquire the bacteria by animal bites (dogs and cats) or by dried animal fecal inhalation.
2. Causes cellulitis but can progress into osteomyelitis, meningitis, joint infections, and pneumonia.
3. *Pasteurella multocida* causes most human infections.
4. **Identifying Characteristics**
   a. Grows well on most agars.
   b. **Colonies** produce a brown color with a "mushroom smell."
   c. Oxidase, catalase, indole, and nitrate positive.
   d. Very susceptible to penicillin.
   e. Nonmotile, pleomorphic, Gram negative coccobacilli that may show bipolar staining.

F. *Legionella spp.*

1. First discovered in 1976 as the cause of pneumonia in people attending an American Legion convention in Philadelphia.
2. Aquatic organisms that may be found in various water systems including humidifiers, whirlpools, and air conditioning ducts. *Legionella* bacteria are resistant to commonly used concentrations of chlorine.
3. Most human disease is caused by *Legionella pneumophilia* serogroup.
4. Causes **Legionellosis** which can be asymptomatic, or mild to severe pneumonia. **Legionnaire's disease** is the severe form of legionellosis. **Pontiac fever** is the mild form, causing flulike symptoms.
5. **Identifying Characteristics**
   a. Gram stain: thin, poorly staining Gram negative bacilli.
   b. Grows on **buffered charcoal yeast extract agar (BCYE),** but does not grow on blood agar; produces tiny colonies on chocolate agar.
   c. **Most biochemical tests are negative,** but *Legionella* is weakly positive for catalase and oxidase.
   d. Other identifying tests: DFA, urine antigen test, and nucleic acid probs.

G. *Chromobacterium spp.*

1. *Chromobacterium violaceum* is found in water and soil.
2. Produces a purple or violet pigment on nutrient agar.
3. Causes wound infections acquired from contaminated soil or water.
4. Produces hydrogen cyanide gas.

key concepts

Summarize growth requirements, biochemical reactions, habitat, and pathology of *Vibrio* and related bacteria.

VIII. VIBRIO AND RELATED SPECIES: CURVED GRAM NEGATIVE BACILLI

A. General Characteristics of Vibrio and Related Curved Gram Negative Bacilli

1. **Oxidase and indole positive.**
2. Some species cause GI disease.

B. *Vibrio spp.*

1. The genus contains 12 species that are inhabitants of salt water.
2. All species are **halophilic** (salt loving) **except** *V. cholerae* and *V. mimicas.*
3. Grows on **thiosulfate citrate bile agar (TCBS)** and enriched blood agar (must add alkaline peptone water), but will not grow on Mac-Conkey agar.
4. Most labs use serology based on somatic O antigens to identify these bacteria.
5. *Vibrio cholerae*
   a. Causes cholera
   b. **0-1 Vibrio** serological type causes cholera, **non-0-1** type does not cause cholera.
   c. *V. cholerae* 01 is subdivided into three serotypes: **Inaba, Ogawa,** and **Hikojima.** *V. cholerae* 01 has two biotypes: **classical** and **El Tor.**
   d. Cholera infections are acquired during travel to endemic areas, including Africa and South America.
   e. Cholera is caused by an enterotoxin that alters ion transport of intestinal mucosa, resulting in a massive release of water and fluids.
   f. Produces **rice water stools.**
   g. In addition to causing cholera, *V. cholerae* can also cause bacteremia, wound infections, and otitis media.
6. *Vibrio parahaemolyticus*
   a. Causes a mild to moderate choleralike diarrhea disease.
   b. Acquired by eating raw shellfish, especially from the Chesapeake Bay region of the Eastern United States.
7. *Vibrio vulnificus*
   a. Is very virulent, causing septicemia and wound infections.
   b. Causes a very quickly progressive wound infection after exposure.
8. *Vibrio alginolyticus*
   a. Causes otitis media, bacteremia, and wound infections.

C. *Aeromonas spp.*

1. Found in fresh and salt water.
2. Infects humans and fish.
3. Causes cellulitis and diarrhea.
4. Species include *A. hydrophilia, A. caviae,* and *A. veronii biovar sobria.*
5. Is a self-limiting infection not usually requiring treatment; however, wound infections may require antibiotic therapy.

D. *Plesiomonas shigelloides*

1. Acquired by eating raw shellfish.
2. Causes gastroenteritis, meningitis, and wound infections.
3. Is a self-limiting infection. Treatment is only required in the immunosuppressed patient or other severe cases.

E. *Campylobacter spp.*

1. Major cause of food poisoning. Causes gastroenteritis, diarrhea, and septic arthritis. Part of many routine stool culture workups
2. Acquire infection by eating un- or undercooked contaminated poultry or other meat products.
3. *C. jejuni* causes most infections.
4. **Identifying Characteristics**
   a. Microaerophilic and **capnophilic.**
   b. **Curved bacilli** that may appear S-shaped or spiral on Gram stain.
   c. **Catalase and oxidase positive.**
   d. Nonfermentative.
   e. Grows on *Campylobacter agar* at **42–43°C,** but will grow very slowly at 37°C.
   f. On wet mount will show **darting** motility.
   g. Resistant to cephalothin, but sensitive to nalidixic acid.

F. *Helicobacter pylori*

1. Causes **peptic** and **duodenal ulcers.**
2. Oxidase, rapid urease, and catalase positive.
3. Although difficult to culture, the organism can be isolated from gastric biopsy on blood agar, *Brucella,* Skirrow's, and modified Thayer-Martin agar. Incubated in increased CO_2.

IX. SPIROCHETES

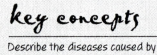

key concepts

Describe the diseases caused by spirochetes and their serological identification characteristics.

A. Three genera cause human disease. *Treponema* (slender with tight coils), *Leptospira* (hooked ends), and *Borrelia* (thicker with few coils).

1. Most spirochetes are obligate intracellular parasites.
2. Spirochetes are long, slender, helically curved bacilli that cannot be shown on Gram stain.
3. Special stains such as silver and Giemsa will stain spirochetes (silver for all spirochetes, and Giemsa only for *Borrelia*).
4. Spirochetes can be observed by dark-field or phase-contrast microscopy.

B. *Treponema pallidum*

1. Causes **venereal syphilis,** which cannot be cultured in the laboratory; must use tissue culture to grow.
2. Diagnosed by serology **VDRL** (venereal disease research lab), dark-field microscopy (corkscrew motility), or **RPR** (rapid plasma reagin).
   a. Nontreponemal tests include the VDRL and RPR, which detect lipid antibodies and are not specific due to biological false-positives caused by Lyme disease, various viruses, autoimmune disorders, and pregnancy.
   b. Treponemal tests include fluorescent treponemal antibody absorption (FTA-ABS) test and microhemagglutination assays for *T. pallidum* (MHA-TP), which are specific and confirmatory.
3. Transmitted by sexual contact, direct blood transmission, or transplacental (congenital syphilis).

4. 4 stages of syphilis:
   a. Primary: skin chancre at the site of inoculation
   b. Secondary: skin rash
   c. Latent: absence of clinical symptoms
   d. Late: CNS disorders (neurosyphilis), skin, liver, and bone disorders
5. Other species include *T. pertenue* (yaws) and *T. oralis* (nonpathogenic oral flora, but may cause Vincent's gingivitis).

C. *Borrelia spp*

1. *Borrelia recurrentis*
   a. Causes **relapsing fever,** which is characterized by recurrent high fever, muscle pain, and confusion.
   b. Carried by body lice.
   c. Is very difficult to culture but can be grown on BSK-II or Kelly's media.
   d. Serological tests are not sensitive. Diagnosis is based on observing the bacterium in the peripheral blood via the Giemsa or special silver stains (difficult to stain due to very low bacterial numbers).
   e. May show increased titers to **proteus OXK antigen.**
   f. Serological tests are currently in the development phase.

2. *Borrelia burgdorferi*
   a. Causes **Lyme disease.**
   b. Is the most common tickborne disease in the United States, carried by the deer tick (Ixodes damninii).
   c. Three clinical stages of the disease:
      1) Rash at the bite site (**erythema migrans**) produces a characteristic target skin rash pattern in many patients.
      2) Enters the blood, which then can go to the bones (arthritis), central nervous system (meningitis, paralysis), or heart (palpitations, carditis).
      3) Characterized by chronic arthritis and may continue for years
   d. **Diagnosis**
      1) Serological tests are sensitive in diagnosing Lyme disease.
      2) Culture: **Barbour-Stoenner-Kelly II medium.**

D. *Leptospira spp.*

1. *L. interrogans* causes leptospirosis (Weil's disease).
2. Infection of rodents, dogs, and cattle.
3. Humans acquire the infection by contact with **contaminated animal urine** (contaminated water or food).
4. The infection can produce fever, kidney, liver, and CNS involvement.
5. **Diagnosis** of leptospirosis:
   a. Direct examination via darkfield microscopy, or silver stain methods.
   b. Cultures: Tween 80 and Fletcher's media.
   c. Serology: varies in sensitivity.

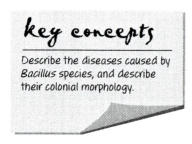

key concepts

Describe the diseases caused by Bacillus species, and describe their colonial morphology.

X. AEROBIC GRAM POSITIVE SPORE FORMING BACILLI (BACILLUS SPP.)

A. General Characteristics

1. *Bacillus* spores can survive adverse conditions for prolonged periods of time and are frequent contaminants of laboratory cultures.
2. Most are nonpathogenic and only genus identification is necessary.
3. *B. anthracis* (anthrax) and *B. cereus* (food poisoning) are pathogenic species.
4. The majority of the species will grow on blood agar and phenylethyl alcohol (PEA).
5. Straight bacillus with square ends (boxcar morphology) appearing in chains and singly. Spores can be central or terminally located.
6. Motile, oxidase positive.
7. Cultures show large, flat colonies.

B. Differentiation of Bacillus Species

1. Cell morphology.
2. Spore shape and location.
3. Aerobic or facultative anaerobic oxygen requirements.
4. Reactions positive for motility, hemolysis, and penicillin susceptibility.

C. *Bacillus anthracis*

1. Causes anthrax, which is **rare in the United States.**
2. Three types of anthrax include:
   a. Cutaneous anthrax: most common form in the world, which produces skin necrotic lesions called **black eschars.**
   b. Pulmonary anthrax: "Wool-Sorter's Disease," spread by inhalation of spores from sheep's wool.
   c. Gastrointestinal anthrax: rarest form.
3. *Bacillus anthracis* spores are centrally located.
4. Susceptible to 10μg of pencillin, and nonmotile.
5. **Colony:** produces large, nonhemolytic colonies with filamentous projections, which are sometimes known as **Medusa-head** colonies.

D. *Bacillus cereus*

1. Important cause of food poisoning but also a common lab contaminant.
2. May also cause opportunistic eye, bone, and brain infections.
3. **Colony:** large, flat, beta-hemolytic colonies with irregular edges.
4. Motile and resistant to 10μg of penicillin

XI. AEROBIC NON–SPORE FORMING GRAM POSITIVE BACILLI

A. *Listeria monocytogenes*

1. Causes spontaneous abortion and meningitis in animals (sheep).
2. Listeriosis causes a variety of infections in neonates, pregnant women, and the immunosuppressed. Meningitis is a common outcome of the infections.

3. Found in the environment (soil and water) and are normal flora of the vagina and intestines in humans.
4. **Identifying Characteristics**
   a. Isolate on most media, **colonies** are small gray beta-hemolytic (narrow zone) colonies.
   b. Closely resembles Group B Streptococci on blood agar.
   c. Listeria demonstrates both **umbrella motility** at room temperature, and end over end motility in a wet mount.
   d. Hippurate, CAMP, esculin, and catalase positive.

B. *Erysipelothrix rhusiopathiae*

1. Mostly infects animals, but humans become infected through contact with infected animals or by consuming infected meat.
2. Humans acquire the infection in the form of cellulitis (erysipeloid lesions), but may also get bacteremia or endocarditis.
3. **Identifying Characteristics**
   a. Pleomorphic Gram positive bacilli.
   b. Nonmotile.
   c. Catalase negative.
   d. Hydrogen sulfide positive.

C. *Corynebacterium spp.*

1. *Cornebacterium diphtheriae* causes **diphtheria.**
   a. Characterized by a pseudomembrane formed by dead cells and exudate.
   b. Bacterial toxins damage all major organs resulting in a high death rate.
   c. Treatment: antitoxin.
   d. Found **only** in humans.
   e. **Identifying Characteristics**
      1) Gram stain: diphtheroid morphology arranged in "picket fences" or "Chinese letters"; can be very pleomorphic.
      2) Staining with methylene blue will show **metachromatic granules,** which are red to purple intracellular granules.
      3) Urease negative, and catalase positive, nonmotile.
      4) **Elek** is the test for toxin production which places *C. diphtheriae* into two catagories:
         a) **Toxigenic *C. diphtheriae*** are strains infected with a bacteriophage that is responsible for the diphtheria toxin gene.
         b) **Nontoxigenic *C. diphtheriae*** are strains that do not produce the diphtheria toxin.
      5) Types of Media
         a) Cystine-tellurite (black colonies).
         b) Tinsdale's Agar (brown to black colonies with halos).
         c) Loeffler Agar supports growth and enhances pleomorphism. Most colonies show small, white gray, to yellow colonial morphology.
         d) Will grow on blood agar.

2. *Corynebacterium jeikeium*
    a. Extremely virulent, causes infections after prosthetic device implants and infections in the compromised patient.
    b. Resistant to most antibiotics.
3. *Corynebacterium urealyticum*
    a. Cause UTIs.
    b. Is rapid urease positive and grows very slowly.

D. *Nocardia asteroides*
    1. Generally found in compromised patients with chronic pulmonary disorders.
    2. **Identifying Characteristics**
        a. Pleomorphic Gram positive bacilli in chains that produce a beading arrangement, appearing **fungal-like** in appearance.
        b. **Partially acid fast, catalase positive, nonmotile.**
        c. Requires up to 6 weeks for growth.
        d. Produces a musty/soil odor.
        e. Exudate contains masses of filamentous organisms with pus that appear like sulfur granules.
        f. Nonmotile and catalase positive.
    3. Other species include *N. brasiliensis* and *N. otitidiscaviarum.*

E. *Lactobacillus spp.*
    1. Is normal flora of the oral cavity, GI, and female genital tract.
    2. Is a rare pathogen.
    3. Catalase negative and nonmotile bacilli.

key concepts

Describe the various anaerobes, including pathology, isolation methods, and identifying characteristics.

XII. ANAEROBES

A. General Characteristics
    1. Anaerobic bacteria comprise most normal flora of the skin, mucus membranes, and intestines.
    2. Suspect anaerobic bacteria in the following situations:
        a. Foul odor
        b. Anaerobic body sites, abscesses, and wounds
        c. Surgical specimens

B. **Anaerobic Media**—contains supplements that enhance anaerobic growth and inhibits other growth. **Vitamin K1** is added to enhance growth of *Provotella* and *Porphyromonas,* and **Hemin** is an enhancement for *Bacteroides* and *Prevotella.*
    1. **Anaerobic Blood Agar:** general growth media.
    2. *Bacteroides* **bile esculin agar (BBE):** used to culture and presumptive identify *Bacteroides fragilis.*
    3. **Kanamycin Vancomycin-laked Blood (KVLB)** enhancement for *Prevotella* and *Bacteroides spp.*
    4. **Phenylethyl alcohol agar (PEA):** used to grow most anaerobes.
    5. **Columbia blood agar with colistin (CAN):** used to grow most anaerobes.
    6. **Egg yolk agar (EYA):** useful in detecting proteolytic enzymes produced by *Clostridium* species.

C. Gram Stain Morphology

1. *Bacteroides* and *Prevotella spp.:* pale, pleomorphic Gram negative cocobacilli with bipolar staining.
2. *Fusobacterium spp.:* long, thin, filamentous Gram negative bacilli with tapered ends, which are arranged end to end.
3. *Actinomcyces spp.:* branching Gram positive bacilli.
4. *Clostridium spp.:* spore location is important in species identification, which may be terminal, central, or subterminal. Gram positive bacilli.

D. Important Biochemical Reactions—Most anaerobic biochemical tests include **catalase, nitrate, urease,** and **indole.** Can also use antibiotic susceptibility disks to ID anaerobes.

E. Anaerobic Gram Negative Bacilli

1. *Bacteroides fragilis*
   a. Nonpigmented bacilli that are responsible for most anaerobic infections, and are becoming resistant to many antibiotics.
   b. Major normal flora of the colon and oral cavity.
   c. Causes infections by gaining entry into normally sterile body sites, especially after surgery, trauma, or disease.
   d. **Identifying Characteristics**
      1) Nonmotile Gram negative bacilli with rounded ends, and may be pleomorphic with tiny vacuoles.
      2) Nonhemolytic on anaerobic blood agar.
      3) Biochemistry: growth in 20 percent bile, catalase positive, lipase negative, bile-esculin positive, lecithinase negative, and gelatinase negative.
      4) Resistant to penicillin, kanamycin, and vancomycin.
      5) Susceptible to rifampin.
      6) Grows on *Bacteroides* **bile-esculin (BBE)** agar, producing brown to black colonies.
      7) Other species include *B. ureolyticus,* which is susceptible to penicillin and kanamycin, but resistant to vancomycin.
2. *Prevotella melaminogenicus*
   a. Pigmented saccharolytic Gram negative bacilli.
   b. Is normal flora of the oropharynx, nose, GI, and urogenital tract.
   c. Causes head, neck, and lower respiratory infections.
   d. **Identifying Characteristics**
      1) Requires up to 3 weeks to grow.
      2) **Young colonies** appear tan; **older colonies** appear brown to black.
      3) Brick-red fluorescence under ultraviolet (UV) light.
      4) Biochemistry: ferments glucose and many other carbohydrates, and is inhibited by 20 percent bile.
      5) Susceptible to rifampin and resistant to kanamycin.
3. *Porphyromonas spp.*
   a. Asaccharolytic pigmented Gram negative bacilli.
   b. Normal flora of the oropharynx, nose, GI, and urogenital tract.

    c. Causes infections of the head, neck, oral cavity, and urogenital tract.

    d. **Identifying Characteristics**

       1) Brick red fluorescence under UV light.

       2) Will not grow on KVLB agar, inhibited by vancomycin, bile, penicillin, and refampin. However, susceptible to kanamycin.

       3) Requires vitamin K and hemin for growth.

4. *Fusobacterium spp.*

    a. Asaccharolytic pigmented Gram negative bacilli.

    b. Normal flora of the upper respiratory tract, GI, and urinary tract.

    c. Causes pulmonary, blood, sinus, and dental infections in addition to brain abscesses. Many infections are associated with metastatic conditions.

    d. Two important species are *F. nucleatum* (causes serious pulmonary infections) and *F. necrophorum* (lung and liver abscesses, and arthritis).

    e. **Identifying Characteristics**

       1) **Colonial morphology:** opalescent with speckles.

       2) Indole positive, nitrate and catalase negative.

       3) Considered to be relatively biochemically inactive.

       4) In addition to the above characteristics, *F. necrophorum* is lipase positive

       5) Inhibited by kanamycin and colistin, resistant to vancomycin.

F. **Anaerobic Gram Positive Spore-Forming Bacilli**

1. *Clostridium* **(General Characteristics of the Genus)**

    a. Anaerobic or aerotolerant.

    b. **Catalase negative.**

    c. Produce **true toxins,** which are excreted from living bacteria.

    d. Some species are normal GI flora of humans and animals, and are found in the soil, water, and dust.

    e. Gram Stain: Gram positive boxcar bacilli.

2. **Group I:** *Clostridium perfringes*

    a. Causes **gas gangrene** (myonecrosis), food poisoning (meats and gravy), postabortion sepsis, abdominal infections, enterocolitis, and antibiotic-associated diarrhea.

    b. Acquire the bacteria through wound punctures or any situation that places the bacteria into an anaerobic environment.

    c. Secretes enzymes and exotoxins that cause severe tissue damage.

    d. Diabetics and patients with circulatory disorders are more prone to infection.

    e. *C. perfringes* is normal flora of the female genital tract, and can result in postabortion infections.

    f. A major cause of food poisoning resulting in a mild to moderate diarrhea without vomiting.

g. Treatment for gas gangrene includes amputation, and hyperbaric oxygen chambers.

h. **Identifying Characteristics**

1) Shows a double zone of hemolysis on anaerobic blood agar.

2) Positive for lecithinase, glucose, lactose, maltose, and fructose.

3) Spores are subterminal and difficult to see.

4) Nonmotile.

5) **Nagler plate:** streak half of a plate with *C. perfringes* type A antitoxin and streak with unknown at right angles to the antitoxin.

6) Reverse CAMP positive.

3. **Group II: *Clostridium tetani***

a. Causes **tetanus.** Tetanospasmin toxin is produced, which is a neurotoxin that affects the anterior horn cells of the spinal cord resulting in involuntary muscle contractions. Contractions begin with the neck and jaw (**"lock jaw"**) and progresses in a backward arching of the back muscles.

b. Bacteria and spores gain entry into the host by puncture wounds, which may include gunshots, burns, or animal bites. The bacteria create necrotic cells that produce the required anaerobic environment.

c. Treatment and prevention: antitoxin and vaccine (DPT) booster every 5 years.

d. **Identifying Characteristics**

1) Gram stain: Gram positive bacillus with round/terminal spores that resemble **drumsticks.**

2) Biochemical: gelatinase, indole and motility positive, lecithinase and lipase negative.

3) Generally not cultured.

4. **Group III: *Clostridium botulinum***

a. Causes botulism and infant botulism.

b. Botulism toxin is a neurotoxin that binds the synapse of nerve fibers, resulting in acute (flaccid) paralysis and death.

c. Botulism is usually from spoiled home-canned foods where the spores are not destroyed.

d. Infant botulism is the most common type of botulism, where it grows in the infant GI tract. The disease was first diagnosed in 1976, and is usually fatal.

e. **Identifying Characteristics**

1) Biochemistry: lipase, lecithinase, glucose, and motility positive.

2) Indole negative.

3) Spores are oval/subterminal that look like tennis rackets.

5. **Group IV: *Costridium difficile***

a. Causes antibiotic-associated pseudomembranous colitis.

b. Until 1975 *C. difficile* was considered nonpathogenic.

c. Is normal GI flora in small percentage of the population, and as many as 30 percent of hospitalized patients may carry the bacteria.

    d. Intestines of patients when broad-spectrum antibiotic use has eliminated their normal intestinal flora.

    e. Produces enterotoxin A, and cytotoxin B.

    f. **Identifying Characteristics**

      1) Biochemistry: negative for lecithinase, lipase, and indole and positive for glucose, fructose, and motility.

      2) Spores are oval and subterminal.

G. Anaerobic Non–Spore Forming Gram Positive Bacilli

1. **Anaerobic *Actinomyces***

    a. Normal flora of animal and human mucosal linings.

    b. *A. israelii* is the most common pathogen which causes abdomen, chest infections, and pelvic actinomycosis in women with IUDs.

    c. **Identification:**

      1) Gram positive bacilli with a beaded appearance; often filamentous.

      2) Exudate will show sulfur granules.

      3) **Colony:** wool to raspberry morphology; colony colors vary from white to red to gray.

2. *Propionibacterium*

    a. Species include *P. acnes* and *P. propionicus.*

    b. Often called anaerobic diphtheroids.

    c. Normal flora of the skin, mouth, and intestinal tracts.

    d. Infections include osteomyelitis, endocarditis, acne, meningitis, and prosthetic implant infections.

    e. Catalase and indole positive.

3. **Mobiluncus**

    a. Causes bacterial vaginosis, pelvic inflammatory disease (PID), and abdominal infections.

    b. Motile, catalase, and indole negative.

    c. Curved bacilli.

    d. Inhibited by vancomycin.

4. **Bifidobacterium:** mostly nonpathogenic normal oral and intestinal flora.

5. **Eubacterium:** mostly nonpathogenic normal oral and intestinal flora.

H. Anaerobic Cocci (Both Gram Negative and Positive)

1. **General Characteristics of Anaerobic Cocci**

    a. Normal flora of the intestines, female genital tract, oral cavity, skin, and respiratory tract.

    b. Associated liver and brain abscesses and wound infections.

2. **Anaerobic Gram Positive Cocci**

    a. **Peptococcus** "anaerobic Staphylococcus"; the only species is *P. niger.*

      1) Catalase positive

      2) Produces black colonies on anaerobic media

    b. *Peptostreptococcus*

      1) Inhibited by sodium polyanethol sulfonate.

      2) Species includes *P. anaerobius, P. magnus,* and *P. asaccharolyticus.*

3) Indole positive.
3. **Anaerobic Gram Negative Cocci**
   a. *Veillonella parvula*
      1) Small, Gram negative cocci
      2) Nitrate positive
      3) Red fluoresence under UV light
      4) Inhibited by kanamycin and colistin, but resistant to vancomycin.

XIII. MYCOBACTERIUM SPP

A. General Characteristics

1. Cause tuberculosis and other diseases.
2. Mycobacteria are very slender, nonmotile, non–spore forming, slow-growing, acid-fast, obligate aerobes.
3. Mycobacteria resist Gram staining due to their cell wall lipids that prevent penetration of crystal violet and safranin.
4. There are 50 species of *Mycobacterium,* 14 of which are pathogenic to humans.
5. Nonpathogenic species are put into the **Runyon** groups.
6. It is necessary to decontaminate most samples before culturing, and sputum must be digested. Specimens from normally sterile sites (CSF, blood, etc.) do not require decontamination.
7. Mycobacteria are **acid fast** and are known as acid-fast bacilli (AFB).
8. All *Mycobacterium tuberculosis* produce **niacin (nicotinic acid),** and most species are **catalase positive.** Some species will convert ferric ammonium citrate to iron oxide.
9. **Specimens**
   a. Lungs (sputum) and bronchial washings, usually 3 to 5 samples are collected on different days.
   b. Urine: 3 to 5 different morning voids.
   c. Blood, may also include bone marrow.
   d. Tissue and body fluids.
   e. Feces are only collected from HIV patients, and collected when *M. avium* is suspected of causing gastrointestinal disease.
10. **Media:** must contain egg components for growth.
    a. Lowenstein-Jensen
    b. Petragnami
    c. American Thoracic Society Agar
    d. Middlebrook Agars
11. **Mycobacteria groups:** mycobacteria are grouped according to their **growth rate, colonial morphology,** and **photoreactivity.**
    a. Growth rate: fast or slow growers.
    b. Colonial morphology: many mycobacteria produce a unique and characteristic colonial appearance.
    c. Photoreactivity: divided into 3 classes:
       1) **Photochromogens** produce yellow to orange pigment when exposed to light.
       2) **Scotochromogens** produce yellow to orange pigment in the light and in the dark.

key concepts

Compare the identifying characteristics of Mycobacterium and their isolation methods.

3) **Nonchromogens** do not produce pigment.

B. Mycobacterium Species

1. *Mycobacterium tuberculosis*

   a. Causes tuberculosis, a chronic disease found only in humans.

   b. Is spread by person to person contact via infected droplets, dust, etc.

   c. Only a few bacteria are necessary to cause disease.

   d. **Primary Tuberculosis**

      1) Begins in the middle or lower lungs. This is a slowly, progressing disease.

      2) The bacteria may spread to the lymphatic system, spine, heart, and meninges.

      3) Macrophages begin phagocytosis that form multinucleated cells surrounded by epithelial cells. Together they form **granulomatous lesions** called **tubercles** which show up on chest x-rays.

      4) Important to note that primary tuberculosis may not lead to active TB in people with healthy immune systems.

   e. **Reactivation or Secondary Tuberculosis (TB)**

      1) Occurs in people who have had primary TB.

      2) Reactivation can be due to poor nutrition, alcoholism, or hormonal factors associated with pregnancy and diabetes.

      3) Requires long-term drug therapy which can last up to 24 months.

         a) Drugs include isoniazid, rifampin, and pyrazinamide.

         b) Streptomycin is also used in combination with other drugs.

   f. **MDRTB** (multidrug resistant *M. tuberculosis*) was first discovered in 1991 and indicates a poor prognosis for recovery.

   g. **PPD** (purified protein derivative) **skin test** for exposure to *M. tuberculosis:*

      1) Composed of heat-killed, filtered, ammonium sulfate precipitated organism.

      2) Is injected intradermal, and is read at 48 hours for redness/swelling.

      3) A positive skin test indicates previous exposure to the bacteria, but not necessarily active disease.

   h. **Colonies** on LJ media appear tan and unpigmented in 14–21 days at 35–37°C, and appear dry and granular.

   i. Acid fast stain often shows ropelike formations from broth culture.

   j. Biochemistry: niacin and nitrate positive, NAP susceptible.

2. *Mycobacterium leprae:* agent of **Hansen's disease** (leprosy).

   a. Cannot be cultured in the laboratory but will grow in cell cultures, mouse footpads, and in armadillos.

   b. Diagnosis is based on characteristic skin lesions and acid-fast staining of lesions.

3. *M. avium* and *M. intracellulare:* *M. avium* may cause disease in the immunosuppressed patient causing lung infections, lymphadenitis, and intestinal infections in HIV patients.

4. *M. fortuitum, M. chelonae, M. abscessus:* each may cause abscesses, osteomyelitis, wound and lung infections.
5. *M. kansasii:* causes pulmonary infections.
   a. Cells show a banded staining area resembling cross bars.
   b. Is nitrate positive and catalase positive.

XIV. MISCELLANEOUS BACTERIA

A. *Bartonella quintana* (Gram Negative Curved Bacilli)

key concepts

List isolation methods, identifying procedures, and define cell structure as related to antibiotic action.

1. Agent of **Trench fever** which is characterized by a 5-day fever period.
2. Also causes growth of neoplastic blood vessels in various parts of the body (bacillary angiomatosis) and other infections such as endocarditis.
3. Spread by human lice.

B. *B. henselae* causes **cat-scratch disease** producing skin lesions. Also causes bacillary peliosis hepatitis and bacillary angiomatosis.

C. *Gardnerella vaginalis* (Gram Variable Pleomophic Coccobacilli)
1. Implicated in **bacterial vaginosis,** UTIs, PID, postpartum sepsis, and may infect the newborn.
2. Is considered normal nonpathogenic vaginal flora in low numbers.
3. Causes the formation of **clue cells,** which are squamous epithelial cells with numerous bacteria attached.
4. Differs from *Lactobacillus* (large Gram positive bacilli). *Gardnerella* are very small Gram-variable coccobacilli.
5. Is catalase negative.

D. **Spirillum minus:** causes rat bite fever.

XV. *CHLAMYDIA, MYCOPLASMA,* AND *RICKETTSIA*

A. *Chlamydia*
1. Obligate intracellular, nonmotile parasite.
2. Cannot produce ATP.
3. Gram negative-like cell wall.
4. Contains both DNA and RNA, and is susceptible to antibiotics.
5. Classified as a bacteria in the family **Chlamydiae.**
6. Diagnosis: cytological methods showing epithelial chlamydia inclusions, requires cell culture to grow, mostly diagnosed by serology (lipopolysaccharide and outer membrane proteins antigens).
7. Includes 3 important species:
   a. *Chlamydia psittaci* (new genus name)
      1) Causes **psittacosis** (ornithosis) or parrot fever, a disease of parrots, parakeets, cockatoos, and other birds such as turkeys and chickens.
      2) Humans get infections by the inhalation of bird fecal dust; uncommon in the United States.
      3) 1–2 weeks incubation period: chills, fever, malaise, can progress to pneumonia (can be fatal).

4) Occupational hazard to farmers, pet shop employees, and bird owners.

5) Diagnosis is by serology.

b. *Chlamydia pneumoniae*

1) Mild respiratory tract infections producing flulike symptoms, also may cause Guillain-Barré syndrome.

2) Has no animal vectors, spread by human to human contact.

3) Also known as **TWAR.**

4) Can be cultured in human cells.

5) Diagnosis is by fluoresence labeled *C. pneumoniae* antibodies.

c. *Chlamydia trachomatis*

1) Causes lymphogranuloma venereum, endemic trachoma, nongonococcal urethritis, conjunctivitis, and infant pneumonia

2) The leading cause of blindness in the world

3) Diagnosis: cell cultures, direct fluorescent antibody tests, EIA, DNA probes, and other serological procedures

B. Mycoplasma

1. Smallest free-living organisms, about the size of a large virus, which makes them difficult to impossible to see with light microscopes.

2. Very pleomorphic with no cell wall, which makes them resistant to all antibiotics that inhibit cell wall synthesis (beta lactams).

3. Contains both RNA and DNA, and can self-replicate.

4. Diagnosed by serology.

5. Can grow on laboratory media, including special media (A7, E, and U agar). Will also grow on blood agar and chocolate agar. Produces a **fried egg** colonial morphology.

6. Species include:

a. *Mycoplasma pneumoniae* "Eaton Agent"

1) Causes tracheobronchitis and community acquired primary atypical (walking pneumonia) pneumonia, resulting in a dry unproductive cough.

2) Spread by direct respiratory contact.

3) Mostly seen in teenagers and young adults.

b. *M. hominis*

1) Opportunistic pathogen linked to PID in sexually active adults.

2) May cause infant meningitis and postpartum fever.

c. *M. fermentans.* Found in the tissue of HIV-infected patients, known as **AIDS-associated** *Mycoplasma.*

d. *Ureaplasma urealyticum*

1) Causes nongonococcal urethritis and may cause other genital tract infections.

2) Urea positive.

C. Rickettsiae

1. Nonmotile, Gram negative intracellular bacteria.
2. Contains RNA and DNA.
3. Infections are spread by insect vectors (ticks, mites, and lice).
4. All rickettsiae (except *Coxiella*) need a host to survive
5. Diagnosis: clinical symptoms, patient history, Weil-Felix serology, immunohistology, and polymerase chain reaction tests.
6. Is cultured in embryonated eggs and tissue cells, and is a biosafety level 3 pathogen.
7. ***Rickettsial* groups:**
   a. Spotted-fever group
   b. Typhus group
   c. Scrub typhus group
8. Species:
   a. ***R. rickettsii:*** causes **Rocky Mountain spotted fever,** is carried by ticks. A very serious disease where death rates are approximately 25 percent.
   b. ***R. prowazekii:*** causes **typhus** (also called epidemic or louse-borne typhus); carried by human lice. Also known as Brill-Zinsser disease, which is a reemergence of the original infection.
   c. ***R. typhi:*** causes **endemic or murine typhus.** Transmitted by fleas.
   d. ***R. felis:*** causes **murine type typhus** and is carried by fleas.
   e. ***R. tsutsugamushi:*** causes **scrub typhus** and is transmitted to humans by mite larvae.
   f. ***Coxiella burnetii:*** causes **Q fever.**
   g. ***Ehrlichia:*** causes ehrlichiosis.

XVI. CLASSES OF ANTIBIOTICS AND ANTIMICROBIAL SUSCEPTIBILITY TESTING

A. Terms

1. **Antibiotics:** chemicals produced by microorganisms that inhibit the growth of other microorganisms. Can also be synthetic.
2. **Antibacterial:** inhibits the growth of bacteria.
3. **Cidal:** kills microorganisms
4. **Static:** inhibits the growth of microorganisms.
5. **Superinfection:** a new infection resulting from the treatment of the primary infection.
6. **Synergy:** when two or more antibiotics are used and the combined effect is greater than what would be expected for the simple additive effect of the agents.

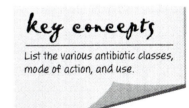

key concepts

List the various antibiotic classes, mode of action, and use.

B. Spectrum of Action

1. **Narrow-spectrum antibiotics:** limited mode of action.
2. **Broad-spectrum antibiotics:** mode of action against a wide range of bacteria.

C. Classes of Antibiotics and Their Mode of Action

1. **Beta-lactam antibiotics:** inhibits cell wall synthesis.
2. **Aminoglycosides:** inhibits protein synthesis at 30S ribosomal subunit, action against Gram negatives and positives. Dosage should be monitored using peak and trough values.
3. **Tetracycline:** inhibits protein synthesis at the 30S ribosomal subunit. A broad-spectrum antibiotic used to treat Gram positive and negative bacteria, *Mycoplasma* and *Chlamydia* infections.
4. **Chloramphenicol:** inhibits protein synthesis by binding to the 50S ribosomal subunit. Used to treat serious Gram negative infections such as typhoid fever and salmonellosis.
5. **Sulfonamides:** inhibits folic acid synthesis by forming nonfunctional analogs of folic acid.
6. **Macrolides:** inhibits protein synthesis.
7. **Glycopeptide:** inhibits cell wall formation by inhibiting peptidoglycan synthesis.
8. **Quinolones:** inhibits DNA activity.
9. **Miscellaneous Agents**
   a. **Polymyxins:** disruption of cell membranes, used for Gram negatives.
   b. **Nitrofurantoin:** inhibits bacterial enzymes, used for UTIs
   c. **Rifampin:** inhibits RNA polymerase, used for TB and *Neisseria* infections.

XVII. PLATING CLINICAL SPECIMENS—Plating protocols will vary between institutions. The plating scheme provided here includes media most often used in many clinical laboratories. However, there are acceptable variations that will occur from one institution to the next.

A. Blood

1. Blood is normally sterile containing no bacteria.
2. Terms and Characteristics
   a. Bacteremia: bacteria in the blood.
   b. Septicemia: bacteria in the blood causing harm to the patient.
   c. Drawing blood cultures: avoid skin contamination and collect sample (if possible) before antibiotic therapy.
   d. Bacteria are in highest numbers in the blood before fever spikes; must collect several specimens at different times for greatest potential bacterial yield.
   e. Culture
      1) Many blood collection bottles contain media.
      2) Incubate one aerobically and one anaerobically.
      3) Most aerobic bottles contain 5 to 10 percent CO_2.
      4) Blood culture bottles contain **SPS,** sodium polyanethol sulfonate, which inhibits complement and inactivates neutrophils and antibiotics.

B. Cerebrospinal Fluid (CSF)

1. CSF surrounds the brain and spinal cord, carries nutrients and waste from these structures, is normally sterile.
2. Meningitis is inflammation of the meninges.

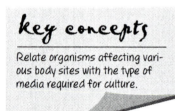

key concepts

Relate organisms affecting various body sites with the type of media required for culture.

3. Encephalitis is inflammation of the brain.
4. Most common isolates in CSF include *H. influenzae, Streptococcus pneumoniae, Streptococcus agalactiae, N. meningitides, E. coli, Staphylococcus aureus,* and *Listeria monocytogenes.*
5. Perform a direct Gram stain and culture on BAP, MAC, and chocolate agar.

C. Throat

1. Usually only check for Group A *Streptococcus.* Screening for other pathogens may occur upon request.
2. Culture on blood agar. Other media as needed by special request.
3. Throat cultures are used to confirm rapid strep tests.

D. Sputum

1. Used to diagnose lower respiratory tract infections (pneumonia).
2. Perform a direct Gram stain and determine the quality of the specimen. Culture acceptable specimens on BAP, MAC, and chocolate agar.
3. Acceptable specimens: There are several methods used to determine specimen acceptability. In general, squamous epithelial cells are an indication of contamination with oral flora, whereas neutrophils indicate a good quality specimen from a patient with a true infection. A good general rule might be: **<10 squamous epithelial cells/low power and >25PMNs/low power** for an acceptable specimen. *Note:* This does not pertain to neutropenic or atypical pneumonia samples, which often have nonpurulent sputum.
4. Most Common Sputum Isolates
   a. *Streptococcus pneumoniae* is a community acquired pneumonia, and is the most common cause of pneumonia in geriatric patients.
   b. *Klebsiella pneumoniae* causes Gram negative pneumonia.
   c. *Staphylocccoccus aureus* causes community acquired and nosocomial pneumonia.
   d. *Pseudomonas aeruginosa* causes nosocomal and severe pneumonia in cystic fibrosis patients.
   e. *H. influenza* causes infection in infants, children, and the immunosuppressed.
   f. *Legionella pneumophilia* primarily infects middle-age males.
   g. *Mycoplasma pneumoniae* causes primary atypical pneumonia, which is mostly seen in young adults.

E. Urine

1. Urine is normally sterile.
2. Voided urine passes over the superficial urogenital membranes and can become contaminated by normal flora. Bacteriuria is bacteria in the urine, but may not indicate a UTI.
3. To help differentiate between contamination by normal flora and true infection, use calibrated loops and perform colony counts after growth has occurred.
4. Culture on BAP and MAC.

5. Most common urine isolates: *E. coli, Klebsiella spp., Enterobacter spp., Proteus spp., Staphylococcus aureus, Staphylococcus saprophyticus, Enterococcus spp., Pseudomonas spp.,* and yeast.

F. Stool

1. Contains many species of anaerobic and aerobic normal flora.
2. Generally only concerned with bacteria that produce gastroenteritis including *Shigella spp., Salmonella spp., Campylobacter spp., E. coli (O157:H7), Yersinia enterocolitica, Clostridium difficile* (must do test for cytotoxin), and *Vibrio spp.*.
3. Plating protocols vary widely but in general include selective and differential media for the isolation and screening of specific pathogens.

G. Genital Tract

1. Usually look for *Neisseria gonorrhoeae* or *Chlamydia trachomatis.*
2. Types of Genital Tract Infections
   a. Cervicitis can be caused by *C. trachomatis, N. gonorrhoeae,* HSV, and *Trichomonas vaginalis.*
   b. Urethritis: *N. gonorrhoeae* and *C. trachomatis.*
   c. Nonspecific vaginitis: caused by an overgrowth of *Gardnerella vaginalis* or a decrease in normal flora.
   d. Pelvic inflammatory disease (PID) is a complication of infection caused by *N. gonorrhoeae* or *C. trachomatis* of the endometrium or fallopian tubes.
   e. Prostatitis: caused by enterics.
3. Plating protocols for *N. gonorrhoeae* include specific selective media (*see* III, B.6). Molecular techniques are commonly used for both of these pathogens.

H. Wounds/Abscesses

1. Superficial skin infections: *S. aureus* and *S. pyogenes*
2. Folliculitis (hair follicle infection): *S. aureus* and *P. aeruginosa*
3. Boils, bedsores, etc.: *S. aureus*
4. Impetigo: *S. pyogenes*
5. Erysipelis: *S. pyogenes*
6. Deep and surgical wounds and abscesses: anaerobes out of the normal body sites

XVIII. BIOCHEMICAL TESTS USED FOR BACTERIAL IDENTIFICATION

A. Catalase Test—Catalase is an enzyme that frees water and oxygen from hydrogen peroxide. Several drops of H_2O_2 are added to a bacterial smear. If the catalase enzyme is present, **bubbles** will form.

B. Coagulase Test

1. **Slide coagulase:** most slide coagulase tests use rabbit coagulase plasma. **Clumping** indicates a positive reaction.
2. **Tube coagulase test** uses the same reagents as the slide method, but is incubated at 37°C for up to 24 hours (reference method).

C. Oxidase Test—detects cytochrome oxidase in the nitrate metabolic pathway. Several drops of oxidase reagent placed on filter paper containing bacterial colonies or directly on plate colonies. A positive

oxidase test is indicated by a color change (color depends on reagent used).

D. Spot Indole Test—detects bacterial **tryptophanase** productions. Tryptophane is broken down by tryptophanase into pyruvic acid, ammonia, and indole. Of the 3 by-products of tryptophane, indole is detected by an aldehyde indicator (**Ehrlich's reagent**), yielding a red color, or **Kovac's reagent** yielding a bright pink.

E. Urease Test—Urease breaks down urea to form NH_3. Organisms to be tested may be inoculated on a urea slant and incubated at 37°C for 18–24 hrs. A bacterial suspension is added to a urease tube and incubated for up to four hours at 37°C. A positive urease test is indicated by a bright pink color.

F. PYR Test—detects L-pyroglutamyl aminopeptidase. A colony is placed on filter paper with the PYR reagent. A positive PYR test forms a **red color.**

G. Bile Solubility Test—colonies of *S. pneumoniae* are soluble in sodium deoxycholate (bile). In the presence of the reagent at 37°C, the colonies dissolve within 30 minutes.

H. Hippurate Hydrolysis Test—shows bacteria that have hippuricase, which hydrolyzes hippurate. A positive hippurate will give a **purple color.**

I. Thermonuclease Test—shows the prodution of heat stable deoxyribonuclease (DNAse). One method uses DNAse test media and a positive reaction yields a pink to red halo around the media holes. Other testing methods are also available.

J. Fermentation Test—shows bacteria that ferment various carbohydrates to produce organic acids. Positive and negative reactions depend on the pH indicators used.

K. Amino Acid Degradation Test—indicates bacterial enzymes that break down various amino acids. The color of positive and negative reactions depends on the pH indicator used in the system.

L. Nitrate Reaction Test—determines the ability of an organism to reduce nitrate to nitrite. After the addition of reagents, a pink result is positive, a colorless reaction requires the addition of zinc dust to confirm. Pink after zinc indicates a true negative. Colorless after zinc indicates a positive nitrate reductase test as nitrate was reduced to nitrite and completely reduced to nitrogen gas.

M. Multitest Systems

1. Most biochemical tests are performed using multitest methodologies.
2. Multitest systems include:
   a. MIC/combination plates
   b. Minitek System
   c. API
   d. Enterotube
   e. Micro-ID

DIRECTIONS Each of the questions or incomplete statements below is followed by suggested answers or completions. Select the **one answer** that is best in each case.

1. Which biochemical test is not consistent with the following bacterial characteristics: Gram positive cocci in clusters, colonies are β hemolytic, smooth, opaque, and circular, and show a golden yellow pigment?
   a. growth on MSA
   b. thermonuclease positive
   c. catalase negative
   d. coagulase positive

2. Which statement is NOT CORRECT for bacteria that cause strep throat?
   a. susceptible to bacitracin
   b. catalase negative
   c. susceptible to SXT disk
   d. colonies are beta hemolytic

3. *Neisseria meningitidis* is positive for which of the following biochemical tests?
   a. oxidase and glucose
   b. catalase and nitrate
   c. maltose and DNAse
   d. catalase and maltose

4. Most members of the Enterobacteriaceae family have which of the following characteristics?
   a. glucose positive, oxidase positive, nitrate negative
   b. glucose positive, oxidase negative, nitrate positive
   c. oxidase positive, nitrate negative, coagulase negative
   d. hippurate negative, indole negative, oxidase negative

5. What enteric would fit the following profile: TSI = alk slant/acid deep, H_2S negative, methyl red positive, nonmotile, citrate negative, urease negative, lactose negative, green colonies on hektoin enteric agar, IMViC (+/−, +, −, −). Infection incubation period is between 1 to 7 days, and is not normal flora of humans.
   a. *Shigella*
   b. *Salmonella*
   c. *Yersinia*
   d. *Proteus*

6. *Moraxella* is a genus that resembles *N. gonorrhoeae;* therefore, which biochemical tests will differentiate the two?
   a. *N. gonorrhoeae* is glucose negative, *Moraxella* is glucose positive.
   b. *N. gonorrhoeae* is glucose negative, *Moraxella* is glucose negative.
   c. *N. gonorrhoeae* is oxidase negative, *Moraxella* is oxidase positive.
   d. *N. gonorrhoeae* is glucose positive, *Moraxella* is glucose negative.

7. On sheep blood agar, which bacterium is β hemolytic with a fried egg appearance, is normal flora of humans but cause infections in children such as skin lesions and septic arthritis, and can isolate from joint fluid?
   a. *Capnocytophaga*
   b. *Kingella*
   c. *Chromobacterium*
   d. *Franciella*

8. A positive test is indicated by a bright pink color change. Positive organisms include *Crytococcus neoformans, Citrobacter, Haemophilus,* and *Proteus* is rapidly positive:
   a. urease
   b. indole
   c. glucose
   d. hippurate

9. Which bacterium is NOT worked up from a stool sample?
   a. *Campylobacter*
   b. *Vibrio*
   c. *E. coli* O547:H7
   d. *Klebsiella*

10. Which 2 organisms are ALWAYS cultured for in a stool sample?
    a. *Proteus* and *Pseudomonas*
    b. *Shigella* and *Salmonella*
    c. *E. coli* and Group A streptococcus
    d. *Listeria* and *Neisseria*

11. Determines slow or fact lactose fermentation:
    a. Gelatin hydrolysis
    b. Voges-Proskauer
    c. Indole
    d. ONPG

12. Which is the best test to differentiate *E. coli* from *Shigella?*
    a. lactose
    b. glucose
    c. citrate
    d. indole

13. Which of the following pattern is CORRECT for *H. influenzae?*
    a. X factor positive, V factor positive, beta hemolysis negative, ALA negative
    b. X factor positive, V factor positive, beta hemolysis negative, ALA positive
    c. X factor negative, V factor negative, beta hemolysis negative, ALA positive
    d. X factor negative, V factor positive, beta-hemolysis positive, ALA negative

14. *Legionella pneumophilia* will grow best on:
    a. glucose-cystine-blood agar
    b. EMB
    c. XLF
    d. buffered charcoal yeast extract agar

15. Identifying characteristics include: grows well on most agars, colonies produce a brown color with a mushroom smell, positive for oxidase, catalase, indole, and nitrates, very susceptible to penicillin.
    a. *Chromobacterium*
    b. *Actinobacillus*
    c. *Capnocytophaga*
    d. *Pasteurella*

16. For the genus Vibrio, which statement is NOT CORRECT?
    a. all species are halophilic
    b. positive for oxidase and indole
    c. curved bacillus
    d. grows well on thiosulfate citrate bile agar

17. Which of the following is rapid urease positive, can isolate on blood, Brucella, Skirrow's and modified Thayer-Martin agar, can show in gastric material using the Warthin-Starry stain, is a major cause of peptic and duodenal ulcers?
    a. *Helicobacter*
    b. *Campylobacter*
    c. *Aeromonas*
    d. *Proteus*

18. Which organism is partially acid-fast with a fungal-like appearance?
    a. *Lactobacillus*
    b. *Nocardia*
    c. *Erysipelothrix*
    d. *Corynebacterium*

19. This anaerobic non–spore forming Gram positive bacillus is often called anaerobic diphtheroids; is catalase and indole positive; considered normal flora of the skin, mouth, and intestinal tract; infections can cause osteomyelitis, acne, and prosthetic implant infections.
    a. *Propionibacterium*
    b. *Mobiluncus*
    c. *Bifidobacterium*
    d. *Anaerobic actinomyces*

20. Which of the following is used to treat Gram positive cocci infections, MRSA, and *Clostridium difficile* by inhibiting cell wall formation by blocking peptidoglycan synthesis?

a. trimethoprim
b. erythromycin
c. vancomycin
d. penicillin

Clinical Parasitology

➤ COMPREHENSIVE KEY CONCEPTS

1. Summarize the various groups of parasites that infect humans according to symptoms of disease, specimen sources, regions of the world where they are endemic, isolation/concentration, and staining procedures.

2. Describe the life cycles of important disease producing parasites and their diagnostic stages in humans.

3. Recognize key morphological structures of parasites and visually identify them in various specimens including stool, blood, and human tissue.

4. Discuss factors that predispose humans to parasitic infections including foreign travel, water/food contamination, intermediate host contact, and environmental habitat.

---

key concepts

Discuss parasite collection procedures and body sites where parasites can be found.

I. INTRODUCTION

A. Parasitic Disease Risk Factors

1. Unsanitary food handling/preparation (contaminated meat and vegetables).
2. Contaminated water, which can be for drinking or recreational use.
3. Immunocomprised resulting from disease states or poor dietary balance.
4. Parasitic transmission by insect sting or bite.
5. Blood transfusion and organ transplantation.
6. Foreign travel to endemic regions of the world.

B. Parasitic Disease Characteristics

1. **Diarrhea is the most frequent symptom,** which is associated with abdominal cramping.
2. Other symptoms depending on parasite type may include:
   a. Intestinal obstruction, weight loss, and bloating.
   b. Organ involvement with ulcers, lesions, and abscesses.
   c. Blood parasites can cause bleeding, anemia, fever, chills, encephalitis, and meningitis.

C. Specimen Collection and Processing

1. Diagnosis of parasite infections often depends on observing parasite stages that may include ova, larva, or adult forms.
2. Specimen types include stools (most common), tissue, and blood.
   a. Stool samples should be free of antibiotics, barium, or other substances that inhibit parasite growth.
      1) 3 grams of sample are required for most parasite analysis.
      2) Stool should be free of urine, because urea inhibits some parasites.
      3) **Fresh stools** are needed for amoebae and flagellate **trophic forms.**
      4) **Liquid stools** are best to detect trophozoites, whereas **formed stools** are best to detect ova and cyst forms.
      5) Stools should not be frozen or allowed to stand at room temperature.
      6) **Polyvinyl alcohol (PVA)** and **sodium acetate formalin (SAF)** can be used to preserve stool samples.

       7) Gross examination of stool may detect **adult forms.**

   b. **Ova and parasite (O & P)** examinations require the sample to be **concentrated.**

      1) Concentration procedures remove fecal debris that could obscure parasites.

      2) Concentration methods include:

        a) Sheather sugar flotation

        b) Formalin-ethyl acetate concentration

        c) Zinc sulfate flotation

      3) **Blood concentration** Methods:

        a) The **knott** method uses low speed centrifugation to concentrate blood samples suspected of containing minimal parasite amounts.

        b) **Buffy coat** slides are used for *Leishmania* or *Trypanosoma* detection.

3. Various stains are used for microscopic detection of stool, tissue, and blood parasites.

   a. Saline wet mounts are quick and easy to perform, and will allow troph motility to be seen.

   b. Permanent stained smears are used to enhance parasite morphology, and to allow for future study.

      1) **Iron hematoxylin stain** is used when enhanced detail is needed; however, the stain procedure is difficult to perform.

      2) **Trichome stain (Wheatley or Gomori)** is the most commonly used stain for parasite study.

      3) **Modified acid-fast stain** is used to detect *Cryptosporidium*.

4. Collection methods

   a. The **Cellophane tape** method is used to collect *Enterobius vermicularis* eggs.

   b. The **Enterotest** (string test) is used to obtain duodenal contents for parasitic examination.

   c. The sigmoidoscope is used to collect colon material.

5. Sample types and associated parasites (genus):

   a. Blood: *Leishmania, Trypanosoma,* and *Onchocerca*

   b. Skin: *Onchocerca*

   c. Vaginal or urethral: *Trichomonas*

   d. Oral (mouth or nasal): *Entamoeba, Trichomonas,* or *Naegleria*

   e. Eye scrapings: *Acanthamoeba*

   f. Tissue: *Naegleria, Acanthamoeba,* and *Leishmania*

   g. Urine: *Schistosoma* and *Trichomonas*

   h. Sputum: *Ascaris, Strongyloides,* and *Entamoeba*

D. Diagnostic Tests

1. Direct fluorescent antibody (DFA): used to identify *Trichomonas vaginalis.*

2. Direct agglutination test (DAT): used to diagnose leishmaniasis and Chagas' disease.

3. ELISA: used to identify *Toxoplasma gondii.*

4. Complement fixation (CF): used to diagnose leishmaniasis, Chagas' disease, and pneumocystosis.

5. Gel-diffusion precipitin (GDP) test: used to detect amoebic infections.

6. Indirect immunofluorescent antibody (IFA): used to diagnose amoebic, malarial, toxoplasmosis, and schistosome infections.

7. DNA probes, flow cytometry, and polymerase chain reactions are being developed for parasite diagnostic use.

II. PARASITE TERMINOLOGY

A. Parasitology has a unique series of terms that are used when discussing or identifying parasitic infections. The following is a selective group of the most commonly used terms.

1. **Carrier:** an asymptomatic host that harbors a parasite and is capable of transmission to others.

2. Cestodes: tapeworms.

3. Ciliates: motile protozoans.

4. **Commensalism:** host-parasite relationship that is beneficial to one member, and harmless to another.

5. Cyst: thick walled stage of amoeba that is resistant to adverse conditions.

6. **Definitive host:** required for adult or sexual phase of a parasitic life cycle.

7. Ectoparasite: external parasites.

8. Egg: also called oocyst, ovum, or zygote.

9. Endoparasite: internal parasites.

10. Filariae: blood or tissue roundworms requiring an insect vector for transmission.

11. Flagellates: protozoans that have flagella.

12. Gravid: pregnant.

13. Helminths: include nematodes (roundworms), cestodes (tapeworms), and trematodes (flukes).

14. Hermaphroditic: tapeworms capable of self-fertilization.

15. Host: any living organism that harbors a parasite.

16. Hydatid cyst: larval stage of *Echinococcus granulosus.*

17. Intermediate host: host containing the asexual phase of a parasite.

18. Larvae: juvenile stage of a parasite.

19. Schizont

   a. Immature schizont: early stage of the asexual sporozoa trophozoite.

   b. Mature schizont: developed stage of the asexual sporozoa trophozoite.

20. **Mutualism:** beneficial to both parasite and host.

21. Nematode: roundworms.

22. Oocyst: encysted form of an egg.

23. Parasite: an organism that that obtains its nutrients from another organism; may be harmful, beneficial, or neutral.

24. Parasitic life cycle: stages in the development of a parasite; may require multiple hosts and specific nutrients.

25. Parasitism: host-parasite relationship where one member benefits at the expense of another member.

26. **Symbiosis:** an association between two organisms.

key concepts

Describe parasite structure using parasitology terminology.

27. Trematodes: flukes.
28. **Zoonosis:** an animal parasite infection that humans can accidentally acquire.

III. INTESTINAL PROTOZOA (AMOEBAE, FLAGELLATES, CILIATES, COCCIDIA)

A. Intestinal Amoebae

1. General characteristics
    a. Unique to the group: **pseudopods,** and **trophozoite** and **cyst** stage are required in the amoebae life cycle.
    b. Most amoebic infections are spread to humans through contaminated water.
    c. Amoebic **cyst** is the infective stage, whereas the trophozoite stage is destroyed by stomach acid.
    d. Laboratory identification: microscopic analysis of cysts (formed stools) and trophozoites (liquid stools), size, nuclear characteristics, and inclusions.
    e. Clinical: the most common outcome is diarrhea.
    f. **Morphological terms** associated with amoeba.
        1) **Trophozoites:** developmental stage of the amoebae.
        2) **Karyosome:** area of chromatin within the nucleus.
        3) **Excystation:** development of the cyst into the trophozoite.
        4) **Encystation:** development of the trophozoite into the cyst.
        5) **Chromatoid bars:** rod-shaped, RNA-containing structures found in the cytoplasm.

2. *Entamoeba histolytica*
    a. Is the only pathogenic amoeba that causes several mild to serious disorders.
        1) **Amoebic colitis** is characterized by abdominal cramping, anorexia, fatigue, and diarrhea. Amoebic colitis can also cause ulcers and amoebic dysentery.
        2) Extraintestinal amebiasis is an infection of the liver by trophozoites.

> *key concepts*
>
> Describe and identify diagnostic stages of amoeba.

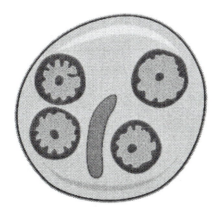

Size Range: 8 – 22 μm
Average Size: 12 – 18 μm

FIGURE 8-1. Entamoeba cyst

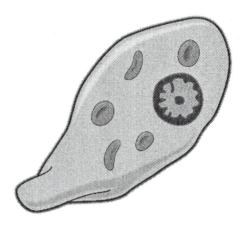

Size Range: 8 – 65 μm
Average Size: 12 – 25 μm

FIGURE 8-2. Entamoeba histolytica

    a) Additional conditions include infections of the spleen, skin, brain, penile/vaginal amebiasis, and lungs.
  b. Life cycle: cysts are infective when ingested. The excystation site is the small intestines. Infective cysts are passed in stools and are resistant to environmental stress.
  c. Morphology
    1) **Cyst characteristics**
      a) Size ranges from 8 to 22μm, and is spherical to round.
      b) Nucleus has 1 to 4 nuclei; peripheral chromatin is fine and uniformly distributed.
      c) Karyosome: centrally located.
      d) Cytoplasm is finely granular with chromatoid bars with round ends.
    2) **Trophozoite characteristics**
      a) Size ranges from 5 to 70μm, and is motile with pseudopodia.
      b) Nucleus has one nucleus; peripheral chromatin is fine and uniformly distributed.
      c) Karyosome: centrally located.
      d) Cytoplasm is finely granular with RBC inclusions.
3. ***Entamoeba coli***
  a. *Entamoeba coli* is generally nonpathogenic but may cause intestinal problems in the immunosuppressed.
  b. Can indicate the presence of other pathogenic organisms.
  c. Needs to be differentiated from *Entamoeba histolytica* for purposes of treatment.
  d. Morphology
    1) **Cyst characteristics**
      a) Size ranges from 8 to 40μm and is spherical shaped.
      b) Nucleus: contains one to eight nuclei, peripheral chromatin is coarse and unevenly distributed.
      c) Karyosome: eccentric and large.

        d) Cytoplasm: coarse with thin chromatoid bars with pointed ends.

    2) **Trophozoite characteristics**

        a) Size ranges from 10 to 60µm, and is motile with short/blunt pseudopods.

        b) Nucleus contains a single nucleus with coarse, unevenly distributed chromatin.

        c) Karyosome: eccentric and large.

        d) Cytoplasm: coarse and vacuolated, with bacterial inclusions.

4. *Naegleria fowleri*

  a. Causes amoebic meningoencephalitis, which is **often fatal within 3 to 6 days.**

  b. *N. fowleri* is found in lakes, ponds, and swimming pools where the water is warm.

  c. Life cycle: trophozoites are the infective stage. *N. fowleri* does not need a host to survive and is considered to be **free-living,** spending its entire life cycle in the external environment.

  d. The amoebae is contracted from contaminated water where trophozoites enter the body through the nasal mucosa and migrate to the brain.

  e. Diagnosis: finding the organism (any stage) in **CSF.**

  f. Morphology (**shows three stages**)

    1) **Cyst characteristics**

        a) Size ranges from 10 to 13µm, and is round.

        b) Nucleus is single, without peripheral chromatin.

        c) Karyosome: centrally located and large.

        d) Cytoplasm: granular and vacuolated.

    2) **Trophozoite characteristics**

        a) Size ranges from 10 to 23µm, and is motile with blunt pseudopods.

        b) Nucleus is single, without peripheral chromatin.

        c) Karysome: centrally located and large.

        d) Cytoplasm: granular and vacuolated.

    3) **Flagellate characteristics**

        a) Size ranges from 7 to 15µm, **pear**-shaped, and is motile with two **flagella.**

        b) The nucleus is indented.

        c) Karyosome: centrally located and large.

        d) Cytoplasm: granular with vacuoles.

5. **Acanthamoeba Species**

  a. Causes amoebic encephalitis and amoebic keratitis (cornea infection).

  b. Life cycle: unknown.

    1) The eye is directly invaded by trophozoites.

    2) Skin, respiratory tract, or CNS infections are caused by the cyst or trophozoite stage (unknown entry route).

  c. Diagnosis: finding the cyst or trophozoite stages in **CSF.**

    d. Morphology
      1) **Cyst characteristics**
        a) Size ranges from 8 to 25μm with a jagged-edge, round shape.
        b) Single nucleus without peripheral chromatin.
        c) Karyosome: centrally located and large.
        d) Cytoplasm is granular and vacuolated.
      2) **Trophozoite characteristics**
        a) Size ranges from 15 to 45μm; motility is by spinelike pseudopods.
        b) Single nucleus without peripheral chromatin.
        c) Karyosome: centrally located and large.
        d) Cytoplasm is granular and vacuolated.
6. **Other Amoebas**
    a. *Entamoeba gingivalis:* causes asymptomatic mouth and genital tract infections.
    b. *Iodamoeba butschlii:* a nonpathogenic intestinal parasite.
    c. *Endolimax nana:* nonpathogenic intestinal parasite.
    d. *Entamoeba polecki:* may cause diarrhea in some patients.
    e. *Entamoeba hartmanni:* nonpathogenic intestinal parasite.

IV. INTESTINAL FLAGELLATES

A. General Characteristics

1. Flagellates are a subclass of protozoa that have one or more flagella that provide the structure for motility.
2. All flagellates have the trophozoite stage but many do not show the cyst stage.
3. Most flagellates live in the small intestines and related intestinal structures.
4. *Giardia lamblia* is the only pathogenic flagellate that causes mild to moderate diarrhea.
5. Other flagellates are considered nonpathogenic but may cause disease in the immunosuppressed.
6. Diagnosis is by microscopic analysis of stool for trophozoites (liquid stool) or cysts (formed stool).
7. Terms Associated with Flagellates
    a. Axostyle: rodlike structures that function in support
    b. Axonemes: the intracellular portion of the flagellum
    c. Undulating membrane: flagella finlike structures that generate a wavelike motion
    d. Cytostome: a very basic or rudimentary mouth

B. *Giardia lamblia*

1. Causes giardiasis (**traveler's diarrhea**), which is characterized by acute diarrhea, abdominal pain, and weight loss.
    a. Self-limiting infections run between 10–15 days, following a 10–35-day incubation period.
2. Infection is due to exposure to contaminated water and food (mostly wild animal stool). Campers and hunters are especially prone to infestation following drinking from streams.

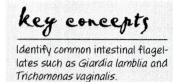

key concepts

Identify common intestinal flagellates such as *Giardia lamblia* and *Trichomonas vaginalis*.

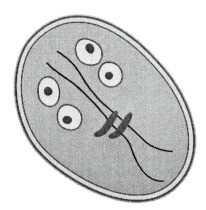

Size Range: 8 – 17 µm by 6 – 10 µm
Average Length: 10 – 12 µm

FIGURE 8-3. Giardia lamblia cyst

   a. Cysts are the infective stage.
   b. Cysts enter the stomach and will excyst in the duodenum.
   c. Resulting trophozoites attach to the duodenum mucosa.
   d. Encystation occurs in the large intestines, and the cysts will pass in the stool.

3. Diagnosis: microscopic analysis of **multiple** stool samples (due to irregular shedding) for trophozoites or cysts.
   a. Other diagnostic tests include the Enterotest and immunology (CIE, ELISA, etc).

4. Morphology
   a. **Cyst characteristics**
     1) Average size ranges from 12µm long to 8µm wide, and is oval shaped.
     2) The nucleus contains no peripheral chromatin.

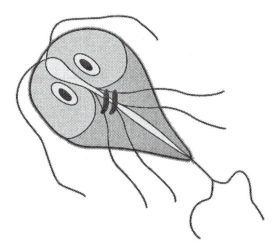

Size Range: 8 – 20 µm by 5 – 16 µm
Average Length: 10 – 15 µm

FIGURE 8-4. Giardia lamblia trophozoite

3) Karyosome: centrally located.

4) Cytoplasm is retracted from the cell wall, and may contain 2 to 4 median bodies (posterior comma shaped structure).

b. **Trophozoite characteristics**

1) Average size ranges from 15μm long to 10μm wide, motile, and pear-shaped. Bilaterally symmetric with two nuclei on each side of a central axostyle ("monkey face" appearance).

2) Nucleus: contains two oval shaped nuclei, contains no peripheral chromatin.

3) Flagella: contains 4 pair of flagella.

4) Contains 2 median bodies, 2 axonemes, and a sucking disc.

C. *Chilomastix mesnili*

1. Is nonpathogenic to humans but has been associated with disease in the immunosuppressed.

2. Transmission is from contaminated food or water containing the cyst stage, which is infective.

3. Diagnosis is by microscopic analysis of stool samples.

4. Morphology

a. **Cyst characteristics**

1) Size ranges from 5 to 10μm in length and is oval shaped.

2) Single nucleus without peripheral chromatin.

3) Karyosome: large and centrally located.

4) Cytostome is defined.

b. **Trophozoite characteristics**

1) Size ranges from 5 to 25μm in length and 5 to 10μm in width, motile, and pear-shaped.

2) Single nucleus without peripheral chromatin.

3) Karyosome: eccentric and small.

4) Flagella: 3 anterior and 1 posterior.

5) Cytostome is very large; a spiral groove is present.

D. *Trichomonas vaginalis*

1. Causes vaginitis (association with cervical cancer) in women, and urethritis in men.

2. *T. vaginalis* is a sexually transmitted disease (STD) and can be congenital.

3. Trophozoites are the infective stage where they infect the epithelial or mucosal lining of the vagina, urethra, and prostate gland.

4. Treatment is Flagyl or metronidazole.

5. Diagnosis: trophozoites are usually detected with a routine urinalysis.

6. Morphology

a. **Trophozoite characteristics**

1) Size averages around 30μm in length, motile (**undulating membrane**), and is pear-shaped.

2) Single nucleus.

3) Flagella: 3 to 5 anterior and one posterior.

4) Large axostyle with granules.

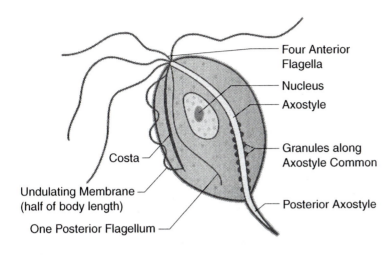

Size Range: up to 30 μm long
Average Length: 8 – 15 μm

FIGURE 8-5. Trichomonas vaginalis

E. *Dientamoeba fragilis*

1. Causes diarrhea, abdominal pain, and anal pruritus.
2. Many cases of *D. fragilis* diarrhea are from individuals living in close quarters, such as inmates, college students, or military recruits.
3. *D. fragilis* infects the mucosal lining of the large intestines. The life cycle is not well defined.
4. Diagnosis: microscopic analysis of trophozoites in the stool. Multiple samples are required. *Note*: The parasite is very delicate and stains very poorly.
5. Morphology
   a. **Trophozoite characteristics**
      1) Size ranges from 5 to 19μm, motile with hyaline pseudopods, and is round-shaped.
      2) Nucleus: two nuclei without peripheral chromatin, but has clumps of chromatin in 4s and 8s.
      3) Cytoplasm: vacuolated with bacterial inclusions.

V. HEMOFLAGELLATES

A. General Characteristics

1. Hemoflagellates inhabit the blood and tissues of humans.
2. Characterized by 4 stages of development: amastigote, promastigote, epimastigote, and trypomastigote.
3. Transmission to humans is by arthropod bites.
4. Diagnosis is by morphology characteristics, patient history, and symptoms.
5. Terms associated with hemoflagellates
   a. Amastigote: nonflagellated and oval form; found in tissue.
   b. Promastigote: stage found in the vector, is flagellated. Rarely seen in the blood. Is seen when cultured, or immediately after transmission.

    c. Epimastigote: long slender form that is flagellated. Found in arthropod vectors.

    d. Trypomastigote: has an undulating membrane running the length of the body, found both in the vector and human. Found in the blood.

6. **Trypansoma species**

    a. Diagnosis is by microscopic analysis of blood and CSF and serological testing.

    b. Disease in rare in the United States, mainly occurring in Africa and South America.

    c. Species that cause disease:

       1) ***Trypansoma brucei***

         a) Causes African trypanosomiasis or sleeping sickness.

         b) Transmission of the infective trypomastigote is by the bite of the tsetse fly.

         c) The disease will affect the lymphatic system and CNS.

         d) The final stage results in coma (hence the name sleeping sickness) and death.

         e) Species **gambiense** and **rhodesiense** are named according to the geographic location of trypanosomiasis.

       2) ***Trypansoma cruzi***

         a) Causes Chagas' disease, which is characterized by lesion formation (chagoma), conjunctivitis, edema of the face and legs, and heart muscle involvement leading to myocarditis.

         b) Transmission of the infective trypomastigote is by the bit of the reduviid bug.

         c) Mostly found in South America.

7. **Leishmania species**

    a. Causes two forms of human leishmaniasis.

       1) Disseminated leishmaniasis: liver, spleen, and reticuloendothelial involvement.

       2) Cutaneous leishmaniasis: causes skin and mucous membrane ulcers.

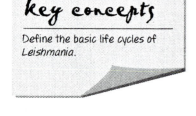

key concepts

Define the basic life cycles of Leishmania.

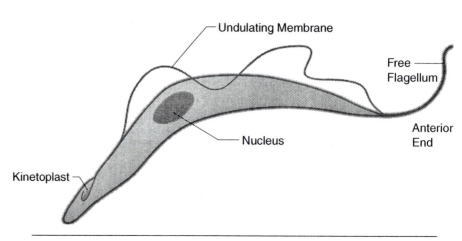

FIGURE 8-6. Trypanosoma

b. Transmission of the infective promastigote is by the bite of Phlebotomus sandflies.

c. The promastigote invades the skin and mucous membrane areas and may spread to the body's organs.

d. Diagnosis: finding the amastigote in the blood or tissue and serological testing.

e. Species that cause leishmaniasis include ***Leishmania braziliensis, Leishmania donovani***, and ***Leishmania tropica.***

f. Mainly a disease of Africa, Eastern Europe, and South/Central America.

VI. SPOROZOA (*PLASMODIUM*)

A. Introduction to **malarial parasites**

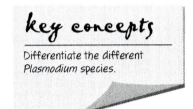

key concepts

Differentiate the different Plasmodium species.

1. Causative agents of malaria.

2. Plasmodium species have two life cycle phases:

   a. **Sporogony:** sexual phase that occurs within the intestinal tract of the mosquito.

   b. **Schizogony:** asexual phase that occurs in the human host.

3. Transmission to humans occurs with the bite of a **female Anopheles** mosquito that harbors the infective **sporozoites** in the salivary gland.

   a. Other forms of transmission include contaminated blood products, contaminated needles, and congenital malaria.

4. Diagnosis is by clinical symptoms and by microscopic analysis of blood smears.

5. *Plasmodium* parasites (characteristics vary as to species) show 3 distinct morphologies:

   a. **Trophozoites** or **ring forms**

      1) Erythrocytic intracellular ringlike appearance.

      2) Giemsa or Wright stain will show a blue cytoplasmic ring connected to a red chromatin dot.

      3) **Mature trophozoites** will loose the ring appearance, but will contain remnants of the cytoplasmic ring and chromatin dot.

   b. **Schizonts**

      1) Active chromatin activity that causes the parasite to increase in size.

      2) Pigmented granules are numerous and brown in color.

      3) **Merozoites:** forms containing developed asexual trophozoites. Number and arrangement depend on species.

   c. **Gametocytes**

      1) Characterized by a chromatin mass staining pink to purple.

      2) Round to oval in shape.

      3) Pigmentation varies as to species.

6. Diagnosis: microscopic analysis of Giemsa (stain of choice) or Wright's smears and serological testing.

7. **Life cycle terminology**

   a. **Sporozoites:** infective stage transmitted to human by Anopheles (saliva) bites.

b. **Schizogony** (asexual phase) occurs in the liver's parenchymal cells.

c. **Exoerythrocyte cycle:** growth and reproduction of the parasite (8–25 days, varies with species).

d. **Merozoites:** contain developed asexual trophozoites that invade erythrocytes.

e. **Erythrocyte cycle:** growth of the merozoites within the erythrocyte; also the parasite will undergo each developmental stage within the erythrocyte.

f. **Gametocyte:** stage that is transmitted back to the mosquito (human blood meal) for completion of the life cycle (sexual phase).

8. Treatment is specific to species. Common antimalarial drugs include quinidine, chloroquine, pyrimethamine, mefloquine, and tetracycline. Drug resistance is emerging.

9. *Plasmodium vivax*

a. Erythrocyte appearance: enlarged and pale, prominent Schuffner's dots.

b. Trophozoites: ring stage is one-third the size of a RBC, mature trophozoites fill the entire RBC.

c. Schizonts: contain 12 to 24 merozoites.

d. Gametocytes: round to oval and almost fills the RBC. Has a large chromatin mass.

e. Miscellaneous characteristics: asexual cycle (**fever cycle**) lasts 48 hours.

f. Causes **benign tertian malaria** following a 10- to 17-day incubation period.

10. *Plasmodium falciparum*

a. Erythrocyte appearance: normal size, usually without Maurer's dots or clefts.

b. Trophozoite: ring stage is one-fifth the size of the RBC, numerous multiple rings.

c. Schizonts: may contain 24 or more.

d. Gametocytes: **crescent** and **banana** shapes are diagnostic.

e. Miscellaneous characteristics: asexual cycle is 24 hours, high ratio of infected RBCs to normal RBCs.

f. Causes **malignant tertian malaria (black water fever)** following a 7- to 10-day incubation period.

11. *Plasmodium malariae*

a. Erythrocyte appearance: normal size without dots or clefts.

b. Trophozoite: Similar to *P. vivax,* but stains more intense blue. Mature trophozoites form **ribbons or bands.**

c. Schizonts: averages 8 to 12 merozoites arranged in **rosettes.**

d. Gametocytes: resemble *P. vivax.*

e. Miscellaneous characteristics: asexual cycle is 72 hours. Diagnosis involves ruling out *P. vivax* and *P. falciparum.*

f. Causes **quartan or malarial malaria** following an 18- to 40-day incubation period.

12. ***Plasmodium ovale***
   a. Erythrocyte appearance: enlarged with thicker ring forms; contains Schuffner's dots.
   b. Trophozoite: maintains its ring appearance as it develops.
   c. Schizonts: averages 4 to 8 merozoites arranged in rosettes.
   d. Gametocytes: resembles *P. vivax* but slightly smaller.
   e. Miscellaneous characteristics: causes the RBC to become crenated.
   f. Causes **benign tertian** or **ovale malaria** following a 10- to 20-day incubation period.

VII. OTHER PROTOZOANS

A. Includes 4 groups of parasites; all are unicellular.
   1. **Ciliates:** *Balantidium coli.*
   2. **Sporozoa** (excluding *Plasmodium*): *Isospora belli* (coccidial parasite), *Cryptosporidium parvum, Toxoplasma gondii,* and *Babesia microti.*
   3. **Blastoccystea:** *Blastocystis hominis.*
   4. **Unique Classification:** *Pneumocystis carinii.*

B. General Characteristics of "Other" Protozoans
   1. ***Balantidium coli***
      a. Causes balantidiasis, characterized by diarrhea to dysentery.
      b. Transmission of the infective cyst is through contaminated (pig feces) water or food.
      c. Diagnosis: microscopic analysis of stool for cysts or trophozoites.
      d. Morphology
         1) **Cyst characteristics**
            a) Ranges in size from 43 to 65µm, is round in shape.
            b) Nucleus: contains 2 kidney-shaped, very large nuclei.
            c) Cytoplasm: contains a double cyst cell wall with numerous cilia between the two cell walls.

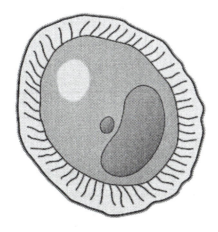

Size Range: 43 – 66 µm
Average Size: 52 – 55 µm

FIGURE 8-7. Balantidium cyst

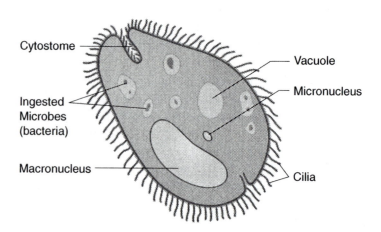

Cytostome

Vacuole

Micronucleus

Ingested
Microbes
(bacteria)

Macronucleus

Cilia

Size Range: 28 – 152 μm by 22 – 123 μm
Average Size: 35 – 50 μm by 40 μm

FIGURE 8-8.   Balantidium coli trophozoite

2) **Trophozoite characteristics**
a) Range in size up to 150μm in length and 125μm in width, and are motile.
b) Nucleus: contains 2 kidney-shaped, very large nuclei.
c) Cytoplasm: one or two contractile vacuoles with cilia around the cell.

2. *Isospora belli*
a. Causes isosporiasis, which is characterized by mild diarrhea to severe dysentery.
b. Transmission is by ingestion of the infective oocyst in contaminated food and water.
c. Humans are the definitive host; there are no intermediate hosts.
d. Diagnosis: microscopic analysis of stool for oocysts.
e. Morphology
1) **Oocyst characteristics**
a) Ranges in size from 25 to 40μm in length, is oval shaped, and is transparent.
b) Cytoplasm is granular containing 2 sporoblasts that contain 4 sporozoites.

3. *Cryptosporidium parvum*
a. Causes cryptosporidiosis, which is characterized by moderate to severe diarrhea.
b. In AIDS patients, *Cryptosporidium* **infections** are the primary cause of death.
c. In the immunosuppressed patient, the parasite causes a wide range of debilitating problems, including malabsorption, stomach, liver, and respiratory disorders.
d. Transmission of the infected oocyst is through contaminated food or water (cow, pig, or chicken feces). Human to human transmission has been documented in **day care centers.**
e. Diagnosis: microscopic analysis of **acid-fast oocysts** from stool or small bowel mucosa epithelial cells.

    f. Morphology

       1) **Oocyst characteristics**

         a) Size ranges from 4 to 6μm, and is round.

         b) Contains 4 sporozoites enclosed within a thick cell wall.

         c) Cytoplasm: may contain several dark granules.

4. *Toxoplasma gondii*

    a. Causes **toxoplasmosis,** is characterized by a broad spectrum of symptoms depending on the individual's state of health. *T. gondii* has a predilection for **CNS** infections.

       1) Healthy individuals: toxoplasmosis often resembles infectious mononucleosis producing fatigue, swollen lymph glands, fever, and myalgia. The disease can become chronic affecting the heart and liver.

       2) Congenital toxoplasmosis: occurs in premature or antibody-deficient infants where symptoms include splenomegaly, jaundice, and fever. CNS infections can lead to developmental problems including vision and hearing problems, hydrocephalus, and mental retardation.

       3) Immunosuppressed and **AIDS toxoplasmosis:** the parasite becomes localized in the CNS with symptoms of encephalitis and brain lesions, which often result in death.

    b. Humans acquire the infective oocyst in 3 ways:

       1) **Cat feces** contaminated food and water.

       2) Ingestion of undercooked meat (**lamb and pork**) containing viable tissue cysts. Estimates that 25 percent of all lamb and pork sold at supermarkets are contaminated.

       3) Transplacental transmission from the infected mother to the newborn.

    c. Diagnosis: serological testing for the *Toxoplasma* antibody, increased IgM titers, and high CSF protein levels.

    d. Because trachyzoites and bradyzoites are very small and thus hard to detect, microscopic analysis of tissue samples is not practical.

    e. Morphology

       1) **Tachyzoite characteristics**

         a) Size range from 1 to 3 μm, bradyzoites are smaller.

         b) Shape: crescent to round.

         c) Single nucleus.

5. *Babesia microti*

    a. Causes babesiosis, which can infect the spleen, liver, and kidneys. Can also cause hemolytic anemia (*B. microti* is an **erythrocytic intracellular parasite**).

    b. Babesiosis is a self-limiting infection; death is a rare outcome.

    c. The infective sporozoite is transmitted to humans by a tick bite (*Ixodes scapularia*).

    d. Most cases in the United States have been in southern New England.

    e. Diagnosis: blood smear analysis and serological testing. Difficult to differentiate from *Plasmodium* species.

f. Morphology

1) **Ring form characteristics**

a) Size range from 3 to 5μm, and is round.

b) Cytoplasm: minimal with 2 or more chromatin dots.

c) 2 to 4 rings per RBCs are noted, often appearing like Maltese crosses.

6. *Blastocystis hominis*

a. Associated with diarrhea and abdominal pain.

b. Transmission is through contaminated food and water.

c. Diagnosis: stool sample analysis.

d. Morphology: a large central vacuole that is 90 percent of the cell with a ring of cytoplasm around it.

7. *Pneumoncystis carinii* **(reclassified and placed into the fungal class Ascomycetes)**

a. Causes pneumocystosis, which is a common cause of nonbacterial pneumonia in immunocompromised patients.

b. Is a major cause of death in AIDS patients.

c. Other high-risk groups include malnourished children and cancer patients.

d. Pneumonocytosis can be congenital.

e. Diagnosis: histology.

f. The life cycle remains undefined.

g. Morphology

1) Trophozoites are very small (2–3μm), oval in shape, and contain a single nucleus.

2) Cysts are round, 5–10μm in size, and contain 4 to 8 nuclei.

VIII. TREMATODES

A. General Characteristics

1. Trematodes (**flukes**) are a class of helminths that are pathogenic to humans.

2. Trematodes are leaflike and flat, hermaphroditic (except the schistosomes), and have two suckers (one opens into the digestive tract, and one is for attachment).

3. The life cycle of trematodes is characterized by the following:

a. Eggs are passed with feces into the water where they hatch.

b. Free-swimming miracidia are released, which are then ingested by **snails (intermediate host)**.

c. Sporocytes (schistosomes) or redia (trematodes) develop in the snail, resulting in the replication of hundreds of cercariae.

d. Cercariae are infective to humans where they are acquired by swimming in infested water.

e. Diagnosis: fecal analysis for egg or adult forms or blood/urine analysis for schistosomes.

f. Can infect many organs, but especially the intestines, liver, and lungs.

4. Terms associated with trematodes

a. **Cercariae:** final stage of development occurring in the snail; are motile by means of a tail.

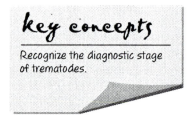

key concepts

Recognize the diagnostic stage of trematodes.

b. **Metacercariae:** encysted form occurring in the second intermediate host (fish or crayfish).

c. **Miracidium:** first larval stage that emerges from the egg in fresh water.

d. **Sporocyst:** emerges from the miracidium as a saclike structure containing the larva.

e. **Rediae:** intermediate larval stage occurring in the sporocyst.

f. **Schistosomule:** resulting form when the cercaria enters human skin and looses its tail.

B. Trematodes

1. **Schistosoma (mansoni, haematobium, japonicum)**

a. Causes schistosomiasis or swamp fever, which is characterized by abdominal pain and bloody diarrhea. Can also cause intestinal lesions and blockage.

b. Prevalent in Africa, but also seen in Puerto Rico and South America.

c. Humans acquire the infective cercaria from contaminated water when the parasite penetrates the skin.

d. Diagnosis: microscopic analysis of eggs found in the stool. Adult forms are rarely seen in human samples.

e. Morphology: the different species of eggs are diagnostic.

   1) *S. haematobium:* large terminal spine
   2) *S. mansoni:* large lateral spine
   3) *S. japonicum:* small lateral spine

2. *Paragonimus westermani* (lung fluke)

a. Causes pulmonary infections, which is characterized by chest pain, cough, bronchitis, and sputum with blood. The parasite in rare cases can migrate to the brain where it causes neurological problems.

b. The infective egg is transmitted in undercooked crabs and crayfish, and they develop in human lung tissue.

c. Most infections occur in Africa, India, and South America.

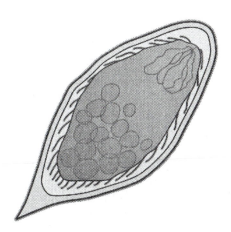

Size Range: 110 – 170 μm by 38 – 70 μm

FIGURE 8-9. Schistosoma haematobium egg

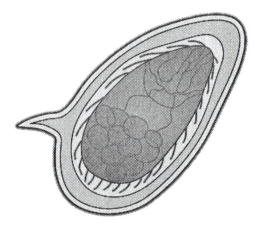

Size Range: 112 – 182 μm by 40 – 75 μm

FIGURE 8-10. Schistosoma mansoni

    d. Diagnosis: microscopic egg analysis in bloody stools.
    e. Morphology: eggs range in size from 72 to 130μm in length with a prominent operculum.

3. ***Clonorchis sinensis* (liver fluke)**
    a. Causes liver problems characterized by fever, abdominal pain, and diarrhea.
    b. Found mainly in China and the Far East.
    c. Humans acquire the disease by eating undercooked fish containing encysted metacercariae.
    d. Diagnosis: egg analysis from stool samples.
    e. Morphology: eggs contain miracidiums showing small knobs opposite the operculum.

4. ***Fasciolopsis buski* (intestinal flukes)**
    a. Causes intestinal problems, including diarrhea and ulceration of the intestines and possibly the stomach.
    b. Found in China and the Far East.

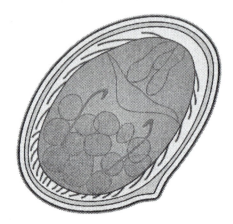

Size Range: 50 – 85 μm by 38 – 60 μm

FIGURE 8-11. Schistosoma japonicum

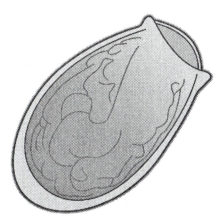

Size Range: 78 – 120 μm by 45 – 60 μm

FIGURE 8-12. Paragonimus westermani egg

    c. *F. buski* is transmitted to the small intestines from contaminated water.
    d. Diagnosis: egg analysis in stool.
    e. Morphology: eggs are large, oblong, and contain an operculum.
    f. ***Fasciola hepatic* (liver fluke)** is a closely related species that resides in the liver.

IX. FILARIAE (FILARIAL NEMATODES)
A. General Characteristics of the Filarial Parasites
    1. Filarial parasites are an order of nematodes consisting of adult threadlike worms.
    2. Filariae inhabit the circulatory and lymphatic system, and are also found in muscle, connective tissue, and serous cavities.
    3. 4 primary species cause disease in humans: *Wuchereria bancrofti, Brugia malayi, Loa loa,* and *Onchocerca volvulus.*

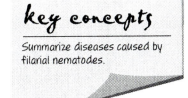

key concepts

Summarize diseases caused by filarial nematodes.

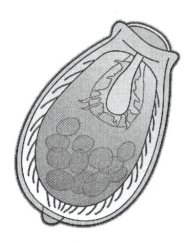

Average Size: 30 μm by 15 μm

FIGURE 8-13. Clonorchis egg

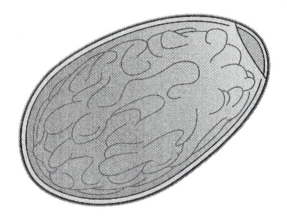

Fasciolopsis Size Range: 128 – 140 μm by 78 – 85 μm
Fasciola Size Range: 128 – 150 μm by 60 – 90 μm

FIGURE 8-14. Fasciola hepatica

4. Transmission of the filariae parasites occurs after the bite of mosquitoes or flies.
5. Diagnosis is by microscopic examination of blood or tissue for microfilariae.
6. Most filarial disease occurs in Africa and South America.

B. Filariae

1. *Loa loa*
   a. Causes subcutaneous tissue infections and infections of the conjunctival lining of the eye.
   b. The skin reaction at the site of worm migration is called Calabar swellings.
   c. Transmission of the parasite is through the bite of the Chrysops (deer) fly.
   d. Diagnosis: blood smear analysis of microfilariae.
   e. Most infections occur in Africa.
   f. Morphology
      1) **Microfilariae characteristics**
         a) Size ranges from 250 to 300μm in length.
         b) Nucleus: contains a row of nuclei that extends to the tail of the parasite.
         c) A sheath is present.

2. *Brugia malayi*
   a. Causes Malayan filariasis, a condition that produces lesions in the lymphatics. **Elephantiasis** may result.
   b. Has the same life cycle as *W. bancrofti,* and is transmitted by the Anopheles or Aedes mosquito.
   c. Diagnosis is by microscopic analysis of microfilariae (night samples offer the largest yields) in blood smears.
   d. Most infections are in the Far East, Japan, and China.
   e. Morphology
      1) **Microfilaria characteristics**
         a) Size ranges from 200 to 300μm in length.

    b) Nucleus: two nuclei are located in the tail.

    c) A sheath is present.

  3. *Wuchereria bancrofti*

    a. Causes Bancroftian filariasis, a condition that produces lesions in the lymphatics. **Elephantiasis** may result.

    b. Vectors for disease transmission are the Culex, Aedes, and Anopheles mosquitoes.

    c. Disease occurs in the tropics and subtropics.

    d. Diagnosis: blood smear analysis of microfilariae.

    e. Morphology

      1) **Microfilaria characteristics**

        a) Ranges in size from 250 to 300μm in length.

        b) Nucleus: no nuclei are found in the tail.

        c) A sheath is present.

  4. *Onchocerca volvulus*

    a. Causes **river blindness;** eye infections may lead to blindness.

    b. Transmission of the infective microfilariae is by the bite of the Simulium (blackfly).

    c. Most infections occur in Africa, South America, and Mexico.

    d. Diagnosis: tissue or ophthalmologic analysis for microfilariae.

    e. Morphology

      1) **Microfilaria characteristics**

        a) Size ranges from 150 to 360μm in length.

        b) Nucleus: no nuclei are located in the tail.

        c) A sheath is present.

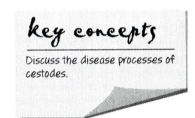

key concepts

Discuss the disease processes of cestodes.

X. CESTODES (TAPEWORMS)

A. General Characteristics

  1. Cestodes are a subclass of helminths comprising true tapeworms.

  2. The adult cestode contains 2 major parts.

    a. Strobilia: consists of a **scolex** and the **proglottids.**

      1) The scolex is the anterior portion of the body containing hooklets or suckers. The crown of the scolex is called the **rostellum.**

      2) Proglottids make up the major portion of the body, containing male and female reproductive structures.

  3. Cestodes have 3 life cycle stages: egg, larval stage(s), and the adult worm.

  4. Cestodes have several intermediate hosts.

  5. Diagnosis: microscopic analysis of stool samples for eggs.

  6. Transmission of infective eggs occurs with contaminated food and water. Contamination can come from the feces of cows, pigs, fish, and humans.

B. Cestodes

  1. *Taenia saginata* **and** *Taenia solium* **(beef and pork tapeworms)**

    a. Causes beef or pork tapeworm infections that are rather mild infections causing abdominal pain and mild diarrhea.

    b. The **ova of** *T. solium* **(in rare cases when humans are the intermediate host)** can cause a lethal larval form of extraintestinal disease called **cysticercosis,** which causes lesions in the cerebral cortex.

c. Infection is by the ingestion of **undercooked beef (*T. saginata*)** or **pork (*T. solium*)** that is contaminated with larva.

d. Diagnosis: egg analysis (the eggs of the two species are identical) in stool samples. Species identification relies on proglottid or scolex analysis.

e. The parasite is found worldwide.

f. Morphology (Taenia eggs are identical):
1) Range in size from 30 to 40μm.
2) 3 pairs of hooklets.
3) Have radial striations.

2. ***Diphyllobothrium latum* (fish tapeworm)**
a. Causes intestinal pain, diarrhea, and vitamin B12 deficiency when the adult worm infects the jejunum.

b. Acquire the infection by eating raw, infected (contains the **pleurocercoid**) fish.

c. Infections occur in populations that eat raw fish, such as northern Europe and Japan. Individuals with pernicious anemia are predisposed to more moderate symptoms.

d. Diagnosis: egg analysis from stool samples.

e. Morphology
1) **Eggs**
a) Range in size from 50 to 80μm in length, and are oblong in shape.
b) The shell is smooth and color is yellow to brown.
c) Terminal knob at one end of the operculum.

3. ***Dipylidium caninum* (dog/cat tapeworm)**
a. Causes diarrhea, abdominal discomfort, and indigestion.

b. Acquire the larval stage from water or food contaminated with infected dog or cat feces.

c. Diagnosis: egg or gravid proglottid analysis in stool samples.

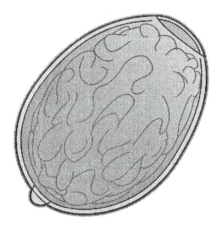

Size Range: 55 – 75 μm by 40 – 55 μm
Average Size: 65 μm by 48 μm

FIGURE 8-15. Diphyllobothrium latum

    d. Morphology
      1) **Eggs**
        a) Range in size from 30 to 65μm in diameter.
        b) Each egg packet may contain 10 to 40 eggs.
        c) Each egg contains 6-hooked onchospheres.

4. *Hymenolepsis nana*
    a. Causes abdominal pain and diarrhea.
    b. Humans get the parasite from rat and house mice feces or human feces. At high risk of infections are nursery school children and college students (close quarters).
    c. **Most common tapeworm in the United States.**
    d. Diagnosis: egg analysis in stool samples.
    e. **Egg morphology**
      1) Average size is 40μm, and is round.
        a) Contains 3 pairs of hooklets.
        b) Polar thickening of the shell is common.

5. *Echinococcus granulosus* **(dog tapeworm or hydatid tapeworm)**
    a. Causes the development of a hydatid cyst in many areas of the body. As the cyst grows, surrounding tissue is destroyed. Depending on cyst location, death can result. The release of hydatid cyst fluid may cause anaphylactic shock to the patient.
    b. Most common where **sheep** (intermediate host) are raised, including England, South America, and Australia. Some cases have been reported in Alaska.
    c. Humans acquire the infection from contaminated dog feces. The dog acquires the parasite by consuming infected sheep meat.
    d. Diagnosis: analysis of hydatid cyst fluid containing cysts and other parasite components, and serological testing.
    e. Egg morphology: the egg contains a cyst wall containing fluid. Other structures within the egg are daughter cysts, brood capsules, and hydatid sand.

XI. NEMATODES (ROUNDWORMS)
A. General Characteristics
1. Nematodes are a class of heminths that includes roundworms.
2. Adult nematodes have a tapered, cylindric body with a esophagus and longitudinal muscles.
3. Diagnosis is based on adult, larvae, ova, or egg morphology.
4. Nematode life cycles are varied as to species, and can be quite complex.
    a. Most require an intermediate host to develop an infective form.
      1) Some nematodes transmit disease through the ingestion of eggs.
      2) Other nematodes transmit disease by larvae, which must gain entry through the skin on its way to the intestines.
      3) All nematodes inhabit the human intestines as part of their life cycle.
5. Cause disease associated with the intestines and the skin, including diarrhea, vomiting, and skin ulcers.

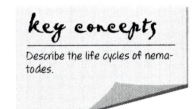

key concepts

Describe the life cycles of nematodes.

6. Nematodes are placed into 2 groups: the intestinal nematodes and the intestinal-tissue nematodes.
   a. Intestinal nematodes include
      1) *Enterobius vermicularis*
      2) *Trichuris trichuria*
      3) *Ascaris lumbricoides*
      4) *Strongyloides stercoralis*
      5) *Necator americanus*
   b. Intestinal-tissue nematodes include
      1) *Trichinella spiralis*
      2) *Dracunculus medinenis*

B. Enterobius vermicularis (Pinworm)

1. Causes pinworm (**enterobiasis**) infections, which are usually self-limiting, characterized by itching and inflammation of the anus. Enterobiasis can be asymptomatic.
2. Pinworm infections are very common in the United States, especially in school-age children.
3. Infective eggs are ingested (found in human stool), then migrate from the digestive tract to the small intestines.
   a. The eggs hatch and release larvae in the small intestines.
   b. Larva develop into adult worms in the colon.
   c. Gravid females migrate to the perianal region where eggs are laid.
   d. The eggs are then infective following a 6-hour incubation period.
   e. Eggs are then spread from the perianal region through scratching.
   f. The eggs will be infective for several weeks and can be found in dust, clothing, etc.
   g. The eggs are very sticky so they easily attached to almost any object.
4. Diagnosis: identification of the egg from a tape preparation in which the sticky side of tape is pressed on the perianal skin.
   a. Yield is best in children if the test is done in the morning, because the gravid female deposits eggs in the perianal folds during the late evening hours.

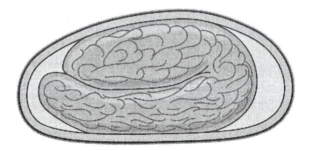

Size Range: 48 – 60 μm long by 20 – 35 μm wide

FIGURE 8-16. Enterobius vermicularis

      b. Itching results from the irritation caused by the deposition of eggs.
5. Treatment is mebendazole or pyrantel pamoate.
6. **Egg morphology**
      a. Ranges in size from 50 to 60μm in length and 30μm in width, is oval shaped with 1 side being flat.
      b. The shell is thick and double-walled.
      c. The egg contains a developing embryo.

C. *Trichuris trichuria* (Whipworm)

1. Causes whipworm infection, which in children presents as colitis and dysentery. In adults symptoms include abdominal pain and bloody diarrhea.
2. Most infections occur in Africa and South America, but infections occur in the deep south of the United States.
3. Eggs (from human feces) are infective to humans where they become adult forms in the intestines.
4. Diagnosis: egg and adult forms in stool samples.
5. Treatment: mebendazole.
6. Morphology of Trichuris eggs
      a. The eggs range in size from 50 to 60μm in length and 25μm in width, and are football shaped with plugs at each end.
      b. The shell is smooth and color is yellow to brown.
      c. The egg contains a developing embryo.
7. Morphology for the adult form
      a. Range in size up to 5cm in length.
      b. The anterior end resembles a whip handle.
      c. The posterior end resembles a whip and is gray in color.

D. *Ascaris lumbricoides* (Roundworm)

1. Causes roundworm (Ascariasis) infections, resulting in intestinal tissue destruction and obstruction leading to death. The worms can also migrate to the lungs where they cause pulmonary disorders.
2. Affect over 1 billion people per year, including in the United States.
3. The Ascaris eggs (infective stage) are contained in human feces and contact will cause disease, especially in children in the Blue Ridge Mountain area of the United States.
4. Diagnosis: analysis of stool for eggs and adult forms.
5. Treatment: surgery, pyrantel pamoate, and piperazine citrate.
6. Morphology of Ascaris eggs
      a. Size ranges up to 75μm in length, and 50μm in width, round shaped.
      b. The shell is thick and contains a developing embryo.
7. Morphology of adult forms
      a. Size: up to 35μm in length.
      b. Color is white to pink.
      c. Female bodies are thinner than males.

E. *Strongyloides stercoralis*

1. Causes threadworm infections, characterized by diarrhea and abdominal pain.

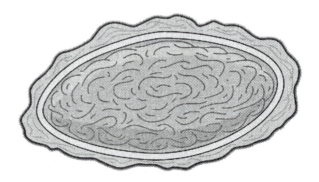

Size Range: 85 – 95 µm by 38 – 45 µm

FIGURE 8-17. Ascaris lumbriocoides

2. Most infections occur in the tropics but have been reported in the Appalachians of the United States.
3. Skin contact with contaminated soil (rhabditiform larvae) is the transmission route for humans.
4. Diagnosis: stool analysis for rhabditiform larvae and the Enterotest.
5. Treatment is thiabendazole.
6. Morphology of rhabditiform larvae
    a. Ranges in size up to 700µm in length.
    b. The tail is notched.

F. *Necator americanus* (hookworm)

1. Causes hookworm infections, depending on the infected body site; symptoms can include coughing (lung infection) and headaches.
2. The parasite is common throughout the world, including North America.
3. Humans acquire the **filariform larvae** through skin penetration. The larvae then enter the lungs or intestines.
4. Diagnosis: larvae identification from sputum or adult worm identification from stool.
5. Morphology of larvae
    a. Size ranges from 250 to 700µm in length.
    b. Long buccal cavity.
6. Morphology of Adult Worm
    a. Ranges in size from 5 to 10mm in length, with the female being larger.
    b. Color is white to pink.
    c. Buccal capsule contains a pair of cutting plates.

G. *Trichinella spiralis*

1. Causes trichinosis, symptoms range from diarrhea to blurred vision, muscle edema (mostly **striated muscle**), cough, and death.
2. The parasite is found worldwide, mainly in pigs and deer.
3. Humans acquire by eating contaminated **undercooked pork**
4. Diagnosis: tissue analysis for encysted larvae. Laboratory values show eosinophilia, leukocytosis, and increased creatine kinase (CPK) and lactate dehydrogenase (LDH).
5. Treatment: most drugs are ineffective.

6. Morphology of encysted larva
   a. Size: up to 125μm in length and 7μm in width (juveniles); adults range up to 1mm in length, are coiled shaped.
   b. Many encysted forms are found in striated muscle tissue.

H. *Dracunculus medinenis* (Guinea Worms)

1. Causes guinea worm infection; symptoms include allergic reactions and painful ulcers.
2. Most infections occur in Africa, India, and Asia.
3. Copepods carry the parasite where they shed the larvae into water.
4. Diagnosis: observing worms emerging from ulcerated areas of the body.
5. Treatment: surgery, slow removal of the worm by pulling it out of the ulcer, or metronidazole.
6. Morphology of adult forms
   a. Adults range in size up to 1.5mm in length for females and 0.4mm in length for males.
   b. Females have rounded anterior ends whereas males have coiled anterior ends.

review questions

DIRECTIONS Each of the questions or incomplete statements below is followed by suggested answers or completions. Select the **one answer** that is best in each case.

1. Which statement is CORRECT for specimen collection and processing?
   a. Liquid stools are best for detecting amoeba and flagellates.
   b. Stool samples can contain urine but does not inhibit parasites.
   c. Fresh stool is needed for amoeba and flagellate detection.
   d. Stools can be frozen without affecting parasitic structure.

2. Cysts are the infective stage, is a self-limiting infection running between 10 to 15 days, exposure is from contaminated water (wild animal stool), campers and hikers are prone to acquiring the infection:
   a. *Giardia lambia*
   b. *Chilomastix mesnili*
   c. *Dientamoeba fragilis*
   d. *Enteromonas hominis*

3. RBC: enlarged and pale, prominent Schuffner's dots; trophozoites: ring stage is one-third the size of the RBC; schizoints: contain 12–24 merozoites; gametocytes: round to oval which fills the RBC; the fever cycle is 48 hours in duration.
   a. *P. vivax*
   b. *P. falciparum*
   c. *P. malariae*
   d. *P. ovale*

4. This parasite often resembles infectious mononucleosis in healthy individuals, humans can acquire the oocyst through contaminated food or water (cat feces) or contaminated undercooked lamb or pork:
   a. *Toxoplasma gondii*
   b. *Babesia microti*
   c. *Balantidium coli*
   d. *Blastocystis hominis*

5. Causes pulmonary distomiasis, often migrates to the brain where it causes neurological problems, the egg is transmitted in undercooked crabs and crayfish whey they develop in human lung tissue, diagnosis is microscopic egg analysis in bloody stool, eggs range in size from 72–130μm in length with a prominent operculum:
   a. *Schistosoma mansoni*
   b. *Clonorchis sinensis*
   c. *Paragonimus westermani*
   d. *Fasciolopsis buski*

6. Which statement is NOT CORRECT when characterizing Trematodes?
   a. They infect the intestines, liver and lungs.
   b. Mosquitoes are the intermediate host.
   c. Eggs are passed with the feces into the water where they hatch.
   d. Diagnosis is by fecal analysis for egg or adult forms or blood analysis for schistosomes.

7. Which *Schistosoma* species has a large terminal spine?
   a. *S. haematobium*
   b. *S. mansoni*
   c. *S. japonicum*
   d. none of the above

8. Which 2 parasites can cause Elephantiasis?
   a. *Loa loa* and *Brugia malayi*
   b. *Brugia malayi* and *Onchocerca volvulus*
   c. *Wuchereia bancrofti* and *Brugia malayi*
   d. *Wuchereia bancrofti* and *Onchocerca volvulus*

9. All nematodes inhabit this human organ site as part of their life cycle:

   a. intestines
   b. liver
   c. esophagus
   d. skin

10. This parasitic infection may result in vitamin B12 deficiency; humans acquire the infective pleurocercoid from fish; individuals with pernicious anemia are predisposed to more moderate symptoms:
    a. *Hymenolepis nana*
    b. *Diphyllobothrium latum*
    c. *Dipylidium caninum*
    d. *Echinococcus granulosus*

9 Clinical Mycology

Contents

➤ COMPREHENSIVE KEY CONCEPTS

1. Correlate unique identifying structural characteristics of fungal groups with specific cultural and growth requirements necessary in cultural and microscopic analysis used in identifying procedures.

2. Relate mycoses to body site and sample collection with environmental and physiological factors that contribute to acquiring a fungal infection.

3. Name the various fungi according to group (cutaneous, opportunistic, etc.) and list the diseases they cause.

I. INTRODUCTION AND GENERAL CHARACTERISTICS

A. Fungal Structure

1. **Hyphae** are long, branching filaments that come together to form the **mycelium.** There are 2 types of hyphae.
   a. **Aseptate hyphae** contain no cellular separations or cross walls. Aseptate hyphae range in diameter from 5 to 15 μm.
   b. **Septate hyphae** have cellular separation or cross walls. Septate hyphae range in diameter from 3 to 6 μm.

2. Hyphae are classified as **vegetative** or **aerial.**
   a. Vegetative hyphae function in food absorption, and are the portion that extends under the surface of the agar or nutrient substrate.
   b. Aerial hyphae extend above the agar or nutrient substrate, and their function is to support reproductive structures called **conidia.**

3. **Conidia** are sporelike structures that function in asexual reproduction. **Conidia are only formed in imperfect fungi.**
   a. Conidia shape is important in fungal identification.
   b. Conidia classification is based on conidia morphological development.
   c. **Microconidia** are single-celled, small conidia.
   d. **Macroconidia** are multicellular, large conidia.

4. Types of conidia
   a. **Arthroconidia:** conidia resulting from the fragmentation of hyphae into individual cells.
   b. **Blastoconidia:** conidia that form as the result of budding.
   c. **Chlamydoconidia:** conidia resulting from terminal cells in the hyphae that enlarge and have thick walls. These conidia can survive adverse environmental conditions.
   d. **Porocondidia:** conidia formed by being pushed through a small pore in the parent cell.
   e. **Phialoconidia:** conidia that are tube-shaped, and can be branched.
   f. **Annelloconidia:** conidia that are vase-shaped; the remaining parent outer cell wall takes on a saw-toothed appearance as the conidia are released.

5. **Mycology Terms**
   a. Molds: multicellular fungi.

key concepts

Describe fungal structure, including hyphae, conidia, spores, and reproduction.

    b. Yeasts: single cell fungi.

    c. Mycoses: fungal infections.

    d. Systemic mycosis: multiorgan infections.

    e. Opportunistic mycoses: fungi infecting the immunocompromised.

    f. Dimorphic fungi: fungi that show both a yeast and mold phase.

B. Sexual and Asexual Reproduction

1. **Sexual reproduction**

    a. a Requires the formation of specialized fungal structures called **spores.**

    b. Fungi that undergo sexual reproduction are termed **perfect fungi.**

    c. Types of spores

      1) **Ascospores:** spores contained in a saclike structure.

      2) **Basidiospores:** spores contained in a club-shaped structure.

      3) **Oospores:** spores resulting from the fusion of cells from two different hyphae.

      4) **Zygospores:** spores resulting from the fusion of two identical hyphae.

2. **Asexual reproduction**

    a. Asexual reproduction only involves division of the nucleus and cytoplasm.

    b. Fungi that undergo asexual reproduction are termed **imperfect fungi.**

    c. **Imperfect fungi are the only fungal group to produce conidia.**

II. CULTURE AND ISOLATION

A. Types of Fungal Media

1. **Sabouraud brain heart infusion agar (SABHI)**

    a. A nonselective media for general isolation.

    b. Contains dextrose, peptone, and brain heart infusion.

    c. Will grow most fungi (and bacteria).

2. **Brain heart infusion agar with blood (BHIB)**

    a. Used to grow most fungi, especially those from sterile body sites.

    b. Contains brain heat infusion and sheep blood.

3. **Sabouraud dextrose agar (SDA)**

    a. Used to grow most fungal pathogens.

    b. The agar has an acidic pH and is nutritionally poor which inhibits most bacteria.

4. **Selective agars** contain various antibiotics that will enhance the growth of specific fungal pathogens and will inhibit bacteria and other undesired growth.

    a. **Inhibitory mold agar (IMA)**

      1) Used to grow most fungal pathogens.

      2) Contains gentamicin.

    b. **Dermatophye test medium (DTM)**

      1) Used to grow skin fungi (dermatophytes).

key concepts

Discuss the different types of fungal media in terms of uses, composition, and inhibition properties.

2) Contains antibiotics and phenol red indicators.
c. Other selective agars include **brain heart infusion with blood, gentamicin,** and **chloramphenicol.**

5. **Differential agars** are used to enhance pigment development, conidia production, and mold to yeast phase enhancement.
   a. **Potato dextrose agar (PDA)**
      1) Used to enhance conidia development.
      2) Enhances pigment development of *Trichophyton rubrum.*
   b. **Birdseed agar:** used to grow *C. neoformans,* produces black to brown colonies.
   c. **Cottonseed agar:** causes *Blastomyces dermatidis* to convert from the mold to yeast phase.
   d. **Cornmeal Tween 80:** Used to differentiate *Candida* species.
   e. **Agars containing rice, casein, and other nutrients** are used to differentiate *Trichophyton* species.

B. Culture Considerations

1. Fungal cultures are incubated at 30°C.
2. Growth requires from several days to several weeks.
3. Cultures should be maintained in a moist environment.
4. Several techniques are used to obtain culture material for slide preparation.
   a. Tease mount method: a dissecting needle is used to pull apart a fungal colony, which is placed on a slide. This method may damage fungal structure, especially conidia.
   b. Cellophane tape method: used to view aerial hyphae.
   c. Slide culture method: contains a fragment of agar containing fungal colonies. This method prevents damage to the fungal structure.

> **key concepts**
> List the temperature and time requirements important in culturing fungus.

C. Direct Examination Methods

1. **Saline wet mount** is used to view fungal elements, such as hyphae, conidia, and budding yeasts.
2. **Lactophenol cotton blue wet mount** is used to stain and preserve fungal elements.
3. **Potassium hydroxide (KOH)** is used to dissolve nonfungal materials in skin, nail, and hair samples.
4. **Gram stains** are used to view yeasts and *C. neoformans.*
5. **India ink** is used to show capsules surrounding *C. neoformans* from CSF.
6. **Calcofluor white stain** shows fungal cell walls; the stain is not absorbed by human tissue. The slide is viewed using fluorescence. Fungi will appear a certain color depending on wavelength.
7. **Wright stain** is used to show yeast forms of *H. capsulatum.*

> **key concepts**
> Discuss the fungal stains used in microscopic analysis.

III. BODY SITES AND POSSIBLE FUNGAL PATHOGENS (MOST COMMON)

A. **Blood**—*Candida spp., Blastomyces dermatitidis, Histoplasma capsulatum,* and *Cryptococcus neoformans.*

> **key concepts**
> Name fungal pathogens associated with various body sites and body specimens.

B. **CSF**—*Cryptococcus neoformans, Candida spp., Histoplasma capsulatum,* and *Coccidioides immitis.*

C. **Hair**—*Microsporum* and *Trichophyton spp.*

D. **Nail**—*Aspergillus, Epidermophyton,* and *Trichophyton spp.*

E. **Skin**—*Candida spp.,* (heavy growth), *Microsporum, Trichophyton,* and *Epidermophyton spp.*

F. **Lungs**—*Candida albicans* (heavy growth), *Aspergillus, Rhizopus,* and *Penicillium spp.*

G. **Throat**—*Candida albicans* (heavy growth) and *Geotrichum candidum.*

H. **Urine**—*Candida albicans* (heavy growth).

I. **Genital (Vaginal, Uterine, Cervix)**—*Candida albicans* (heavy growth).

IV. CUTANEOUS AND SUPERFICIAL FUNGI (DERMATOPHYTOSIS)

A. Introduction
1. Cutaneous and superficial mycoses are infections of the skin, hair, and nails.
2. Superficial mycoses are infections that involve the outer epithelial layers of the skin and top layers of the hair and nails.
3. Cutaneous mycoses involve deeper layers of the skin with more tissue
4. **Dermatophytes** is the term used to group the various fungi that cause infections of the skin, hair, and nails.
   a. Dermatophytes contain 3 genera.
      1) *Trichophyton*
      2) *Epidermophyton*
      3) *Microsporum*
5. Superficial and cutaneous fungi are rarely invasive to other areas of the body.

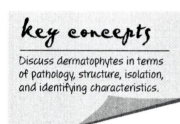

key concepts

Discuss dermatophytes in terms of pathology, structure, isolation, and identifying characteristics.

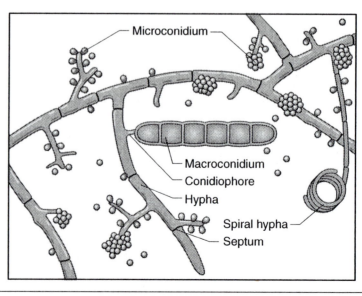

FIGURE 9-1. Trichophyton

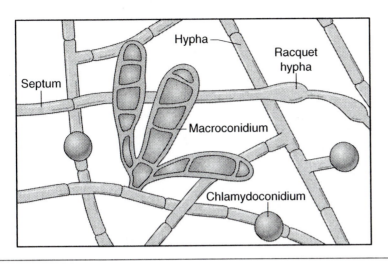

FIGURE 9-2. Epidermophyton

6. All fungal skin infections are termed **Tinea.**
7. **Types of Tinea infections and their causative agents**
   a. *Tinea pedia* or **athlete's foot:** is an infection of the spaces between the toes.
      1) Caused by *Trichophyton* species and *Epidermophyton* species.
      2) Characterized by itching and scaling.
   b. *Tinea corporis* or **ringworm:** an infection of smooth skin.
      1) Caused by *Microsporum* species and *Trichophyton* species.
      2) Characterized by circular patches of scaly skin.

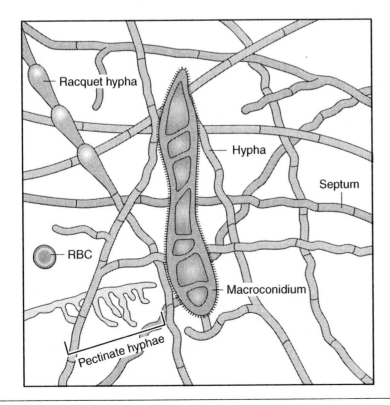

FIGURE 9-3. Microsporum

     c. *Tinea unguium* or **onychomycosis:** an infection of the nails.
       1) Caused by *Epidermophyton* species and *Trichophyton* species.
       2) Characterized by discoloration, thickening, and progressive destruction of the nails.
     d. *Tinea capitis*: an infection of the scalp.
       1) Caused by *Microsporum* species and *Trichophyton* species.
       2) Characterized by circular bald patches on the scalp.
     e. *Tinea barbae* or **barber's itch:** an infection of beard hair.
       1) Caused by *Microsporum* species and *Trichophyton* species.
       2) Characterized by skin lesions.
     f. *Tinea cruris* or **jock itch** is an infection of the groin.
       1) Caused by *Trichophyton* species and *Epidermophyton* species.
       2) Characterized by itching and scaling of the groin area.

B. **General Culture and Microscopic Characteristics of Dermatophytes**—the following are only general characteristics of the genera, individual species may show additional characteristics.
  1. **Trichophyton**
    a. **Culture** characteristics: 2 colony types will be seen between 7 to 10 days on SABHI at room temperature.
      1) Buff granular colonies, rose to tan colored, with a yellow, brown, or red reverse.
      2) White fluffy colonies with a colorless to yellow reverse.
    b. Microscopic characteristics
      1) Macroconidia are smooth /thin walled, pencil shaped, contain 3–7 cells, and are few in number.
      2) Microconidia are round to club shaped in grape-like clusters, and are few to numerous in number.

  2. **Epidermophyton**
    a. **Culture** characteristics: on SABHI at room temperature, colonies will appear yellow with a tan reverse within 10 days.
    b. Microscopic characteristics
      1) Macroconidia are smooth/thin walled, club shaped, contain 2 to 5 cells, and are numerous in number.
      2) Microcondia are not present.

  3. **Microsporum**
    a. **Culture** characteristics: on SABHI at room temperature, colonies will be light tan, with a salmon-colored reverse. Microsporum are very slow growers.
    b. Microscopic characteristics
      1) Macroconidia are rough/thin to thick walled, spindle shaped, contain 4–8 cells, and are numerous in number.
      2) Microconidia are club shaped, single, and are few in number.

V. YEASTS
A. Introduction
  1. Yeasts are common causes of UTIs (urinary track infections) in women, and can cause a number of other diseases in healthy and

immunosuppressed individuals. In addition, yeast can cause new-born infections and meningitis. The 2 most common causes of yeast infections are **Candida albicans** and **Cryptococcus neoformans**.

2. Methods for Identification
   a. Microscopic
      1) Saline wet mounts and Gram stains will show budding yeast.
      2) Yeasts are discovered in routine urinalysis.
      3) **India ink** preparations are used to show the capsule surrounding **Crytococcus neoformans**.
   b. Culturing
      1) Yeasts are grown on SABHI at between 25–30° C.
      2) Yeasts will form cream-colored, mucoid to smooth colonies within several days. On blood agar, yeast colonies will appear like *Staphylococcus* colonies.
   c. **Yeast agars**
      1) **Cornmeal agar with Tween 80**
         a) Used to differentiate *Candida* species by enhancing the formation of fungal elements such as hyphae and conidia.
         b) **C. albicans** will show chlamydospores with clusters of blastoconidia along the hyphae.
   d. **Germ tube production**
      1) **Germ tubes** are hyphaelike extensions of young yeast cells showing parallel sides, nonseptate (showing no cell wall division), and will not constrict at their point of origin. **Note: Pseudohyphae** look like germ tubes but are septate and constricted at their point of origin.
      2) Germ tube procedure: incubate yeast with serum at 37° C for 2 hours and look for germ tube production.
      3) **Candida albicans** are positive for germ tube production.
         a) **Candida tropicalis** is use for the negative control.
   e. **Carbohydrate assimilation test**
      1) Used for identification of yeasts based on carbohydrate utilization.
      2) Different carbohydrates are impregnated in agar. Growth around the different carbohydrates indicates a positive result for that particular carbohydrate.
   f. **Urease Test**
      1) Used to identify **Cryptococcus neoformans** which is urease **positive.**
      2) **C. albicans** is used for the negative control.
      3) A positive urease is indicated by a pink to purple color.
   g. **Serological** testing is available for *Cryptococcus neoformans* and for *Candida albicans*.

B. Clinically Significant Yeasts
1. **Candida albicans**
   a. The most common yeast isolate, and the causative agent for candidiasis (a general term for *Candida* infections).

b. Normal flora of the mucus membranes lining the respiratory, GI, and the female urogenital tract.

c. **Types of candidiasis**
   1) Thrush (mouth)
   2) Vulvovaginitis (vagina)
   3) Onychomycosis (nail infections)
   4) Paronychomycosis (cuticle infections)

d. *C. albicans* can also cause systemic infections, including meningitis, UTIs, heart, and lung infections.

e. Predisposition to *Candida* infections includes burns, wounds, diabetes mellitus, antibiotic therapy, pregnancy, leukemia, and immune problems.

2. *Cryptococcus neoformans*

a. Causes cryptococcosis, which can produce a mild-to-moderate pulmonary infection; however, in the immunocompromised patient, cryptococcois can lead to meningitis. Cryptococcosis is also associated with prostate and tissue infections.

b. *C. neoformans* can be acquired by contact with pigeon, bat, or other bird droppings, in addition to contaminated vegetables, fruit, and milk.

c. Identifying characteristics for direct specimens
   1) India ink will show the capsule surrounding the organism.
   2) On Gram stain the yeasts appear in spherical form, and are not of uniform size.
   3) Biochemical tests include:
      a) Positive for urease and phenol oxidase
      b) Inositol utilization
      c) Negative for nitrate reduction
   4) Hematoxylin and eosin (HE) stains are used to show capsules in tissue.

d. Culture characteristics: Niger seed agar: brown to black colonies.

VI. OPPORTUNISTIC FUNGI

A. Introduction

1. Many fungi rarely cause disease in healthy individuals, but can cause disease in individuals with medical conditions and in the immunosuppressed.

2. General Characteristics of Opportunistic Fungi
   a. Most form colonies within several days (rapid-growers).
   b. Humans acquire through inhalation of the conidia.
   c. Most opportunistic fungi live on organic matter (**saprophytic fungi**) found in the soil.
   d. **Are very common in the environment.**
   e. Laboratory identification
      1) Opportunistic fungi are inhibited by many antibiotics; therefore, media should not contain these substances.
      2) **Must be repeatedly isolated in patients** in significant numbers because they are frequent contaminants and are found in high numbers in the environment.

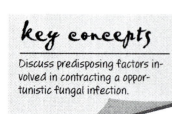

key concepts

Discuss predisposing factors involved in contracting a opportunistic fungal infection.

3) Identification is based on microscopic morphology.

4) Enhancement media should be used for conidia formation.

B. Clinically Significant Opportunistic Fungi

1. *Aspergillus Spp.*

   a. Causes **aspergillosis,** which can infect the skin, heart, lungs, and CNS. Pulmonary aspergillosis affects the bronchi, lungs, or sinuses.

   b. *Aspergillus fumigatus* is the most common cause of aspergillosis.

   c. General identifying characteristics of the genus:

      1) Colony: granular/fluffy, or powdery growth within 2 days on SABHI. Pigmentation varies according to species.

      2) Microscopic: hyphae are septate that terminate in a large, spherical conidiophore.

   d. *Aspergillus* species with identifying characteristics:

      1) *A. niger:* colonies are yellow to black with a yellow reverse.

      2) *A. flavus:* colonies are green to brown with red brown reverse.

      3) *A. terreus:* colonies are green to yellow with yellow reverse.

      4) *A. clavatus:* colonies are blue to green with white reverse.

      5) *A. fumigatus:* colonies are green to gray with a tan reverse.

2. **Zygomycetes**

   a. Members of the Zygomycetes class include Absidia, Mucor, Rhizomucor, Rhizopus, and Syncephalastrum.

   b. Cause of infections known as zygomycoses and mucormycoses.

      1) Produce allergic reactions in susceptible individuals.

      2) Cause infections of the lungs or paranasal sinuses.

      3) Spores gaining entry into body sites can cause infections to those areas.

      4) Zygomycetes produce toxins that can cause gastrointestinal infections.

      5) Blood infections can lead to CNS disorders.

   c. General class identifying characteristics

      1) Colony: growth after several days is dense, colonies show a cotton candy texture, and pigmentation ranges from white, gray, to brown.

      2) Microscopic: hyphae can be septate or aseptate, and are ribbonlike and thin-walled.

      3) Zygomycetes form **rhizoids,** which resemble tree roots that function in attachment and nutrient absorption.

VII. SUBCUTANEOUS FUNGI

A. Introduction

1. Fungi causing subcutaneous mycoses can gain entry into the skin by means of trauma to the skin.

2. Resulting subcutaneous lesions are characterized by being chronic, hard, crusted, and ulcerated.

3. The feet are commonly affected.

key concepts

Name the subcutaneous fungi and list their unique identifying characteristics.

4. Humans acquire the infections from vegetation contaminated with the fungi.

5. Subcutaneous mycoses are mainly caused by **dematiaceous fungi,** which is a group of slow-growing fungi found in the soil and vegetation.

6. **Types of subcutaneous mycoses**

   a. **Mycetoma:** a granulomatous infection of the subcutaneous tissue, which causes cutaneous abscesses. Exudate from mycetomas will contain red, yellow, or black granules. Most infections are found in Africa. Causative agents include *Pseudoallescheria, Exophilia, Acremonium,* and *Madurella.*

   b. **Chromoblastomycosis:** Chromoblastomycosis is a localized infection characterized by chronic, hard, or tumorlike lesions. Most infections involve the feet or lower legs. Seen mostly in tropical areas of the world. Most infections are caused by *Fonsecaea pedrosoi.* Other fungi causing chromoblastomycosis are *Phialophora, Cladosporium, Exophiala,* and *Wangiella.* Identifying characteristics: Lesions are examined for **sclerotic bodies** (copper colored fungal cells). Colonies are folded or heaped, and are gray to black.

   c. **Phaeohyphomycosis:** Superficial or subcutaneous infections that can become systemic. Resulting systemic infections can cause endocarditis, and brain abscesses. Fungi causing phaeohyphomycosis include *Bipolaris, Curvularia,* and *Phialophora.* Identifying characteristics: Microscopic examination shows yellow septate hyphae that may contain budding yeast cells.

   d. **Sporotrichosis:** a subcutaneous infection, lymph and pulmonary infections can occur. Also known as Rose gardener's disease. Can get the infection from rose thorns. Caused by *Sporothrix schenckii,* which is a **dimorphic** fungus (mold and yeast phase). Identifying characteristics: Colonies will be wrinkled, with a cream to black color. Yeast cells may be seen in segmented neutrophils.

VIII. SYSTEMIC DIMORPHIC FUNGI

A. Introduction

1. This fungal group can disseminate to any of the body's organ systems.

2. Dimorphic fungi exhibit two growth phases, including the yeast (when grown on media with blood) and mold phase (when grown on Sab. dextrose agar).

3. **Most dimorphic fungi will exhibit the yeast phase at 35°–37°C, and the mold (or mycelial) phase at 25–30°C.**

4. Identifying characteristics

   a. Based on temperature/medium requirements, colonial and conidia/hyphae morphology.

   b. Slants are used to culture because the **mold forms are highly infective.**

   c. Colonies are membranous that develop tan aerial mycelia.

   d. Conidia identification is necessary in species identification.

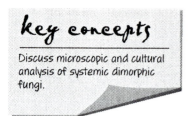

key concepts

Discuss microscopic and cultural analysis of systemic dimorphic fungi.

   e. **Conversion of dimorphic fungi from the mold to yeast phase is confirmation that the fungus in question is dimorphic.**
5. Systemic dimorphic fungi include:
   a. *Blastomyces dermatitidis* (blastomycosis)
   b. *Coccidioides immitis* (cocccidioidomycosis)
   c. *Histoplasma capsulatum* (histoplasmosis) ·
   d. *Paracoccidioides brasiliensis* (paracoccidioidomycosis)
6. Most systemic dimorphic fungi are very slow growers requiring 3–7 weeks to grow.
7. ***Blastomyces dermatitidis***
   a. Causes blastomycosis, which is a respiratory infection that can infect the skin and bones. Can be mild to chronic.
   b. Acquired by conidia or hyphae inhalation.
   c. *Blastomyces* organisms can be cultured from tissue or body fluids.
   d. Identifying characteristics
      1) Microscopic
         a) Mold phase: single smooth-walled, round to oval conidia at the ends of short conidiophores.
         b) Yeast phase: large, round, thick-walled, budding yeasts.
      2) Culture
         a) At room temperature a yeastlike colony develops, and the colony over time will become fluffy white to tan.
         b) Conversion from the mold to yeast phase requires 4–6 days.
8. ***Coccidioides immitis***
   a. Causes coccidioidomycosis, which causes an infection of the lungs, bones, joints, skin, lymph nodes, CNS, and adrenal glands.
   b. Can be acute or chronic, self-limiting or requiring medications.
   c. Most infections are in the southwest, and may be called desert fever or valley fever in the San Joaquin Valley in California where many cases are diagnosed.
   d. Infections can be acquired through spore inhalation from the environment.
   e. Identifying characteristics
      1) Microscopic
         a) Branching thick-walled, rectangular (barrel shaped) conidia.
         b) Tissue phase shows round, thick-walled sporangia filled with small endospores.
      2) Culture
         a) At 37°C on SABHI agar, colonies will appear moist white that turn fluffy white in about a week.
         b) **As with all mold phase fungi, always use a hood to prevent inhalation of spores.**
9. **Histoplasma capsulatum**
   a. Causes histoplasmosis, a fatal pulmonary infection, but can also spread to the spleen, liver, kidneys, and heart.

    b. Infection is acquired by spore inhalation from barns, chicken houses, and bat caves.

    c. Most infections occur in the southern and midwestern United States, and along the Appalachian Mountains.

    d. Identifying characteristics

        1) Microscopic

            a) The mold phase will show conidia at 90-degree angles to hyphae. Macroconidia are smooth with finlike edges. Microconidia are small, round to teardrop shaped.

            b) Yeast will appear as small single-budding cells that are unremarkable in morphology.

        2) Culture

            a) Mature colonies are woolly and velvety appearing tan colored.

10. *Paracoccidioides brasiliensis*

    a. Causes paracoccidioidomycosis, which is a chronic granulomatous disease of the lungs and skin. Can spread to the liver and spleen.

    b. Mostly found in South America.

    c. Acquired by spore inhalation or ingestion.

    d. Identifying characteristics

        1) Microscopic

            a) Yeast cells are thick-walled, multiple budding yeast cells with very narrow necks.

        2) Culture

            a) Colonies are smooth with white to tan aerial mycelium.

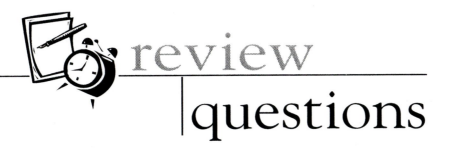

review questions

DIRECTIONS Each of the questions or incomplete statements below is followed by suggested answers or completions. Select the **one answer** that is best in each case.

1. Which characteristic is NOT correct when describing conidia?
   a. Function in asexual reproduction
   b. Only found in perfect fungi
   c. Important in fungal identification
   d. None of the above

2. Fungi that undergo asexual reproduction are termed:
   a. Imperfect
   b. Perfect.
   c. Septate.
   d. Aseptate.

3. Which of the following contains antibiotics and phenol red indicators, used to grow skin fungi?
   a. Inhibitory mold agar
   b. Dermatophye test media
   c. Potato dextrose agar
   d. Birdseed agar

4. Which type of environment will enhance fungal growth?
   a. Dry
   b. Humid
   c. Warm and dry
   d. Cool and dry

5. Calcofluor white stain is used to:
   a. Preserve fungal elements.
   b. Dissolve non-fungal elements.
   c. Stain fungal cell walls without staining human tissue.
   d. Show capsules of *Cryptococcus neoformans* in CSF.

6. Which of the following is caused by Microsporum species and Trichophyton species, and characterized by erythematous lesions?
   a. Ringworm
   b. Oncychomycosis
   c. Barber's itch
   d. Jock itch

7. Which genus produces two colony types at 7–10 days on SABHI, one of which will be rose to tan with a yellow/brown reverse; the other type will show white fluffy colonies with a colorless/yellow reverse?
   a. Trichophyton
   b. Epidermophyton
   c. Microsporum
   d. Mucor

8. Which of the following is the method for producing germ tubes?
   a. Growth on blood agar
   b. Add serum to yeast at 37°C for two hours
   c. Add glucose to yeast, incubate at 37°C for three hours
   d. Growth on horse blood agar

9. Which of the following is correct regarding germ tube production controls?
   a. *Candida tropicalis* is used for the positive control.
   b. *Candida albicans* is use for the negative control.
   c. *Cryptococcus neoformans* is used for the positive control.
   d. *Candida tropicalis* is used for the negative control.

10. Which of the following are CORRECT statements? (select all that apply)

   a. Aspergillus spp. is a very common laboratory contaminant.
   b. Penicillium can cause pulmonary, ear, skin, and bladder infections.
   c. Thizopus can cause rare cases of mycotic keratitis.
   d. Helminthosporium causes onchomysosis.
   e. Tinea capitis is an infection of the scalp.
   f. Blastoconidia are conidia that form as a result of budding.
   g. KOH is used to observe Cryptococcus neoforman capsules in CSF.

10

Clinical Virology

contents

➤ **COMPREHENSIVE KEY CONCEPT**

1. Correlate sample collection, processing, and transport with body site infection and diagnostic methodologies.

_____

I. INTRODUCTION
A. General Characteristics
1. Obligate intracellular organisms.
2. Contains DNA or RNA (single or double stranded); viruses lack ribosomal RNA.
3. Do not have a system to produce ATP.
4. Viruses range in size from 25–270nm.
5. 21 families of viruses cause human disease, 14 of which are RNA viruses, and 7 are DNA viruses.
6. Identification is based on nucleic acid type, size, shape, and if an envelope is present.

B. Viral Structure
1. Viron is the entire viral particle.
2. Capsid is the protein coat that enclosed the genetic material.
3. Capsomer are protein subunits that make up the capsid.
   a. Structure of attachment for entry into the host cell.
   b. Vary in size and shape.
4. Nucleocapsid is composed of the capsid and genetic material.
5. Envelope is the outer membrane, composed of a phospholipid bilayer, which is composed of glycoproteins and matrix proteins. Naked nucleocapsids are viruses with no envelops.

C. Replication
1. Adsorption is attachment of the virus to the host cell.
2. Pentration is entry of the virus into the host cell.
3. Uncoating is the loss of the capsid within the host cell that allows viral genetic material to be exposed.
4. Eclipse is the replication and expression stage of the genetic material.
   a. Viral DNA or RNA serves as the template for mRNA production.
   b. mRNA codes for viral protein synthesis.
   c. Genetic material is assembled into a protein coat, and is further assembled into a whole virus.
   d. Viruses are then released from the host cell.

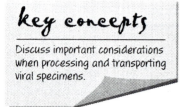

key concepts

Discuss important considerations when processing and transporting viral specimens.

D. Specimen Processing
1. Samples should be collected early in the disease course.
2. Viruses are in highest concentrations during the first several days following symptoms.
3. Samples should come from the infected site.
   a. Skin infections: rash site.
   b. Respiratory infections: sputum or throat swabs.

    c. CNS: stool or throat swabs. CSF is not cultured because CNS viruses shed viruses into the throat or stool where they are cultured.

E. Sample Transport
1. Viral samples must have a cell culture transport medium.
2. Viral transport medium contains:
    a. Buffered saline
    b. Protein stabilizers
    c. Antibiotics that inhibit nonviral growth
3. Viral cultures can be frozen; however, their antigenicity will be diminished.

II. SAMPLE SITES AND ASSOCIATED VIRAL CAUSES
A. Upper Respiratory System
1. Sputum, throat swabs, secretions, and aspirates.
2. Caused by rhinovirus, influenza, parainfluenza, respiratory syncytial virus (RSV), Epstein-Barr virus (EBV), Herpes Simplex virus 1 and 2 (HSV-1, HSV-2), and coronavirus.
3. Croup and bronchitis can be caused by influenza, parainfluenza, RSV, and adenovirus.
4. Pneumonia in children can be caused by RSV, parainfluenza, adenovirus, measles, and varicella-zoster virus (VZV).
5. Pneumonia in adults can be caused by influenza, HSV, VZV, cytomegalovirus (CMV), and RSV.

key concepts

List the causative viral agent responsible for disease by body site and the required specimen for viral identification.

B. Viral Meningitis
1. CSF, throat swabs, stool samples, serum, and urine (mumps).
2. Caused by enterovirus, echovirus, HSV-2, VZV, mumps, and lymphocytic choriomeningitis virus (LCM).

C. Encephalitis
1. Brain biopsy and serum.
2. Caused by HSV-1, VZV, and arbovirus.

D. Cutaneous Rashes
1. Throat swabs, stool samples, serum, and urine (CMV).
2. Caused by HSV-1, HSV-2, echovirus, mealses, rubella, enterovivus, CMV, EBV, and parvovirus B-19.

E. Urogenital Infections (Urethritis, Cervicitis, Penile Infections, etc.)
1. Needle aspirates and endocervical swabs.
2. Caused by HSV-2.

F. Gastroenteritis
1. Stool samples and rectal swabs.
2. Caused by adenovirus and calcivirus.

G. Eye Infections
1. Eye swabs and surface scrapings.
2. Caused by HSV, adenovirus, and VZV.

H. Neonatal Infections
1. Urine, throat swabs, and serum.
2. Caused by rubella, HSV, and CMV.

III. VIRAL IDENTIFICATION
A. Histology and Cytology
1. Cellular inclusions are diagnostic for many viruses.
2. DNA viruses produce nuclear inclusions since they are assembled in the nucleus.
3. RNA viruses produce cytoplasmic inclusions (assembled in the cytoplasm).
4. HSV and VZV cause intranuclear inclusions, and CMV causes "owl eye" inclusions.

B. Cell Culture
1. Cell culture is the primary means of identifying viruses.
2. Primary cell cultures are derived directly from infected tissue.
   a. Diploid cell lines include 75 percent of cells with the same karyotype as the original parent tissue. Used to grow influenze, parainfluenze, mumps, enterovirus, and adenoviruses.
   b. Heteroploid cell lines include greater than 25 percent of cells having an abnormal karyotype from the original parent tissue.
      1) Used to grow HSV, VZV, CMV, adenovirus, and rhinoviruses.
3. Slides are made from cell cultures and examined for cellular changes, including clumping, vacuoles, granules, cell fusion, multinucleated cell development, and cellular destruction.

C. Electron Microscopy
1. Due to size, viral structure can only be seen by electron microscopy.
2. Electron microscopy is the only method to identify Norwalk agent, astrovirus, calicivirus, and coronavirus, as these viral agents cannot be cell cultured.

D. Other Methods for Identification
1. Direct detection of viral antigens.
2. Serological detection of viral antibodies.
3. Viral gene probes.

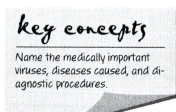

key concepts

Name the medically important viruses, diseases caused, and diagnostic procedures.

IV. MEDICALLY IMPORTANT VIRUSES
A. Adenovirus
1. Identifying Characteristics
   a. Contain DNA, icosahedral shaped, contain no envelope, and their size ranges from 70–90nm.
2. Infections
   a. Respiratory tract infections, especially in young children.
   b. UTIs, GI infections, and pharyngitis.
   c. Eye infections in newborns, immunosuppressed patients, and military recruits (due to congested living environment).
3. Sample collection: throat swabs, eye samples, and stool.

B. Hepatitis A Virus (HAV)

1. Identifying characteristics
   a. Contains RNA, icosahedral shaped, contains no envelope, and size ranges from 24–30nm.
   b. Member of the *Picornaviridae* family and the *Enterovirus* genus.
2. Infections
   a. Infections are spread by the fecal-oral route, and are generally due to poor sanitation and hygiene. Food handling transmission is common. Can also acquire the infection from contaminated shellfish, including shrimp, oysters, scallops, etc.
3. Clinical picture
   a. 15–40-day incubation period.
   b. Liver involvement (jaundice), nausea, anorexia, and malaise.
   c. Mortality rate is less than 1 percent.
4. Diagnosis is by clinical symptoms and serology.
5. Serological indicators
   a. General serology testing includes hepatitis B surface antigen and hepatitis B core antibody.
   b. Anti-HAV IgM is positive in acute infections.
   c. Anti-HAV (positive) and anti-HAV IgM (negative) indicate a past HAV infection.

> **key concepts**
>
> Compare the different antigenic types of hepatitis virus according to spread of infection, clinical picture, and diagnosis.

C. Hepatitis B Virus (HBV)

1. Identifying characteristics
   a. Contains DNA, has an envelope, size range is between 42–47nm, and contains Dane particles (double-shell particles).
   b. Member of the *Hepadnaviridae* family.
2. Infections
   a. Infections are spread by contaminated body fluids, including blood.
   b. Infections are acquired by contaminated blood products, needle sticks, tatoos, body piercing, IV drug abuse, and renal dialysis.
   c. HBV vaccines are available and are recommended for all health care workers.
3. Clinical picture
   a. 50–180-day incubation period.
   b. Liver involvement leading to fatal hepatitis.
4. Diagnosis
   a. Clinical symptoms and serology.
5. Serological indicators
   a. HBsAg: Is the first marker to be positive, but will become negative as the patient recovers. In chronic infections, HBsAg will remain positive.
   b. Anti-HBsAg: indicates total Ab to HBsAg, and is positive for life. Also indicates recovery or immunity after HBV vaccination.
   c. Anti-HBcAg-IgM: indicates recent acute infection.

  d. Anti-HBcAg: total Ab to HBcAg. Is highly positive in acute infection stages. Also indicates current or past infections, but does not indicate recovery or immunity.
  e. HBeAg: is positive in acute and chronic stages of infection; also indicates the level of infections.
  f. Anti-HBeAb: associated with a good prognosis.

D. Hepatitis C Virus (HCV)
1. Identifying characteristics
   a. Contains RNA, has a lipid envelope.
   b. Related to the *Flaviviridae* family.
2. Infections
   a. Causes what used to be considered Non-A, Non-B hepatitis (NANB).
   b. Spread through contaminated blood products, organ transplants, renal dialysis, and IV drug abuse.
3. Clinical picture
   a. 2–25 week incubation period.
   b. Liver involvement, including cirrhosis and liver cancer.
   c. No vaccine currently exists for HCV.
4. Diagnosis
   a. Increased liver enzymes, including ALT.
   b. Serological indicators
      1) HBcAg is positive.
      2) Anti-HBcAg is positive.

E. Hepatitis D Virus (HDV)
1. Also called delta virus.
2. Contains RNA and their size ranges from 35 to 37nm.
3. HBV must be present before HDV is infective.
4. Diagnosis: serology.

F. Hepatitis E Virus (HEV)
1. Contains RNA, size is 32–34nm.
2. Associated with NANB hepatitis.
3. Spread by contaminated water.
4. Diagnosis includes Western blot assays.

G. Herpesviruses
1. General characteristics
   a. Contain DNA, icosahedral shaped, has envelopes, and range in size from 90 to 100nm.
   b. Member of the *Herpetoviridae* family.
   c. Produce latent viral infections.
   d. Sites of latency include leukocytes and peripheral nerves.
   e. Reactivation may result from physiological stress.
   f. Infections are more severe in adults than in children.
   g. Herpesviruses include Herpes Simplex virus (HSV), Varicella-Zoster virus (VZV), cytomegalovirus (CMV), Epstein-Barr virus (EBV) and human herpes virus Type 6 (HHV-6).
   h. Infections are usually more severe in adults.

2. **Herpes Simplex Virus-1 (HSV-1)**
   a. Cause mouth lesions and fever blisters.
   b. Most cases are very mild, and require no treatment.
   c. Other symptoms may include mild fever and general malaise.

3. **Herpes Simplex Virus-2 (HSV-2)**
   a. Is the causative agent of genital herpes, which is a common STD.
   b. Lesions appear on the penis, cervix, and vagina.
   c. Has been shown to have an **association with cervical carcinoma.**
   d. Infant infection acquired during childbirth can cause CNS damage.
   e. Sample collection is from genital lesions.
   f. Diagnosis is by clinical symptoms and DFA or immunological methods.

4. **Varicella-Zoster Virus (VZV)**
   a. Causes two major diseases
      1) Varicella or chickenpox
      2) Herpes Zoster or shingles
   b. **Chickenpox**
      1) Is a childhood illness; however, adults can become infected producing more serious symptoms.
      2) Produces a skin rash with fever.
      3) Infection is spread by respiratory aerosol.
      4) The incubation period is from 1 to 2 weeks.
      5) Individuals are contagious 48 hours before the rash and will remain contagious until scabbing of all lesions.
      6) **Aspirin should not be given due to an association with Reye's syndrome.**
   c. **Shingles**
      1) Reactivation of the chickenpox virus in the peripheral or cranial nerves.
      2) Reactivation is due to physiological stress.
      3) Produces skin vesicles and severe pain around the rash site.
      4) Complications include CNS disorders, eye problems, and facial paralysis.
      5) Occurs mainly in the elderly.
      6) Diagnosis is from clinical symptoms.

5. **Cytomegalovirus (CMV)**
   a. Causes opportunistic infections that produce mild symptoms, but may be asymptomatic.
   b. The virus is transmitted through contact with saliva or blood.
   c. Congenital infections cause developmental problems for the newborn.
   d. Diagnosis is by serological testing of saliva, milk, semen, or blood.

6. **Epstein-Barr Virus (EBV)**
   a. Is associated with **Burkitt's lymphoma, chronic fatigue syndrome,** and **infectious mononucleosis.**
   b. The virus is found in the saliva.

c. Incubation lasts between 1 to 2 months, and will cause fever, enlarged lymph nodes, and swollen tonsils.

d. Diagnosis is by serology.

7. **Human Herpesvirus Type 6 (HHV-6)**

a. Infects T-lymphocytes.

b. The virus is contracted by respiratory contact.

c. Causes exanthem subitum, also known as **roseola or sixth disease.**

d. Sixth disease causes rash, sore throat, and fever in children.

H. Human Papilloma Virus (HPV)

1. Member of the *Papovaviridae* family

2. Contains DNA, icosahedral shaped, has envelopes, and their size ranges from 40–55nm.

3. Causes plantar warts, venereal warts, and other cutaneous lesions. Some HPV are **associated with cervical cancer.**

I. Picornavirus

1. Contains RNA, no envelope, and ranges in size from 20–30nm.

2. The *Picornaviruses* include poliovirus, coxsackie virus, echovirus, enterovirus, and rhinovirus

3. **Poliovirus**

a. Causes polio, which is transmitted by the fecal-oral route.

b. Two types of vaccines have been used against poliovirus.

1) **Salk vaccine** is a formalin-killed vaccine.

2) **Sabin vaccine** is a live, attenuated vaccine (more commonly used).

4. **Coxsackie Virus**

a. Causes meningitis, pharyngitis, and myocarditis.

b. Coxsackie A causes foot and mouth disease.

5. **Echovirus**

a. Associated with causing nonspecific fever, upper respiratory infections, and meningitis.

6. **Enterovirus**

a. Causes gastroenteritis.

b. Usually isolated from stool samples.

7. **Rhinovirus**

a. Causes the **common cold.**

b. Over 100 serotypes are known, therefore, identification is usually not done.

c. Prevention includes adequate hand washing and avoiding hand to nose contact.

J. Orthomyxovirus

1. RNA viruses, helical shaped, contain envelopes, and ranges in size from 75–125nm.

2. The family contains the **influenza viruses.**

3. Influenza viruses have hemagglutinin antigens (HA) and neuraminidase antigens (NA). These antigens allow the viruses to attach to the surface of RBCs and respiratory epithelial cells.

4. Vaccines are available each year, and are derived from viral types causing the most infections in the previous year.

5. Diagnosis is from clinical symptoms and serology.

K. Paramyxoviruses

1. RNA viruses, helical shaped, enveloped, and range in size from 150 to 300nm.

2. Paramyxoviruses contain *Paramyxoviruses, Morbillivirus,* and *Pneumovirus.*

3. ***Paramyxovirus***

   a. Include parainfluenza virus, mumps virus, *Morbillivirus,* and *Pneumovirus.*

      1) Parainfluenze virus causes childhood croup, which is a respiratory infection characterized by fever, and a hoarse cough.

      2) Mumps is an infection of the parotid glands, which causes swelling and difficulty in swallowing.

      3) *Morbillivirus* causes rubeola or measles.

      4) *Pneumovirus* (respiratory syncytial virus or RSV) causes respiratory and ear infections. These are most common in newborns and young children.

L. Rhabdovirus

1. RNA viruses, bullet shaped, enveloped, and range in size from 150 to 350nm.

2. The *Lyssaviruses* cause rabies.

3. The rabies virus gains entry into the human by animal or bat bite where the CNS is infected. The disease progresses to convulsions, coma, and fatal encephalitis.

4. Diagnosis is through medical history of animal bites, and finding **Negri bodies** in infected brain cells.

5. Rabies vaccination is available.

M. Reovirus

1. RNA viruses, icosahedral shaped, no envelope, and range in size from 50 to 80nm.

2. Reoviruses include Reovirus, Rotavirus, and Orbivirus.

3. Reoviruses cause gastroenteritis in infants and young children.

N. Retrovirus

1. RNA viruses, icosahedral shaped, have envelopes, and range in size from 80–130nm.

2. Retroviruses have reverse transcriptase, which transcribes RNA into DNA.

3. Retroviruses includes *Oncornaviruses, Lentiviruses.*

4. **Oncomaviruses**

   a. This subfamily of viruses includes human T-cell lymphotrophic virus type I (HTLV-1) and human T-cell lymphotrophic virus type II (HTLV-2).

   b. These viruses are closely associated with adult T-cell leukemia, hairy cell leukemia, and lymphoma.

5. **Lentiviruses**
   a. Include the human immunodeficiency viruses types 1 and 2 (HIV-1, and HIV-2).
   b. **Is the causative agent of acquired immunodeficiency syndrome or AIDS.**
   c. Transmission is by contaminated blood and blood products.
   d. The virus infects the body's T-cells, which results in a breakdown of the immune system.
   e. Spread of the virus is by sexual contact with infected individuals (homosexual or heterosexual), IV drug use, congenital, or contaminated blood products.
   f. Associated infections include *Pneumocystis carinii* pneumonia, CMV infections, cryptosporidosis, candidiasis, and toxoplasmosis.
   g. Malignant associations include Kaposi's sarcoma, anal cancer, and B-cell lymphomas.
   h. Diagnosis is by clinical history and serology.
   i. Confirmatory diagnosis is by the Western blot method.

6. **Filoviridae**
   a. Includes **Marburg** virus and **Ebola** virus.
   b. Causes hemorrhagic fever with high fatality rates.
   c. Most cases are in Africa.
   d. Mode of transmission is unclear.
   e. Sizes ranges from 800–1000nm.

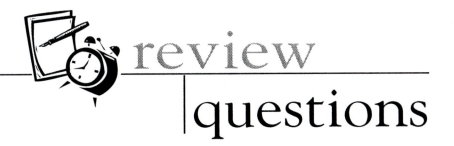
review questions

DIRECTIONS Each of the questions or incomplete statements below is followed by suggested answers or completions. Select the **one answer** that is best in each case.

---

1. Which of the following is NOT a general characteristic of a virus?
   a. Obligate intracellular organisms
   b. Do not produce ATP
   c. Identification is based on size, shape, and type of nucleic acid
   d. Contain both DNA and RNA

2. Identifying characteristics of this hepatitis virus include: contains DNA, infections spread by contaminated body fluids, 50 to 180-day incubation period, and anti-HbcAg-IgM indicates a recent acute infection.
   a. HAV
   b. HBV
   c. HCV
   d. HEV

3. Which of the following is NOT caused by a herpesvirus?

   a. Genital lesions
   b. Shingles
   c. Chronic fatigue syndrome
   d. Fifth disease

4. Which of the following has been declared eradicated by the World Health Organization?
   a. Venezuelan equine encephalitis
   b. Smallpox
   c. Rift Valley fever
   d. Korean hemorrhagic fever

5. The Sabin polio vaccine uses which of the following?
   a. Formalin-killed viruses
   b. Live, attenuated viruses
   c. Synthetic viruses
   d. None of the above

11 Management, Laboratory Principles, Education, and Research

contents

➤ COMPREHENSIVE KEY CONCEPTS

1. Discuss the importance of communication, planning, organizing, directing, and leadership in management.

2. Analyze the role of the manager in change and financial management.

3. Explain principles of laboratory operations and techniques: quality control, microscopic examination, and laboratory safety.

4. Describe specific procedures for various types of phlebotomy.

5. Discuss the importance of competency-based education in clinical laboratory science.

6. Analyze the educational process and the tools used to deliver and assessment knowledge attainment.

7. Contrast and compare experimental designs and qualitative research.

8. Analyze the role of research in clinical laboratory science.

MANAGEMENT

I. NATURE OF MANAGEMENT
   A. The **Information Age** will change management from supervision of "factory" workers to coordination of knowledge workers.
      1. Organizational Structure

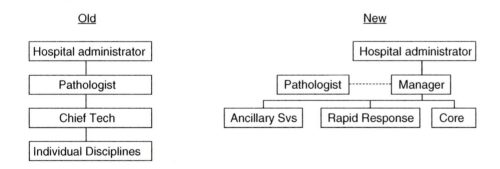

II. MANAGEMENT PROCESSES
   A. Planning
      1. **Definition:** develop a pathway(s) to accomplish the organization's mission and goals using resources and time.
      2. **In order to plan for the future, one must first determine where the organization stands.** A **SWOT** analysis can be performed both internally and externally:
         a. **S**—strengths of the organization
         b. **W**—weaknesses of the organization
         c. **O**—opportunities available to the organization
         d. **T**—threats to the organization
      3. Once the SWOT analysis is complete, the manager can plan a course of action for the organization to follow that will accomplish its goals and mission.

key concepts

Discuss the different types of plans used in an organization and explain the importance and process of goal setting, writing objectives, and performing the SWOT analysis.

4. Formulating goals
   a. Written goals allow all employees to work toward a common result.
   b. Goals should be broad—objectives are written to achieve specific tasks.
5. Writing **objectives**
   a. Objectives are tasks to achieve goals.
   b. Objectives are focused on achieving 1 goal.
   c. Each objective deals with 1 task.
   d. Objectives are very specific.
   e. Objectives are written using action verbs.
   f. Objectives are evaluated against specific and specified numerical criteria.
6. **Types of plans**
   a. **Short range or tactical plans:** cover a 1–5 year period and focus on tasks that can be completed in this time frame.
   b. **Operational plans:** may be for 1 year or 1 budget period. Concerns operations.
   c. **Strategic planning:** maps out the course of an organization for approximately 20 years. Strategic plans involve tactical and operational plans as well as forming alliances and partnerships with key players (sometimes even competitors). This plan is evaluated and modified yearly.

B. Organizing
   1. **Time management**
      a. Laboratorians have their work dictated by the health care system—patient admissions, emergency patients, and outpatients. Managers have more flexibility to plan their work because it is dictated by administration (organization).
      b. Managers have more control over their workload and therefore, they must identify, control, and eliminate or curtail specific situations that rob them of time.
         1) Identify important tasks and make sure these are accomplished first. These tasks may require most of a manager's resources.
         2) Develop skills necessary to facilitate use of manager's time.
            a) **Managerial skills:** organized, able to delegate, knows when to say "no," can take control, effective planning, able to prioritize, conduct effective meetings, and good listening skills.
            b) **Educated:** knows organization or goals, able to see the big picture, meets deadlines, gives good and clear instructions, and understands teams.
            c) **Controls interferences:** avoids lengthy unnecessary phone calls, "drop-in" visitors, reading junk mail, and too much socializing.
            d) **Decision-making capabilities:** controls perfectionism, able to make a decision, appropriately detailed oriented.

key concepts

Discuss the concept of time management and give practical examples of how this is practiced in a laboratory.

e) **Develops resources:** adequate money in budget, functional and up-to-date equipment, adequate staff, and support from the administration.

f) **Self-discipline:** avoids procrastination, inappropriate socializing.

2. **Structure**

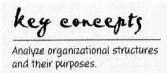

a. The manager develops a structure that allows plans to be carried out and objectives accomplished.

b. The organizational structure is based on authority, responsibility, and accountability.

1) **Authority**

a) Formal: assigned by organization or administration

b) Informal: gained informally through competence or leadership qualities.

2) **Responsibility:** assigned by administration through delegation.

3) **Accountability:** occurs when the person responsible for completing a task is evaluated to determine if the task was completed.

3. **Reengineering**

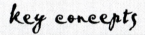

a. **Definition:** reorganizing work processes in an organization.

b. First map the specific work processes to determine if more effective processes could be implemented.

c. Benchmarking is a process whereby the best process in one organization is modified to fit similar processes in another organization.

d. Examples

1) Use of robotics to automate (particularly specimen processing)

2) Computerization

3) Pneumatic tube system to transport specimens

4. **Inventory Management**

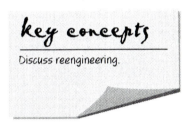

a. Objectives of an efficient laboratory is to experience few shortages in testing reagents, supplies, and materials.

b. Requisitions of contract and purchase orders to obtain necessary quantities of materials, etc., in suitable time frames.

c. Managers are responsible for purchasing laboratory instruments and service contracts to maintain instruments.

d. Instrument selection includes cost comparison of instruments from various instrument manufacturers.

e. Many hospital laboratories contract with outside agencies to provide blood products for patients.

f. Hospitals contract with outside companies to handle biohazardous waste and/or hazardous waste.

C. **Directing**

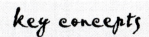

1. **Definition:** persuading employees to perform the tasks that help the organization accomplish its mission and goals.

2. Techniques of directing

a. **Authoritative:** issuing orders, telling someone what to do. Does not allow employee to decide how best to accomplish task.

    b. **Coaching:** instilling confidence and motivation into an employee about accomplishing a task. The employee has more say so in how to accomplish a task.

    c. **Empowerment:** when an employee is allowed to determine what task and how to accomplish the task to help the manager solve a problem or to allow an organization to come closer to accomplishing their mission and goals. Employees are allowed to be creative and innovative to solve problems. Employees are allowed to take risks without fear of admonishment for failing.

3. **Communicating**

    a. **Spoken communication**

      1) **Advantages**

        a) Immediate message conveyed.

        b) Feedback immediate.

        c) Can determine other factors: body language, tone of voice, eye contact, and implied meanings.

      2) **Disadvantages**

        a) Can't save it.

        b) Receiver interpretation of message may be different from that of speaker's intentions.

        c) Body language, tone of voice, eye contact may confuse recipient or sender.

        d) Can't retract spoken words.

        e) Tips: gender, age groups, ethnicity, professional, emotional state, and other barriers exist for effective communication.

    b. **Written communication**

      1) **Advantages**

        a) Can save communication encounter.

        b) Deliver same message to many receivers.

        c) Can add graphics to explain or clarify message.

        d) Readers can review, interpret, then respond to initial message.

      2) **Disadvantages**

        a) Feedback delayed.

        b) Can be impersonal.

        c) Final.

        d) Tips: memos and e-mail considered informal communication; letters are considered formal communication.

    c. **Listening**

      1) Active listening components

        a) Privacy.

        b) Eliminate (reduce) physical barriers.

        c) Listen to words, but look at behavior, and interpret implied meaning.

      2) Restate what you think you've heard to ensure accuracy and capture any implied meanings.

      3) Remain objective, but give signals (nod, keep eye contact, say, "go on") to show speaker that you are listening.

key concepts

Analyze the importance of active listening, the significance and permanence of written communications, and the power of spoken communication.

4) Identify what the sender wants from the listener.

5) Summarize the plan for action and time when action will be complete.

4. **Motivating**

   a. **Definition:** influencing a person to act in a particular way and generate initiative within that person.

   b. **Motivators include:**

      1) Reward (i.e., bonus)

      2) Empowerment

      3) Praise

      4) Recognition

      5) Pay

      6) Encouragement

5. **Delegating**

   a. **Definition:** assigning responsibility and accountability for a task to an employee.

   b. **Effective delegation** occurs when the manager selects the right task for the right person, prepares an overview of exactly what must be done, allows time for task to be completed, then provides recognition for performing the task.

6. **Coaching**

   a. Create an atmosphere of trust.

   b. Allow employees to take risks and not be reprimanded for failures.

   c. Make everyone feel that they are important.

   d. Work through emotions of players.

   e. Seek feedback by asking questions.

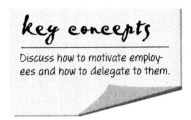

key concepts

Discuss how to motivate employees and how to delegate to them.

D. **Giving Directives and Managing Change**

   1. Managerial function that enables the manager to get his people to do the most and their best.

   2. Work done through employees with development of their skills by managers.

   3. Good directives

      a. **Reasonable:** an employee is able to, desires to, and has resources to do so.

      b. **Understandable:** clear expectations of him or her. The employee can repeat the directive in his/her own works accurately.

      c. **Appropriately worded** and delivered in a nonthreatening tone. A directive can be presented in the form of a suggestion. Avoid giving orders.

      d. **Important** for getting the job done. Requests should not be made for the personal gain of the supervisor.

      e. **Time limits** should be included in directives and should be of reasonable length.

   4. Major techniques for directives

      a. **Autocratic**

         1) Detailed instructions given of exactly how and what is to be done.

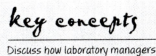

key concepts

Discuss how laboratory managers must manage change.

2) The manager's way is the best and employees need not think of another way to complete the task.

3) Inhibits employees thinking for themselves. They lose interest and initiative. Ambition, imagination, and involvement in daily job will be diminished or lost.

b. **Consultative**

1) Also called participative, democratic, permissive, or empowered management.

2) Views employees as eager to do a good job and equipped with the skills to do so.

3) Believes employees will become more motivated if left alone to do their job.

4) Input is sought from employees to help solve a problem or tackle a project.

5) Employees are consulted about tackling a project. When in angreement, an employee is assigned to the project to complete within a specific time frame. The employee decides how the project is to be accomplished.

6) Information must flow freely between manager and employee. Good ideas need to be explored, no matter who thinks of them.

7) Employees are allowed to think for themselves and make worthwhile contributions to the organization.

8) Atmosphere is created of mutual confidence where the employee can call on the manager when necessary with no fear of reprisal.

9) Similar to active learning that is more effective than passive learning. Employees work out solutions to problems and projects more effectively than giving them the solutions.

c. **Change and influence**

1) Organizations are constantly changing in leadership positions to capture more market share and to meet technological advancements.

2) The degree and complexity of changes varies among departments in organizations.

3) Change is best accepted by employees if presented in a nonthreatening way. Managers must promote change and keep morale high.

4) Explaining the reasons for change may lead to acceptance by many employees.

5) Reasons People Resist Change

a) **Uncertainty**: they do not want to be moved out of their comfort zone because it will take effort on their part to analyze the change, learn new procedures, or perform additional tasks.

b) **Perception**: Everyone brings with them particular life experiences, values, and perceptions. Each individual has a different perception of the same event.

c) **Loss**: Within the organization, there exists relationships between all workers that are built upon respect, trust, and expertise. Change can destroy all those relationships and make people lose status or perceived status among peers.

    d) **Self-interests**: Change disturbs the current state of affairs. Even though it may not be perfect, people have arranged their life so that their need satisfaction is stable. Change produces instability and uncertainty.

    e) **Insecurity**: Job security and being able to earn a wage that will allow an individual to pay the bills and maintain a decent standard of life is why people work. Change usually produces insecurity as people see their jobs threatened or taken away from them.

  6) Overcoming resistance to change

    a) Managers should allow ample time for the change and not expect to follow a rigid timeline for implementing the change.

    b) Employees deserve to know why changes are being made. Managers should give employees plenty of time to have their questions and concerns answered. The manager should also state the desired effects of the change.

    c) Managers should involve employees in planning and implementing the change. When employees take part in making something happen, they are more likely to take ownership and accept the change more readily.

    d) **Change is stressful for everyone.** It is important to include stress management techniques to help decrease the stress of change.

E. Leadership

1. Essential component of every organization.
2. **Purpose**: leadership produces change.
3. The following steps can assist a leader in producing meaningful change in an organization:

  a. **Establish direction**: a vision of the future of the organization is established and strategies are developed and implemented to bring the organization closer to that vision.

  b. **Align people**: communicate the vision and strategies to other people using words and deeds so that the vision and strategies are understood and accepted.

  c. **Motivate and inspire**: energize people to implement the vision and strategy changes by satisfying basic needs (achievement, belonging, recognition, self-esteem, and a control of one's life) that may go unmet.

III. MANAGING FINANCES

A. Principles

  1. **Spreadsheets**

    a. **Income/expense spreadsheet**

      1) Shows income generated and expenses incurred over a period of time (month, quarter, year).

      2) Net revenue = income generated − expenses incurred.

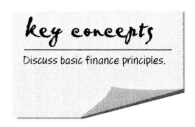

key concepts

Discuss basic finance principles.

b. **Balance sheet**
   1) Shows the financial situation of the organization at a specific point in time.
   2) This sheet contains current assets (cash, patient receivables, inventory), current liabilities (accounts payable, accrued salaries), property and equipment (land, building, equipment, and instruments), and long-term obligations (bonds payable, loans).
   3) Add the assets, subtract the liabilities, and the result is net worth.

c. **Cash-flow statements** show the in-flow and out-flow of cash for a specific period.
   1) Net cash flow from operations.
   2) Net cash flow from investments.
   3) Net cash flow from financial activities.

d. Miscellaneous data needed by managers: test volumes per laboratory section, supply costs, labor costs, cost per billable test, workload, rejection rates, contamination rates, and productivity.

2. **Budgets**
   a. Usually done annually as a plan for spending for the next year.
   b. Incorporates workload data, new programs, test costs, previous year revenues, previous year costs, capital equipment costs, operating expenses, labor costs, and equipment maintenance costs.
   c. Most organizations use data from the previous year, then estimate increased costs for the coming year and add this figure to the budget.
   d. Zero-based budgeting involves starting the budget process from a 0 figure and justifying and researching every cost that will be incurred before arriving at the final budget.

3. **Revenue**
   a. **Medicare and Medicaid**
      1) The federal government pays health care organizations for providing care to beneficiaries using a method called prospective payment system (PPS).
      2) Health care organizations are paid a lump sum for services according to the diagnosis code (ICD-9) for the patient's illness.
      3) The government established a database and derived average costs for many illnesses.
      4) The government develops a payment schedule, and this is the amount an organization is paid.
   b. **Health Maintenance Organizations (HMOs)**
      1) HMOs contract with hospitals to provide services for patients.
      2) The hospital is paid a set fee to provide specific services per HMO enrollee. For example, if an HMO has 300 enrollees (covered lives), they may contract with the hospital to provide x-ray, laboratory, and physical therapy services for their patients at $100/patient per year.

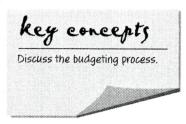

key concepts

Discuss the budgeting process.

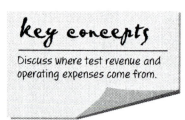

key concepts

Discuss where test revenue and operating expenses come from.

      3) This method is call **capitated reimbursement**; it is based on the number of enrollees at a specific amount per enrollee.

  4. Operating Costs

    a. **Definition:** what it costs to produce test results. This includes direct and indirect costs.

    b. **Direct costs:** costs that are directly associated with producing test results. These include supplies and labor.

    c. **Indirect costs:** costs that indirectly contribute to producing laboratory tests. These include electricity bills, paper towels, soap, bleach, and computer software.

    d. **Fixed costs:** remain the same from month to month no matter how many tests are produced.

    e. **Variable costs:** change with the amount of work performed.

    f. **Capital costs:** related to purchasing equipment or instruments that cost more than $500.

B. Cost Management

1. **Definition:** keeping cost as low as possible without compromising the quality of care delivered to patients.
2. Employees become very valuable sources for suggestions to increase efficiency and effectiveness of work patterns.

C. Cost Analysis

1. **Cost per billable test** entails gathering data on wages, collection and handling fees, reagent cost, controls and references cost, disposables cost, instrument maintenance, depreciation, miscellaneous costs, and indirect costs.
2. **Cost Per Billable Test** Calculation

Cost for testing = Instrument cost + administration costs + supplies + labor

Profit = Revenue per test − cost per test

Revenue per test = Total revenue/total number of tests

key concepts

Discuss how to calculate cost per billable test and breakeven analysis.

D. Breakeven Analysis

1. **Breakeven analysis = where revenues = expenses**
2. Calculation

Breakeven (BE) test volume = annual fixed costs / (test price − variable costs)

BE minimum price per test = annual fixed costs / test volume + variable costs

BE minimum revenue = annual fixed costs / [(test price − variable costs)/test price]

E. Cost Accounting

1. **Definition:** systems that study costs associated with performing tests.
2. Focuses on internal processes

key concepts

Discuss how cost containment is achieved.

F. Cost Containment

1. Focuses on ways of first reducing costs, then secondly maintaining quality.
2. Centralizing services is one way to control costs.

    a. Centralized purchasing

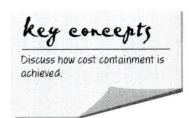

    b. Centralization of jobs
  3. Eliminates unnecessary testing.
  4. Employee retention, retraining, cross training, and flexible wage and benefits programs.

IV. QUALITY MANAGEMENT
  A. Championed by Deming, Juran, Crosby, and Shewhart.
  B. Quality Programs
  1. Components

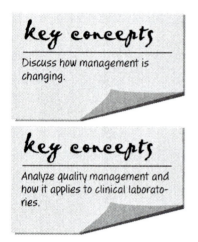

key concepts

Discuss how management is changing.

key concepts

Analyze quality management and how it applies to clinical laboratories.

    a. **Statistical analysis:** especially important in production control. Used to analyze the quality of results. In the lab, statistical analysis includes internal and external quality control.
    b. **Training and education:** employees are not considered the problem. Employees need adequate training and education to perform the best possible job. Inadequate training and education leave an employee unprepared to perform their best.
    c. **Evaluation:** quality programs establish goals or targets to reach. The progress toward accomplishing these goals is assessed. If satisfactory progress toward a goal is not achieved, then the process needs to be changed or modified to achieve satisfactory progress towards a goal.
    d. **Feedback:** this is a continuous process. Monitoring and evaluation takes place for several indicators.

  C. Continuous Quality Improvement (CQI)
  1. Processes
    a. Quality circle: 8–12 employees from various departments who work together using CQI principles to improve a process.
    b. Top management must be committed to CQI for it to work.
    c. The data teams generate is vital and important to the process, but the success of CQI is dependent upon using this data to improve existing processes.

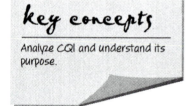

key concepts

Analyze CQI and understand its purpose.

  2. The cycle of quality improvement that was developed by Deming:
    a. **P.D.A.C. Plan → Do → Act → Check**
    b. **Feedback is a crucial step in this cycle.** Without feedback, there is no improvement.
  3. Quality management may use Pareto charts, flowcharts, or cause-and-effect charts to describe processes.

  D. Managerial Roles and Functions
  1. Managerial functions include planning, organizing, directing, decision making/problem solving, coordinating, and communicating.
  2. Managerial roles include:
    a. Represent the organization.
    b. Hold formal authority.
    c. Responsible for strategies to accomplish mission and goals of the organization.
    d. Managing personnel
      1) Evaluations

2) Hiring

3) Promoting

e. Financial responsibility

1) Budget

a) Capital

b) Operating

2) Revenue

3) Expenses

f. Communication: employees, supervisors/team leaders, colleagues, and patients.

g. Motivation: employees, supervisors/team leaders, colleagues, and self.

h. Time management.

i. Oversee customer service.

j. Implement innovative ways to expand services, expand customer base, and fulfill the bottom line.

E. Leadership

1. Different from Management

a. Management involves planning and budgeting, organizing and staffing, and controlling and problem solving.

b. Leadership involves establishing direction, aligning, motivating, and inspiring people.

2. Structure of Leadership

a. Purpose: to create leadership processes and help produce changes needed to cope with a changing environment.

b. Content: can vary: very focused or very broad

c. Assignment: roles are assumed or assigned in a more fluid way in businesses that change often.

3. The Origin of Leadership

a. Personal characteristics: high drive/energy level, good intelligence and thinking skills, good mental and emotional health, and integrity.

b. Career Experiences

1) Promotes leadership: challenging assignments early in a career, visible leadership role models who are very good or very bad, assignments that broaden a person's experience.

2) Inhibits leadership: a long series of narrow and tactical jobs, vertical career movement, rapid promotions, measurements and rewards based on short-term results only.

> ***key concepts***
> ─────
> *Analyze the concept of leadership and how it differs from management.*

LABORATORY PRINCIPLES

I. QUALITY CONTROL

A. Reasons for Quality Control (QC)

1. Determines reportability of patient results

a. Controls must fall within expected range.

b. Use normal, high, and low controls when available.

2. Random patient values accuracy.

3. Data for quality assurance (QA) programs.

4. Data for decision making, especially in taking corrective actions.

B. Types of Quality Control

1. Gaussian Probability Curve

a. Show changes in standard deviations.

b. Caused due to changes in reagent vendors, instrument problems, improper storage of reagents, bad controls, or poor pipetting technique.

2. Levey-Jennings (L-J) QC Graph

a. Plot laboratory QC results by time, day, and month.

b. Show out of control data, sudden changes of data, and gradual changes such as trends.

3. Westgard Rules

a. Used to interpret control charts and to detect error.

b. Controls are rejected (varies from lab to lab) when the following criteria are met:

1) 1_{3s}: Reject results outside $+/- 3SD$.

2) 2_{2s}: Reject 2 consecutive results outside $+/- 2SD$.

3) 4_{1s}: Reject 4 consecutive controls if greater than $+1SD$ or less than $-1SD$ from the mean.

4) 10_x: Reject 10 consecutive controls are on one side of the mean.

5) **Note**: For a more detailed analysis of the Westgard Rules, refer to the quality assurance section found in Chapter 4.

4. Delta Check

a. Show significant differences in lab values of the same patient.

b. Usually the delta check is failed if results show a 10 percent variation. For example, if a patient has a 15.0g hemoglobin at 7A.M. and a 10.5g hemoglobin at 7P.M., the delta check would fail, causing the patient's samples to be rechecked or redrawn.

II. PHLEBOTOMY

A. Patient and collection preparation—Phlebotomy personnel should smile, introduce themselves, explain the procedure, be courteous, and act professional.

1. Identify the patient by wrist or arm-band.

a. Ask his/her name.

b. Use patient identification number.

1) Hospital system number

2) Birth date

3) Phone or social security number

2. Choose a venipuncture site: usually the median cubital vein, cephalic vein, or basilic vein.

3. Assemble necessary equipment, including gloves, alcohol swabs (betadine for blood cultures and alcohol levels), and tourniquets (Velcro or latex band).

a. Remember to never leave the tourniquet on patient more than 1 minute

1) Patient results will be affected due to blood flow stasis.

      b. Needles usually are 20 to 21 gauge.
        1) Higher number means smaller needle diameter
        2) Use each needle **only once**.
      c. Assemble evacuated tube collection devise or syringe (for difficult draw).
    4. After the draw:
      a. Apply pressure to the site.
      b. Cover the needle.
      c. Invert anticoagulation tubes several times.
      d. Label all tubes completely.
    5. Different types of blood drawing equipment include syringes, vacuum tubes, butterfly needles, and lancets.

B. Always Practice **confidentiality** Regarding Patient Information

C. Types of Blood Collection Tubes
    1. **Red** stopper tubes contain no additives.
      a. Used whenever serum is required for a test.
      b. Frequently used in chemistry and blood bank.
    2. **Lavender** stopper tubes
      a. Contain tripotassium ethylenendiaminetetraacetate (EDTA), an anticoagulant.
      b. EDTA ratio is 1.5 mg/1mL of whole blood. Prevent coagulation by forming insoluble calcium salt by removing ionized calcium (chelation).
      c. Used in hematology for CBCs, slide preparation, and other routine hematology procedures.
    3. **Blue** tubes contain **sodium citrate** used for ESR and coagulation studies.
      a. 3.2 percent sodium citrate in a 1:9 ratio (1 part sodium citrate to 9 parts whole blood)
      b. Prevents coagulation by removing calcium.
      c. Used for coagulation testing and ESRs.
    4. **Green** tubes contain **heparin** used for special hematology procedures.
      a. Heparin ratio is 0.2mL/1mL of whole blood.
      b. Prevents coagulation by inactivating thrombin.
      c. Used for osmotic fragility and lupus testing.
    5. **Light blue** tubes contain **thrombin and soy bean trypsin** used for fibrin and degradation product studies.

III. SAFETY
A. Laboratory Safety
    1. **Bloodborne pathogens:** infectious disease that can be spread by contact with infected body fluids. Diseases include HIV, hepatitis, TB, etc.
    2. **Universal precautions:** handle all fluids as contaminated, including avoiding mouth/mucus membrane contact, and wearing protective euipment.

IV. TYPES OF MICROSCOPES

A. Light—most common microscope in the clinical laboratory; used for differentials and bone marrow slides.

B. Phase Contrast—used to view unstained samples, urine sediment, and platelet counts.

C. Polarized—used to view urine sediment and crystals.

EDUCATION

I. FUNDAMENTALS OF EDUCATION

A. Components of Education

1. **Curriculum:** determined by the body of knowledge of the profession.
2. **Competencies** are the skills that must be mastered by students to become an entry-level clinical laboratory scientist.
3. **Objectives** are measurable and observable behaviors that will enable students to master entry-level competencies.
4. **Instruction** is the process of passing knowledge and skills to students. This can include lecture, reading, demonstration, the Internet, and group projects. It includes design of practice to develop psychomotor skills and attitudes in the affective domain.
5. **Testing**: measures the amount of knowledge they have learned. Tests are objective measures of learning.
6. **Evaluating:** measures cognitive, pyschomotor, and behavioral learning. Documents how well students master entry-level competencies.

B. Competency-Based Education (CBE)

1. **Definition**: program curriculum is based on competencies, determined by the profession as entry level.
2. The competencies are set by the National Accrediting Agency for Clinical Laboratory Science (NAACLS) in the Essentials and Guidelines of Accredited Educational Program, the Competency Statements of American Society of Clinical Pathologists (ASCP), and the Competency Assurance Documents, Statements of Competence from American Society for Clinical Laboratory Science (ASCLS).
3. Objectives are action statements that reflect the skill (psychomotor), the behavior (affective domain), and the knowledge (cognitive) to be mastered by a student. The objectives must be measurable so that student progress toward mastering the objectives can be assessed.
   a. Benefits to Students
      1) Clearly states expectations of students.
      2) Helps students capture relevant subject matter.
      3) Gives student self-direction.
      4) Begins lifelong learning process for student.
   b. Benefits to teachers
      1) Expectations of students clearly defined.
      2) Important subject matter identified.
      3) Base for testable material.

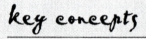

key concepts

Discuss the components of education and the roles of the student.

key concepts

Discuss competency-based education and the benefits for students and teachers.

    4) Holds teacher accountable.

    5) Helps teachers plan course, lectures, labs.

  c. Each objective must contain:

    1) The doer (A = Audience).

    2) The activity (B = behavior, the verb)

    3) The specified conditions (C = conditions, circumstances).

    4) The standard (D = degree that implies mastery.

    5) For example, the *student* (doer) must *classify* the bacteria (the activity) in *5 minutes* (condition) with *100% accuracy* (the standard).

II. PROFESSIONAL COMPETENCY

A. Cognitive Domain

  1. Consists of progressive levels of difficulty

Cognitive Domain	Professional Function
Evaluation	
Synthesis	Problem Solving
Analysis	
Application	Understanding by applying
Comprehension	to new situations
Knowledge	Recall

  a. Knowledge: subject matter—facts.

  b. Comprehension: linking to what you already know.

  c. Application: applying new knowledge to a new situation.

  d. Analysis: breaking down a situation into its components and determining the interrelation of its parts.

  e. Synthesis: take separate components and bring together to produce a meaningful product.

B. Affective Domain

  1. Consists of progressive levels of depth/sophistication.

Affective Domains	Professional Function
Characterization	Identifies with value
Organization	Internalizes and
Valuing	assures value
Responding	
Receiving	Awareness & reaction

  a. Receiving: how students listen; their attitude toward constructive criticism and directions.

  b. Responding: how students reply

  c. Valuing: students assign value to learning opportunities, constructive criticism, and directions.

  d. Organization: application of a student's internalized values.

  e. Characterization: the inherent personality manifested in behavior.

C. Psychomotor Domain

  1. Consists of progressive levels of complexity.

key concepts

Discuss how professional competency results from cognitive, affective, and psychomotor domains.

Psychomotor Domains	Professional Function
Origination	Modify
Adaptation	
Coordination	Experience
Proficiency	
Preparation	Aware and ready to
Observation	respond

a. Observation: watches a procedure being performed.

b. Preparation: organizes work space to perform a test.

c. Manipulation: does the test.

d. Coordination: performs many tasks in a coordinated manner.

e. Adaptation: transfers old skills when performing a new test.

f. Origination: develops new manual dexterity to perform tests easier.

key concepts

Describe various teaching methods.

III. TEACHING METHODS

A. Roles of the Teacher

1. Expert: must be knowledgeable about the subject they are teaching; must be capable of using resources.

2. Authority: teachers are given formal authority over students.

   a. Formal authority includes developing course policies and procedures, grading structure, test and lab structure, cognitive, behavioral and psychomotor objectives.

   b. Must oversee that students develop entry-level competencies.

3. Facilitator: organize and present knowledge to students in an orderly, understandable manner.

   a. The teacher must take into account different student learning styles and different student learning rates.

   b. The teacher is responsible for getting students to apply what they have learned

4. Compliance manager: responsible for ensuring students follow the policies and rules of the program and institution.

5. Responsibilities

   a. Follow OSHA safety regulations

   b. Prepared for class

   c. The rapid turnaround time for assignments, grades, and evaluations

B. Teaching Methods

1. Lesson plan

   a. Plan of details of what should be accomplished, cognitive, affective domain, and psychomotor objectives, lecture notes, handouts, overheads, electronic presentations, kodachromes, demonstrations, etc.

2. Lecture: an expert talks to a group of people about a particular topic.

3. Cooperative learning

   a. small groups learning topics

    b. groups use all members as resources; cooperate in a friendly environment to learn

  4. Problem-based learning: presentation of a problem to students. They work together to find the solution.

  5. Computer-assisted learning: Use of software programs to learn and review topics.

  6. Role play

    a. Students act out situations

    b. Provides nonthreatening learning environment

    c. Identify solutions to difficult/bad scenarios

  7. Distance education: learning from nontraditional delivery to students.

    a. Traditional delivery at specific outreach sites away from a higher learning institution.

      1) Via the Internet for on-line courses

      2) Via video conferencing equipment

C. Assessment

  1. **Definition:** determining how well students understand the subject matter presented to them.

  2. **Types of tests**

    a. Pretest: a test given to students to determine what students already know about a subject.

    b. Posttest: a test given to students to determine what they have learned. The score of the pretest is compared with the score of the posttest to assess learning.

  3. **Test attributes**

    a. Reliability: refers to how stable and consistent a test is from year to year.

      1) Consistency is composed of the quality of the test.

      2) Adequate test questions.

      3) Objective test questions.

    b. Validity: when a test asks questions about specific information.

    c. Objectivity: fairness, adequate to complete, good format (enough space to answer questions), and questions that relate back to stated objectives.

  4. Structure of test **questions**

    a. 3 levels: I (recall), II (interpretation), and III (problem solving)

      1) Recall the simplest question because it asks the student to regurgitate information.

      2) Interpretation: the student is asked to use material learned to tell something about a process, test, or principle.

      3) Problem solving: student is presented with a problem and asked a specific question related to that problem.

IV. STUDENTS

A. Learners/Students

  1. Definition: contracted customers who take classes to earn a degree, diploma, or certification, or learn specific information. Graduates of a program are products of the educational process.

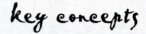

key concepts

Discuss the concept of assessment and the structure of test questions.

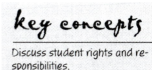

key concepts

Discuss student rights and responsibilities.

2. Responsibilities
   a. Know degree requirements from the school.
   b. Attend all classes and be on time.
   c. Maintain academic honesty.
   d. Maintain a professional demeanor.
   e. Adhere to institution, department, and class rules.
   f. Notify instructor ASAP if absent, tardy from class, or if something prevents completion of an assignment.
3. Rights
   a. Right to a good quality education.
   b. Right to fair assessment in a class.
   c. Right to respect from the instructor.
   d. Right to ask questions.
   e. Right to receive extra help.

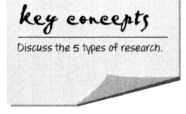

key concepts

Discuss the accrediting agency for clinical laboratory science programs.

B. Clinical Laboratory Science Education

1. ASAHP: American Society of Allied Health Professional Schools. Formed in 1967. Provides interactions among allied health programs. It is a volunteer organization and produces the *Journal of Allied Health*.
2. ASCP (American Society of Clinical Pathologists): professional organization and certifying agency: Board of Registry. Clinical laboratory scientists can be associate members.
3. NAACLS (National Accrediting Agency for Clinical Laboratory Science): organization that accredits medical technology/clinical laboratory scientist and medical/clinical laboratory technician programs.
4. NCA (National Credentialing Agency): organization that prepares and administers the NCA certification examination.

key concepts

Define the following research terms—theory, hypothesis, null hypothesis, statistical significance, and control group.

RESEARCH

I. INTRODUCTION TO RESEARCH METHODS

A. Research Definitions

1. **Theory**: an explanation to a problem, or how variables are related to other variables.
2. **Hypothesis**: a statement regarding supposed relationships among variables, and research will support or not support the hypothesis.
3. **Null hypothesis (H_o)** is a hypothesis that attempts to prove no relationship between variables.
4. **Statistical significance**: used to show differences or similarities that will support a theory or hypothesis.
5. **Control group**: a group that is untreated or receives no special treatment.
6. **Variables**: factors influencing data or outcomes. Must be accounted for in final statistical analysis.

key concepts

Discuss the 5 types of research.

B. Types of Research

1. Experimental-comparison designs
   a. Comparing different groups that have been assigned to receive different treatments.

2. Single-case experimental design
   a. The same subjects receive different treatments, and comparisons or changes are noted.
3. Correlational design
   a. The most common design that is nonexperimental.
   b. 2 or more variables are measured to determine relationships.
   c. Example: Is self-esteem related to grades?
4. Descriptive research
   a. A type of nonexperimental quantitative research.
   b. Describes a group or set of variables as they exist without external or internal interference.
   c. Example: new medical technology/clinical laboratory science (MT/CLS) employees are compared with experienced MT/CLS employees.
5. Questions related to research design development
   a. Is the problem an important one?
   b. Does the theory regarding the problem make sense?
   c. Does the collected data confirm the hypotheses?
   d. Is the study feasible given the available resources?

II. RESEARCH METHODS
A. Experimental—Comparison Design
1. Introduction
   a. Answers questions that involve comparison of 1 treatment or condition with another.
2. Random assignment
   a. One of the most important features of the experimental comparison design is the use of random assignment of subjects to various treatments.
      1) Random assignment solves one of the most critical problems of research design, which is selection bias.
      2) Example: 100 hospital laboratory names are put into a box and 50 are drawn out. 25 of the laboratories are given an in-service in safety while the remaining 25 are not given the safety in-service. Which hospital laboratory will have the best safety record?
   b. Stratified Random Assignment
      1) The process of random assignment in the **same category**.
      2) Example: random selection of labs that are private.

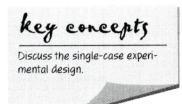

key concepts

Discuss the experimental-comparison research design.

B. Single-Case Experimental Designs
1. Introduction
   a. In single-case experiments, 1 or more subjects are observed over a period of time.
      1) The observations establish a baseline of the variables being observed.
      2) Once the baseline is established, a treatment is started.
      3) The baseline is then analyzed to determine if the treatments have made a difference to the original observations.

key concepts

Discuss the single-case experimental design.

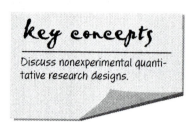

key concepts

Discuss nonexperimental quantitative research designs.

C. Nonexperimental Quantitative Designs

1. Introduction
   a. Uses a series of observations about a subject or group of subjects in order to determine differences or similarities. No treatment is applied to the observed subjects.
   b. Example: Edward Jenner in the 1700s observed dairymaids who had cowpox but did not get smallpox. He determined that people with cowpox would not get smallpox.
   c. Quantitative research is a type of descriptive research where the researcher is observing a subject in relation to determining differences and similarities.
   d. Types of quantitative (descriptive) research
      1) Survey research
         a) Uses questions to study a population or problem.
      2) Assessment research
         a) Typically uses criterion-referenced tests that are constructed to measure skills that are believed to be important.
      3) Historical research
         a) Research that uses historical documents rather than people.
         b) The goal of historical research is to find connections between events in the past rather than between variables in the present.

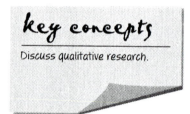

key concepts

Discuss qualitative research.

D. Qualitative Research

1. Introduction
   a. Qualitative research is intended to explore important environmental phenomena by immersing the investigator in the situation for extended periods of time.
   b. Characteristics of qualitative research
      1) Uses the natural setting as the direct source of data and the researcher as the key instrument.
      2) Descriptive.
      3) Concerned with process rather than simply with outcomes or products.
      4) Tends to analyze data inductively.
      5) Meaning is of essential concern to the qualitative approach.
   c. Types of qualitative research
      1) **Naturalistic observations** are those when the observer tries not to alter the situation being observed in any way but simply records whatever is seen.
      2) **Open-ended interviews** attempt to let the person being interviewed tell their story in detail without interference by the interviewer.
      3) Data used in qualitative research include:
         a) Field notes
         b) Documents and photographs
         c) Statistics

III. MEASURES AND SAMPLING
A. Concepts of Critical Importance
1. **Reliability** refers to the degree to which a measure is consistent in producing the same readings when measuring the same things.
    a. In the case of questionnaires, tests, and observations, the goal is to create measures that will consistently show differences between groups that occur in all situations where those measures are used.
2. **Validity** refers to the degree to which a measure actually measures the concept it is supposed to measure.
    a. Types of validity
        1) **Content validity**: the degree to which the content of a test matches some objective criterion.
        2) **Predictive validity**: the degree to which scores on a scale or test predict later scores.
        3) **Concurrent validity**: the correlation between scores on a scale and scores on another scale that has been established to be valid.
        4) **Construct validity**: the degree to which scores on a scale have a pattern of correlations with other scores or attributes that would be predicted to exist.

key concepts

Discuss two measurement constructs and the different types of measures.

B. Types of Measures
1. **Achievement** tests can be constructed to assess a particular content domain, e.g. Iowa Test of Basic Skills.
2. **Standardized** tests can be constructed to cover a wide range of performance levels; most standardized tests use a multiple-choice format.
3. **Criterion-referenced** tests are constructed around a well-defined set of instructional objectives, e.g. ASCP and NCA certification tests.
4. **Questionnaires** can be developed to assess personality, attitudes, and other noncognitive variables.
    a. Characteristics involved in constructing questionnaire:
        1) Questions should be as short and clear as possible.
        2) Double negative questions should be avoided.
        3) Cover all possibilities if multiple choice questions are used.
        4) Include points of reference or comparison when possible.
        5) Emphasize words that are critical to the meaning of the questions.
        6) Ask only important questions.
5. **Interviews** are used to ask individuals specific questions; however, interview data are more difficult to collect and analyze.
    a. Constructing an interview protocol.
        1) Questions must be developed.
        2) Develop notes that will indicate a course of action in response to certain answers.
        3) Be prepared for clarification of questions and responses.
        4) Have a plan to analyze the collected data.

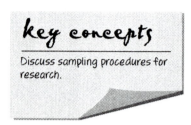

key concepts

Discuss sampling procedures for research.

C. Sampling

1. Introduction to sampling
   a. Sampling is very important in research design; it is designed to assess part of the larger group.
   b. Each member of the population from which the sample is drawn should have an equal and known probability of being selected.
   c. The larger the sample size, the smaller the sampling error.
2. Types of samples
   a. **Cluster samples** include sampling groups rather than individuals.
   b. **Stratified random samples** include random assignment of subjects to 1 or more groups that will ensure that each group has certain characteristics.
   c. **Samples of convenience** include sampling a small group and making the argument that these findings will apply to the larger group.
3. Sample size
   a. A critical element of research design.
   b. If the sample is too small, chances are good that no statistically significant results will be obtained.
   c. The sample size should include **at least 30 in each group.**
   d. Generally the larger the sample size, the better chance will be to observe statistical significance.

IV. PLANNING THE STUDY

A. Criteria for a Research Topic

1. Of interest to you and others.
2. Important.
3. Build on previous research.
4. Timely.
5. Resources (time, money, research tools) available to adequately study the topic.

B. Gather Information

1. Start with a widely focused literature search: Internet searches are a good way to start, along with abstracts, journals, and books.

C. Steps in the Proposal (What You Want to Do and How You Will Do It)

1. **Statement of the problem**: briefly introduces the questions to be answered and discusses the importance of the problem.
2. **Hypotheses**: a statement that summarizes what you expect to find or learn.
3. **Literature review**: a summary of the research relevant to the topic.
4. **Procedures** should include the following:
   a. Subjects and sampling plan
   b. Procedures
   c. Measures
   d. Analysis of the collected data
5. **Time frame** for study completion.

V. INTRODUCTION TO STATISTICAL TERMS

A. Scales of Measurement

1. **Nominal scale**: uses numbers as names for certain categories or groups. Nominal scale numbers have no relationship to one another.
2. **Ordinal scale**: ordinal scale numbers are in a definite order, but without regard to distance between each number.
3. **Interval scale**: scores or numbers differ from one another by the same amount, without regard to a zero point.
4. **Ratio scale** is an interval scale with a true zero point.

B. Measures of Central Tendency

1. **Mean**: average of a set of numbers.
2. **Medium**: the middle score of a set of numbers.
3. **Mode**: the most frequent score.

C. Measures of Dispersion

1. **Standard deviation** (SD) is the dispersion or scatter of a set of numbers. SD is the square root of the variance.
2. **Variance**: the degree of dispersion or scatter of a set of numbers. The variance is the square of the standard deviation.

D. Statistical Comparisons

1. **Statistical significance**: where 2 or more statistics are found to be more different than would be expected by random variation.
2. **t-test**: statistics used to determine if means from 2 different samples are different beyond what would be expected due to sample to sample variation.
3. **t-test for comparisons of 2 means from matched groups**: used to compare the same subjects under 2 different conditions or at two different times.
4. **Analysis of variance (ANOVA)**: used to compare more than 2 samples.
5. **Analysis of covariance (ANCOVA)**: used to compare 2 or more group means after **adjustment** for a control variable.
6. **Chi square**: uses frequency count data, such as the number of individuals falling into a particular category.

VI. WRITING A JOURNAL ARTICLE

A. Format and Style of Journal Articles

1. **Abstract**: brief synopsis (about 150 words) that summarizes the purpose, methods, and study results.
2. **Introduction**: brief review of the literature supporting the topic, describing the purpose and significance of the study.
3. **Methods**: definition of the procedures and methods used in the study.
4. **Results**: description of the findings of the study.
5. **Discussion**: analysis of results and correlation to support the theory and literature discussed in the introduction.
6. **Summary**: 1 or 2 paragraphs capturing key results.
7. **References**: citations of other people's work used in the body of the article; substantiates theory and results.

key concepts

Discuss scales, measures of central tendency, measures of dispersion, and statistical comparisons.

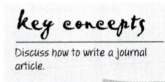

key concepts

Discuss how to write a journal article.

B. Tips for Getting Published

1. Have several people read your manuscript for accuracy, content, etc.
2. Follow the format, style, and other journal requirements very carefully.
3. If your article is rejected, make editorial adjustments and resubmit.
4. Send rejected articles to another journal for possible publication.

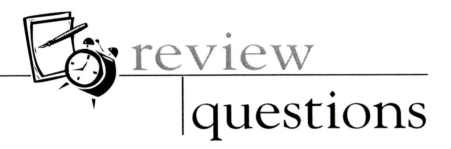

review
questions

DIRECTIONS Each of the questions or incomplete statements below is followed by suggested answers or completions. Select the **one answer** that is best in each case.

---

1. Managers perform all the following roles EXCEPT:
   a. Ordering supplies.
   b. Communicate with employees.
   c. Customer services.
   d. Hold informal authority.

2. Statements written to achieve specific tasks are:
   a. Missions.
   b. Tasks.
   c. Objectives.
   d. Strategic directions.

3. Good management skills consist of all the following EXCEPT:
   a. Ability to Prioritize.
   b. Listening skills.
   c. Disorganized.
   d. Financial acumen.

4. Employees are empowered when they are:
   a. Allowed to determine what task to do and how to do it.
   b. Allowed to do what they want.
   c. Given feedback at regular intervals.
   d. Promoted.

5. Active listening consists of everything EXCEPT:
   a. Identifying what the sender wants from the listener.
   b. Restating what was heard.
   c. Keeping eye contact.
   d. Talking in an area.

6. The quality improvement cycle developed by Deming is:
   a. Act—Check—Do—Plan.
   b. Plan—Act—Feedback—Repeat.
   c. Plan—Do—Act—Check—Do.
   d. Do—Plan—Act—Check.

7. People resist change for all the following reasons EXCEPT:
   a. Self-interest.
   b. Certainty.
   c. Perception.
   d. Insecurity.

8. Budgeting incorporates all the following EXCEPT:
   a. Annual federal inflation figure.
   b. Workload data.
   c. Capital equipment costs.
   d. Operating expenses.

9. Competency-based education is a curriculum based on:
   a. Federal guidelines.
   b. Accreditation standards.
   c. Pathologists' perceptions.
   d. Entry-level competencies.

10. Professional competencies include all the following EXCEPT:
    a. Cognitive.
    b. Affective.
    c. Management.
    d. Psychomotor.

11. 3 levels of test questions are:
   a. Recall, synthesis, interpretation.
   b. Recall, interpretation, problem solving.
   c. Recall, synthesis, problem solving.
   d. Easy, interpretation, case studies.

12. Types of research designs include all the following EXCEPT:
   a. Nondescriptive designs.
   b. Experimental-comparison designs.
   c. Descriptive research.
   d. Correlation design.

13. Stratified random assignment is:
   a. Nonrandom assignment in a different category.
   b. Nonrandom assignment in the same category.
   c. Random assignment in a different category.
   d. Random assignment in the same category.

14. Quantitative research is a type of descriptive research where the researcher observes a subject:
   a. To determine differences.
   b. In relation to determining differences and similarities.
   c. For bad habits.
   d. For characteristic traits.

15. Characteristics of qualitative research include all the following EXCEPT:
   a. Data analyzed statistically.
   b. Uses natural settings.
   c. Focuses on process not just outcomes.
   d. Data analyzed inductively.

16. Which of the following refer to the degree to which a measure is consistent in producing the same reading when measuring the same things?
   a. Concurrent reliability.
   b. Construct validity.
   c. Validity.
   d. Reliability.

17. A questionnaire should have the following characteristics EXCEPT:
   a. Short and clear questions.
   b. Double negative questions.
   c. Ask only important questions.
   d. Reference points or comparisons are included.

18. The larger the sample size, the smaller the:
   a. Population bias.
   b. Sample bias.
   c. Sampling error.
   d. Random sample.

19. Standard deviation is
   a. The dispersion of a set of numbers.
   b. The statistics used to determine if means are from two different populations.
   c. Used to compare more than two samples.
   d. Used for frequency count data.

20. Which of the following describes an interval scale with a true zero point?
   a. Ordinal scale
   b. Nominal scale
   c. Interval scale
   d. Ratio scale

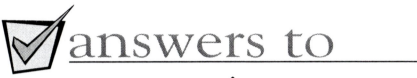

answers to review questions

Chapter 1
1. c
2. b
3. c
4. c
5. b
6. a
7. a
8. c
9. b
10. b

Chapter 2
1. b
2. c
3. c
4. a
5. d
6. b
7. b
8. c
9. b
10. a
11. a
12. c
13. a
14. a
15. d

16. d
17. d
18. c
19. b
20. b

Chapter 3
1. c
2. a
3. d
4. a, b
5. c
6. b, e
7. b
8. c
9. a
10. d

Chapter 4
1. c
2. a
3. b
4. c
5. c
6. b
7. a
8. d
9. c
10. c

11. c
12. b
13. a
14. b
15. b
16. a
17. d
18. c
19. c
20. b

Chapter 5
1. a
2. d
3. b
4. c
5. a
6. a
7. b
8. d
9. c
10. c
11. a
12. b
13. d
14. a
15. d
16. b

17. c
18. a
19. d
20. d
21. b
22. c
23. a
24. d
25. b
26. b
27. c
28. a
29. a
30. c
31. d
32. a
33. b
34. b
35. d
36. a
37. c
38. d
39. c
40. c

Chapter 6
1. c
2. b

3. d
4. b
5. a
6. d
7. d
8. d
9. a
10. b
11. A
B
O—cold
anti-A₁—weak subgroup of A
acquired B
O—elderly patient
12. b
13. b
14. d
15. c
16. a
17. b
18. b
19. a
20. d

Chapter 7
1. c
2. c
3. a
4. b
5. a
6. d
7. b
8. a
9. d
10. b
11. d
12. a
13. a
14. d
15. d
16. a
17. a
18. b
19. a
20. c

Chapter 8
1. c
2. a

3. a
4. a
5. c
6. a
7. a
8. c
9. a
10. b

Chapter 9
1. b
2. a
3. b
4. b
5. c
6. c
7. a
8. b
9. d
10. a, b, e, f

Chapter 10
1. d
2. b

3. d
4. b
5. b

Chapter 11
1. d
2. c
3. c
4. a
5. d
6. c
7. b
8. b
9. d
10. c
11. b
12. a
13. d
14. b
15. a
16. d
17. b
18. c
19. a
20. d

Index